ADVANCES IN

Surgery

Editor-in-Chief
John L. Cameron, MD

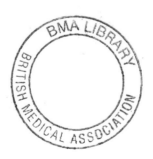
ELSEVIER

PHILADELPHIA   LONDON   TORONTO   MONTREAL   SYDNEY   TOKYO

ADVANCES IN
Surgery

VOLUMES 1 THROUGH 47 (OUT OF PRINT)

VOLUME 51

 litor: John Vassallo
Developmental Editor: Sara Watkins

Editorial Office:
Elsevier
1600 John F. Kennedy Blvd,
Suite 1800
Philadelphia, PA 19103-2899

International Standard Serial Number: 0065-3411
International Standard Book Number: 978-0-323-64227-9

ADVANCES IN
Surgery

CONTRIBUTORS

OLUSEYI AKINTORIN, MD, Department of Surgery, Harvard Medical School, Beth Israel Deaconess Medical Center, Boston, Massachusetts, USA

PETER J. ALLEN, MD, FACS, Murray F. Brennan Professor in Surgery, Department of Surgery, Hepatopancreatobiliary Service, Memorial Sloan Kettering Cancer Center, New York, New York, USA

THOMAS A. ALOIA, MD, Associate Professor, Department of Surgical Oncology, The University of Texas MD Anderson Cancer Center, Houston, Texas, USA

RAMY BEHMAN, MD, Division of General Surgery, University of Toronto, Sunnybrook Health Sciences Centre, Toronto, Ontario, Canada

KARL Y. BILIMORIA, MD, MS, Surgical Outcomes and Quality Improvement Center, Northwestern University, Chicago, Illinois, USA

HERBERT CHEN, MD, FACS, Chairman, Fay Fletcher Kerner Endowed Chair, Professor, Department of Surgery, Biomedical Engineering, The University of Alabama at Birmingham (UAB) School of Medicine, Surgeon-in-Chief, UAB Medicine, Senior Advisor, UAB Comprehensive Cancer Center, Birmingham, Alabama, USA

JAYER CHUNG, MD, MSc, Assistant Professor, Division of Vascular Surgery and Endovascular Therapy, Michael E. DeBakey Department of Surgery, Baylor College of Medicine, Houston, Texas, USA

SUZANNE B. COOPEY, MD, Assistant Professor, Harvard Medical School, Division of Surgical Oncology, Massachusetts General Hospital, Boston, Massachusetts, USA

R. CLEMENT DARLING III, MD, Chief, Division of Vascular Surgery, Professor of Surgery, Albany Medical College, Albany Medical Center Hospital, President, The Vascular Group, Albany, New York, USA

FRANCESCA M. DIMOU, MD, MS, Department of Surgery, University of South Florida, Tampa, Florida, USA

KATHRYN E. ENGELHARDT, MD, Surgical Outcomes and Quality Improvement Center, Northwestern University, Chicago, Illinois, USA; Department of Surgery, Medical University of South Carolina, Charleston, South Carolina, USA

WILLIAM E. FISHER, MD, FACS, Professor, Vice Chair for Clinical Affairs, Chief, Division of General Surgery, George L. Jordan, M.D., Chair of General Surgery, Michael E. DeBakey Department of Surgery, Director, Elkins Pancreas Center, Baylor College of Medicine, Houston, Texas, USA

ELIZABETH B. HABERMANN, PhD, MPH, Robert D. and Patricia E. Kern Scientific Director for Surgical Outcomes Research, Associate Professor of Health Services Research, Departments of Surgery and Health Sciences Research, Mayo Clinic, Rochester, Minnesota, USA

MARY T. HAWN, MD, MPH, Professor and Chair, Department of Surgery, Stanford University, Stanford, California, USA

PETER K. HENKE, MD, Leland Ira Doan Research Professor of Vascular Surgery and Professor of Surgery, Section of Vascular Surgery, Department of Surgery, University of Michigan, Ann Arbor, Michigan, USA

CYRUS JAHANSOUZ, MD, Resident, Department of Surgery, University of Minnesota, Minneapolis, Minnesota, USA

PAUL J. KARANICOLAS, MD, PhD, FRCSC, FACS, Division of General Surgery, University of Toronto, Sunnybrook Health Sciences Centre, Toronto, Ontario, Canada

BRADFORD J. KIM, MD, MHS, Research Fellow, Department of Surgical Oncology, The University of Texas MD Anderson Cancer Center, Houston, Texas, USA; General Surgery Resident, Department of Surgery, Indiana University School of Medicine, Indianapolis, Indiana, USA

LISA M. KODADEK, MD, Fellow, Department of Surgery, Johns Hopkins School of Medicine, Baltimore, Maryland, USA

MARY R. KWAAN, MD, MPH, Associate Professor, Department of Surgery, University of California, Los Angeles, Los Angeles, California, USA

PAMELA A. LIPSETT, MD, MHPE, Warfield M. Firor Endowed Professor of Surgery, Professor of Surgery, Anesthesiology and Critical Care Medicine, Johns Hopkins School of Medicine, Baltimore, Maryland, USA

REEMA MALLICK, MD, Clinical Instructor, Department of Surgery, The University of Alabama at Birmingham, Birmingham, Alabama, USA

CAITLIN A. McINTYRE, MD, Postdoctoral Research Fellow, Department of Surgery, Hepatopancreatobiliary Service, Memorial Sloan Kettering Cancer Center, New York, New York, USA

AVERY B. NATHENS, MD, MPH, PhD, FRCSC, FACS, Division of General Surgery, University of Toronto, Sunnybrook Health Sciences Centre, Toronto, Ontario, Canada

ANDREA OBI, MD, Assistant Professor, Section of Vascular Surgery, Department of Surgery, University of Michigan, Ann Arbor, Michigan, USA

JAN RAKINIC, MD, Professor, Department of Surgery, Southern Illinois University School of Medicine, Springfield, Illinois, USA

TAYLOR S. RIALL, MD, PhD, Professor, Department of Surgery, The University of Arizona, Tucson, Arizona, USA

TEVIAH E. SACHS, MD, MPH, FACS, Assistant Professor, Department of Surgery, Boston University School of Medicine, Boston, Massachusetts, USA

BARBARA L. SMITH, MD, PhD, Professor, Harvard Medical School, Division of Surgical Oncology, Massachusetts General Hospital, Boston, Massachusetts, USA

JOSE M. SOLIZ, MD, Associate Professor, Department of Anesthesiology and Perioperative Medicine, The University of Texas MD Anderson Cancer Center, Houston, Texas, USA

STEVEN C. STAIN, MD, Henry and Sally Schaffer Chair, Professor, Department of Surgery, Albany Medical Center Hospital, Albany Medical College, Albany, New York, USA

JONAH J. STULBERG, MD, PhD, MPH, Assistant Professor of Surgery, Surgical Outcomes and Quality Improvement Center, Northwestern University, Chicago, Illinois, USA

SPENCE M. TAYLOR, MD, President, Greenville Health System, Chair, Board of Managers, GHS Health Sciences Center, Professor of Surgery, University of South Carolina School of Medicine Greenville, Greenville, South Carolina, USA

JONATHAN R. THOMPSON, MD, Vascular Surgery Fellow, Section of Vascular Surgery, Department of Surgery, University of Michigan, Ann Arbor, Michigan, USA

JENNIFER TSENG, MD, MPH, James Utley Professor and Chair of Surgery, Department of Surgery, Boston University School of Medicine, Boston, Massachusetts, USA

JEAN-NICOLAS VAUTHEY, MD, Chief, Hepato-Pancreato-Biliary Section, Professor, Department of Surgical Oncology, The University of Texas MD Anderson Cancer Center, Houston, Texas, USA

TYLER S. WAHL, MD, MSPH, General Surgery Resident, Department of Surgery, The University of Alabama at Birmingham, Birmingham, Alabama, USA

THOMAS WAKEFIELD, MD, Professor, Section of Vascular Surgery, Department of Surgery, University of Michigan, Ann Arbor, Michigan, USA

COURTNEY J. WARNER, MD, Assistant Professor of Surgery, Albany Medical College, Vascular Surgeon, The Vascular Group, The Institute for Vascular Health and Disease, Albany, New York, USA

ADVANCES IN
Surgery

CONTENTS

VOLUME 52 • 2018

Prevention and Treatment of *Clostridium difficile* Enterocolitis
Lisa M. Kodadek and Pamela A. Lipsett

The Management of Venous Thromboembolic Disease: New Trends in Anticoagulant Therapy
Andrea Obi and Thomas Wakefield

Proper Use of Cholecystostomy Tubes
Francesca M. Dimou and Taylor S. Riall

Is Maintenance of Certification Working in Surgery?
Spence M. Taylor

How Should Gallbladder Cancer Be Managed?
Teviah E. Sachs, Oluseyi Akintorin, and Jennifer Tseng

How to Predict 30-Day Readmission
Tyler S. Wahl and Mary T. Hawn

Nipple-Sparing Mastectomy
Barbara L. Smith and Suzanne B. Coopey

Should the Management of a Ruptured Abdominal Aortic Aneurysm Be Regionalized?

Courtney J. Warner, Steven C. Stain, and
R. Clement Darling III

Diagnosis and Management of Hyperparathyroidism

Reema Mallick and Herbert Chen

Management of Aortoenteric Fistula

Jayer Chung

Benign Anorectal Surgery: Management
Jan Rakinic

Intraperitoneal Drainage and Pancreatic Resection
William E. Fisher

How Long Should Patients with Cystic Lesions of the Pancreas Be Followed?
Caitlin A. McIntyre and Peter J. Allen

What Is the Best Pain Control After Major Hepatopancreatobiliary Surgery?
Bradford J. Kim, Jose M. Soliz, Thomas A. Aloia, and Jean-Nicolas Vauthey

Are Opioids Overprescribed Following Elective Surgery?
Elizabeth B. Habermann

Contemporary Management of Critical Limb Ischemia
Jonathan R. Thompson and Peter K. Henke

The Use of Lavage for the Management of Diverticulitis

Cyrus Jahansouz and Mary R. Kwaan

Advances in Surgery 52 (2018) 1–14

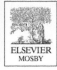

ADVANCES IN SURGERY

ELSEVIER
MOSBY

Surgeon Scorecards
Accurate or Not?

Kathryn E. Engelhardt, MD[a,b], Karl Y. Bilimoria, MD, MS[a],
Jonah J. Stulberg, MD, PhD, MPH[a,*]

[a]Surgical Outcomes and Quality Improvement Center, Northwestern University, 633 North Saint Clair Street, 20th floor, Chicago, IL 60611, USA; [b]Department of Surgery, Medical University of South Carolina, 96 Jonathan Lucas Street, Charleston, SC 29425, USA

Keywords

- Quality indicators • Outcome measurement • Public reporting • Risk assessment
- Access to information

Key points

- There is a public demand for comparative surgeon evaluation and scoring.
- Unintended consequences of surgeon-specific reporting should be understood and mitigated.
- Scoring methodologies should consider data quality, measure selection, sample size, risk adjustment, and report design to optimize usefulness and minimize adverse consequences.

INTRODUCTION

The power of publicly reporting quality data to drive change has been shown repeatedly through well-designed and executed research efforts [1,2], and the concepts of surgeon-specific outcome reporting is not new. In 1990, the Department of Health in New York first publicly reported mortalities for individual surgeons performing cardiac surgery under the Cardiac Surgery Reporting System [3]. Due in part to their efforts, mortalities for common cardiac procedures have fallen from 2.7% in 1992 when the reporting efforts started to 1.8% today with much less variation among hospitals [4]. Driven by a public interest in increased transparency coupled with increasing access to data, interest in surgeon-specific scorecards has grown in recent years. Most recently, public

Disclosures: The authors have nothing to disclose.

*Corresponding author. E-mail address: Jonah.Stulberg@nm.org

https://doi.org/10.1016/j.yasu.2018.03.009

watchdog groups such as ProPublica have developed their own version of surgeon-level comparative quality reports [5].

Accurate quality reports have the capacity to identify poor-quality outliers so that these areas can be targeted for improvement, but transparency is not without unintended and potentially adverse consequences. For example, following release of surgeon-specific cardiac surgery outcome reports in Pennsylvania, many surgeons openly admitted to avoiding higher-risk patients and higher-risk procedures [6]. In this article, the authors briefly explore the history of surgeon-specific quality reporting and elucidate the methodology used to develop currently available scorecards. The authors then identify the major hurdles regarding scorecards' accuracy and discuss current innovations in quality assessment.

SIGNIFICANCE
History of surgeon specific reports
As early as the 1800s, surgeons have been interested in tracking their results [7]. In 1914, surgeon Ernest Codman resigned from Massachusetts General Hospital and started his own hospital based on the "End Results" idea, which Codman described as "[T]he common sense notion that every hospital should follow every patient it treats, long enough to determine whether or not the treatment has been successful, and then to inquire, 'If not, why not?' with a view to preventing similar failures in the future" [8]. Although longitudinal tracking of patient outcomes is now widely accepted, definitions around what outcomes should be tracked and whether these outcomes should be shared at the individual surgeon level is still heavily debated.

In 1990, New York State Department of Heath published the first physician-specific mortality report, the Cardiac Surgery Reporting System [3]. Pennsylvania similarly published the Consumer Guide to Coronary Artery Bypass Graft Surgery [6]. These projects were followed by citywide and statewide projects in Cleveland, Minneapolis, California, Florida, and Oregon [6]. These reports were pioneering an era of transparency that was further fueled by the Institute of Medicine's report on health care quality: Crossing the Quality Chasm [9]. This report raised concern about the marked variation in the quality of medical and surgical care across the United States resulting in exploding interest in measuring and reporting on quality of care.

Currently available report cards
Patients searching for information to compare one surgeon to another now have several options available free on the Internet. Most rely on patient self-reported experience, but a few have started to make use of publicly available administrative data (Table 1). These approaches have different strengths and weaknesses and likely serve different purposes. The authors focus, however, primarily on the use of administrative data used for the purpose of comparing surgeon-level outcomes.

Table 1
Summary of representative scorecards

	Sponsor	Data source	Primary outcomes	Access
Surgeon Scorecard	ProPublica	CMS	"Adjusted complication rate"	https://projects.propublica.org/surgeons/
healthgrades	Healthgrades Operating Company, Inc	Patient Surveys	Likelihood of recommendation, trustworthiness, helpfulness, staff, scheduling	https://www.healthgrades.com/
SurgeonRatings	Consumer Checkbook	CMS, Physician Surveys	Death rates, "other bad outcomes" Recommended most by surveyed doctors	http://www.checkbook.org/surgeonratings/
Top Doctors	Castle Connolly Medical Ltd	Physician Surveys	Recommended most by surveyed doctors	http://castleconnolly.com/
Vitals	MDX Medical, Inc	Patient Surveys	Overall star rating, ease of appointment, promptness, courteous staff, accurate diagnosis, bedside manner, spends time with me, follows up after visit	http://www.vitals.com/

Data from Refs. [5,29–32].

Are scorecards accurate?

Ensuring the accuracy of scorecards is a complex process involving many key concerns: the data source, measure selection, sample selection, sample size, and risk adjustment. Accuracy is the degree to which the results of the measurement, in this case a surgeon-specific outcome, are reflective of the underlying correct value or truth (Fig. 1). In addition to being accurate, report cards are expected to be precise. Precision in this case is defined as the degree to which the estimate from the measurement varies around the actual truth or correct value on repeated measurement. Therefore, an accurate and precise scorecard is desired that repeatedly reflects the truth about the quality of the surgeon with very little variation.

However, this is more difficult to achieve than it may seem. An individual patient's outcome from a surgical episode is the result of a complex interplay of many factors related to patient characteristics, hospital characteristics, and system-level factors in addition to provider quality (Fig. 2). Therefore, any

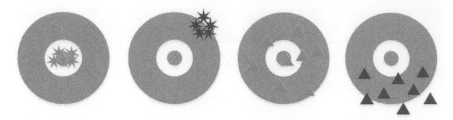

Fig. 1. Accuracy versus precision. Accurate measurement means "hitting the target." Green indicates accuracy, whereas red indicates inaccuracy. Stars indicate precision, and triangles indicate imprecision. Measurements that approximate the true value are accurate. Measurements that have little error among them are precise. An accurate scorecard will reflect a rating that approximates the true value, regardless of whether the measurements resulting in the scorecard are precise.

scorecard that relies on outcomes to estimate surgeon-specific quality needs to attempt to control for variation in these other influences on the outcome. Furthermore, administrative data were not collected with the intent of providing evidence of physician quality, which many investigators have noted decreases the accuracy of these data for the purpose of quality reporting [10,11]. In the following section, each of the major methodologic elements that should be evaluated when determining if an individual scorecard is accurate is discussed.

What factors influence accuracy?
Source data quality
Currently available comparative reports rely on administrative data sets rather than data abstracted directly from the medical record for quality purposes. Administrative data sets are the accumulation of data originally collected for billing purposes and have been shown to have several limitations when compared with data that are collected specifically for quality measurement purposes, including comprehensive collection of comorbidities and accurate collection of complications [10]. Despite these shortcomings, administrative data sets are cost-effective and typically very large. Therefore, if the limitations of administrative data sets can be overcome through other methodological means, they are certainly a tempting resource for development of comparative reports.

To date, the most widely publicized scorecard is ProPublica's Surgeon Scorecard (PPSS) [5,12]. The data set that ProPublica used was the Limited Data Set released by the Center for Medicare and Medicaid Services (CMS) reflecting services provided between 2009 and 2013 [12]. These data reflect inpatient error admissions for all Medicare beneficiaries over the 4-year period. The PPSS developers aggregated 4 years of results to an individual surgeon and presented risk-adjusted outcomes for individual surgeons related to 5 specific procedures.

However, after release of the PPSS, several limitations of administrative data became readily apparent. First, many "surgeons" ranked on the PPSS were not

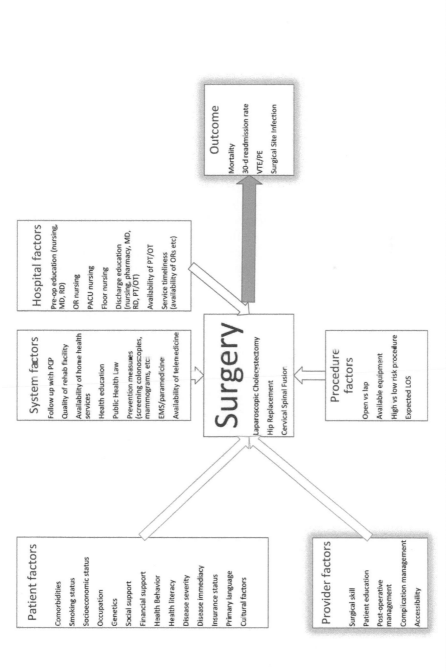

Fig. 2. Association between provider performance and patient outcome. There are many determinants of surgical outcomes; however, scorecards are designed to evaluate the provider factors' direct effect on the outcome measured. EMS, emergency medical services; lap, laparoscopic; LOS, length of stay; MD, medical doctor; OR, operating room; PACU, post-anesthesia care unit; PCP, primary care physician; PT/OT, physical therapy/occupational therapy; RD, registered dietitian; VTE/PE, venous thromboembolism/pulmonary embolism.

actually surgeons but rather internists, hospitalists, and anesthesiologists. This highlighted the lack of granularity and significant inaccuracies in identification of individual providers [11]. Although the next iteration of the PPSS seeks to eliminate the incorrect providers, ProPublica will never be able to overcome the inherent inaccuracies within administrative data: any data not needed explicitly for billing purposes will likely be too inaccurate to be repurposed reliably for comparative quality reporting (Table 2).

Sample selection

Rarely does one have access to the entire population susceptible to a given outcome (eg, every case a surgeon has performed, every patient exposed to flu), so a sample of the population is used to estimate the effect one expects to see within the entire population. A central tenant of sample selection is the representativeness of the sample to the whole population. How well the sample represents the population will determine how accurately the rate of a given outcome within the sample estimates that of the entire population.

ProPublica used CMS data to calculate an individual surgeon's "Adjusted Complication Rate" with the assumption that this rate would be reflective of all patients undergoing that same operation by that same surgeon [12]. However, in order for a case to be included in the ProPublica analysis, all cases were (1) operations associated with an inpatient stay and (2) operations performed on patients 65 years old or older. When compared with data collected in the American College of Surgeons' National Surgical Quality Improvement Project (ACS NSQIP), the administrative data set failed to capture a very large proportion of cases. Almost 96% of laparoscopic cholecystectomies and 93% of anterior spinal fusions were missed using the PPSS methodology (Table 3). When the overwhelming majority of cases performed are missing from the sample, it raises significant concerns about the sample accurately representing the truth. Furthermore, the sample differs in a systematic way from the other cases raising an even greater concern that providers within the PPSS will be judged on a biased sample of their cases [13]. Therefore, accurate and thoughtful sample selection is a vital component of developing an accurate comparative report.

Table 2
Comparison of potential data sources used to compare surgeons

	Administrative	Clinically abstracted	Survey data
Cost	Low	High	Variable
Timeliness	1 y or longer when used for research	Very variable	Variable
Size	Typically large population based	Typically small	Small
Generalizability	High	Project specific	Low
Data collection	Predetermined for billing	Control over the variables collected	Based on reputation or personal experience
Accuracy	Typically low	Typically high	Subjective

Table 3
Decrease in number of eligible patients with successive application of propublica's exclusion criteria

	All cases	Inpatient	Nonemergent	Age ≥65
Laparoscopic cholecystectomy				
N, patients	83,264	12,782	8952	3430
%, patients	100	15.4	10.8	4.1
Radical prostatectomy				
N, patients	19,674	8545	8514	3891
%, patients	100	43.4	43.3	19.8
TURP (transurethral prostate resection)				
N, patients	11,468	3604	3248	2662
%, patients	100	31.4	28.3	23.2
Cervical fusion of anterior column				
N, patients	17,867	5476	5203	1398
%, patients	100	30.6	29.1	7.8
ALIF (lumbar fusion of anterior column), posterior approach				
N, patients	3888	3408	3378	1006
%, patients	100	87.7	86.9	25.9
PLIF (lumbar fusion of posterior column), posterior approach				
N, patients	3623	3118	3082	1178
%, patients	100	86.1	85.1	32.5
Total knee arthroplasty				
N, patients	88,693	85,871	85,477	51,193
%, patients	100	96.8	96.4	57.7
Total hip arthroplasty				
N, patients	57,284	52,597	51,703	28,193
%, patients	100	91.8	90.3	49.2
All operations				
N, patients	1,941,251	940,906	799,121	353,015
%, patients	100	48.5	41.2	18.2

Each column shows the number of eligible cases after the application of that additional exclusion criterion. Successive exclusion criteria were applied moving from left to right, recalculating the number of eligible cases after each step.
From Ban KA, Cohen ME, Ko CY, et al. Evaluation of the ProPublica surgeon scorecard "adjusted complication rate" measure specifications. Ann Surg 2016;264(4):570; with permission.

Selection of measures
Classically in the Donabedian framework, selection of measures are described as either structure items (eg, whether the surgeon is board certified), process items (eg, whether appropriate antibiotics are used at an appropriate time), or outcome items (eg, 30 day readmission rate) [14]. A critical component of a good process measure is whether it links directly and proportionally to an outcome of interest. If comparison of differences in a reported process measure is not representative of differences in a relevant outcome, one questions the utility of measuring and reporting these differences [15].

The outcome measure ProPublica developed for use in their scorecard was "Adjusted Complication Rate (ACR)" [12], defined as any mortality or readmission within 30 days of the index operation. They attempted to select for only related readmissions using the admission diagnosis code and estimating whether that diagnosis could reasonably be attributed to the index operation [12]. To evaluate the accuracy of this newly developed outcome measure, 2 questions need to be addressed: (1) does this new measure reflect a meaningful outcome? And (2) does it reflect underlying quality differences between providers?

Ban and colleagues [13] sought to answer the first of these questions. They found that the methodology described by ProPublica missed 84% of postoperative complications (in part by excluding complications that occur during the index operation) when compared with complications measured in ACS NSQIP. Furthermore, they found that the new ACR measure reported by ProPublica correlates poorly with well-established postoperative outcomes (specifically, all-cause morbidity, death, or serious morbidity, and surgical site infection), which are thought to be important to patients and reflective of quality differences between providers. Therefore, the ACR measure missed common complications that occur while an inpatient, capturing only those events that occur after discharge and lead to a readmission. Understanding what the chosen metric has captured will allow consumers to interpret the findings accurately.

Sample size

The sample size must be large enough to demonstrate a statistically significant difference in the chosen measure when a clinically significant difference exists between surgeons (Table 4). There are many methods for determining the minimum sample size necessary in a given situation, but the salient point is that clinically significant differences vary by the type of metric used. Hall and colleagues [16] recently published their work with the ACS NSQIP data, whereby they attempted to calculate the minimum number of cases needed in order to detect a clinically and statistically significant difference between individual surgeons on a set of outcome measures. They found that in order to detect a difference in surgeon-specific mortality with 70% reliability, each surgeon would need to amass 1985 cases. They concluded that it is not practical to compare surgeon-specific mortality using NSQIP data, and a different metric for comparison needs to be sought. In addition, this theme of requiring very large sample sizes in order to detect meaningful quality differences was echoed by Jaffe and colleagues [17], who found that a sample size of 617 cases would be necessary to detect a 50% difference in ProPublica's "adjusted complication rate" in a laparoscopic cholecystectomy. In general, the rarer an outcome measure occurs, the larger the sample size needed to detect a clinically significant difference between providers.

Risk adjustment

Consumers of physician scorecards expect the results to reflect the physician's effect on his or her patient's outcomes. However, in health care, every patient is unique and they are operated on in a unique setting with a unique team; therefore, in order to compare across all of these contextual variations, a scorecard

Table 4
Results from 3 analyses of the required sample size needed to detect a clinically significant difference in performance for the given outcome with a 95% confidence interval

Procedure	Outcome	Average rate of chosen outcome, %	Sample size needed	Difference detected	Power
Jaffe et al [17], 2016	Laparoscopic cholecystectomy	"Adjusted complication rate"	4.4	617	1.5× the average complication rate	0.8
Walker et al [26], 2013	Esophagectomy or gastrectomy	Mortality	6.1	109	2× the average mortality	0.8
	Bowel resection	Mortality	5.1	132	2× the average mortality	0.8
	Hip fracture surgery	Mortality	8.4	102	2× the average mortality	0.8
	Cardiac surgery	Mortality	2.7	256	2× the average mortality	0.8
Hall et al [16], 2015	Any ACS NSQIP procedure	Morbidity	19.3	140	Statistically significantly different from the average performance	0.7[a]
	Any ACS NSQIP procedure	Surgical site infection	6.1	254	Statistically significantly different from the average performance	0.7[a]
	Any ACS NSQIP procedure	Mortality	2.2	1985	Statistically significantly different from the average performance	0.7[a]

[a]Indicates reliability (not power).
Data from Refs. [16,17,26,33].

reliant on outcomes must perform some risk adjustment in order to attempt to account for this variation [18]. A common criticism of scorecards is that they do not properly account for case mix and that they are biased in favor of surgeons with low-risk patients.

What factors influence usefulness?

Timeliness

For information about surgeon performance to be useful, it must reflect current practice [19]. Unfortunately, administrative data sets are often several years delayed and may not reflect current trends. Even clinically abstracted data such as ACS-NSQIP has a lag time of 6 to 12 months before comparative reports are given back to hospitals for quality improvement. An ideal model would be one that pulls data automatically from an electronic medical record and updates as soon as new data are available. We are far from this scenario, but efforts continue to try to realize this ideal. The Illinois Surgical Quality Improvement Collaborative has begun producing surgeon-specific reports in real time, and research on the ideal measures and risk adjustment model is ongoing [20].

Report format

There is a growing design industry focused on the interaction between consumers and health care services [21]. In general, comparative reports should be easy to interpret (by patients without medical training and all literacy levels), should highlight meaningful differences between providers while clearly demonstrating that some differences are not clinically relevant, and should reflect trends as well as static estimates. The format should be designed with the user in mind so that all intended users reach the same conclusions about the data presented.

Unintended consequences

The intended consequences of publicly reported data are 2-fold: (1) poor performers are incentivized to improve their outcomes through quality improvement because (2) patients will seek out surgeons with better reported outcomes. However, unintended or adverse consequences may occur with both currently available scorecards and poorly designed and executed scorecards. Instead of driving improvement in quality of care, scorecards may result in manipulation of the system on the front end through patient or procedure selection. Surgeons may begin to avoid high-risk patients [22]. This reaction was a well-described consequence of the ratings of cardiothoracic surgeons [23]. As a result of comparative performance reports of cardiac surgeons published starting in 1992, 59% of cardiologists reported increased difficulty in finding surgeons willing to perform coronary artery bypass surgery in severely ill patients who required it, and 63% of cardiac surgeons reported they were less willing to operate on such patients [6]. Therefore, not only must appropriate case-mix adjustment be performed, but surgeons need to believe that the risk adjustment methodology adequately adjusts for their unique patient mix in order to avoid this consequence.

A more subtle issue than patient selection is procedure selection. A patient may have a clinical problem that is amenable to 2 different operations. One procedure may have the chance for durable results but is higher risk in the short term. The other operation may be a straightforward procedure with few risks in the short term but is known to have poor long-term durability. If performance measures focus only on 30-day outcomes, surgeons may shift their practice to performing less complex cases to improve their short-term outcomes at the expense of long-term results.

In addition, providers could improve their reported results on the back end by manipulating the measurement of a chosen outcome. If the chosen outcome is surgical site infection and it is defined as "an infection *requiring opening of a wound*," then a wound may be left open and left to heal by primary intention. In this way, few if any wounds could ever be counted as having an infection because there are no staples or stitches to remove.

Last, public reporting of outcomes may have an unintended effect on training the next generation of surgeons. Surgeons may be less willing to allow trainees to perform cases for fear of damaging their publicly reported outcomes, even if this fear is unwarranted (as most studies support the safety of resident involvement in cases). However, there is a paucity of data exploring this hypothesis [24,25].

In addition to the above consequences, which are magnified by poorly designed or executed reports, patient choice may be inadvertently manipulated by an inaccurate report or by patient misinterpretation of a seemingly accurate report. If a surgeon is falsely reported as being superior or even adequate but actually has terrible outcomes, patients are in danger of receiving substandard care. In addition, this surgeon has a sense of complacency and may not recognize any need for improvement [26]. On the other hand, if a surgeon with good outcomes is falsely reported as being inferior, the public nature of this reporting could irreversibly damage their reputation not only among patients but also among referring physicians [24].

In addition to reports that are inaccurate to begin with, misinterpretation of an accurate report may mislead consumers. Examples of misleading reports are when summary scores are provided without confidence intervals and when surgeons are placed into performance categories (low, medium, high, and so on) without consideration of the confidence interval. In this second scenario, a borderline surgeon with a low sample size (and thus a wide confidence interval) may be misclassified based on an imprecise mean. This inaccuracy is the danger of reports with categories, stars, or other such classification systems [11]. However, a report with bands of confidence intervals without some sort of classification loses its usefulness to consumers if it is uninterpretable. An ideal report should be precise in its measurement and user-friendly in its display.

FUTURE DIRECTIONS

A critical decision point in the design of a comparative reporting system is: who is the audience of this comparative report? For a patient to choose a provider, objective data will likely need to be combined with subjective information. This data may include factors that a practitioner cannot easily change. For example, a woman may prefer a female breast surgeon, or a non-English speaker may prefer a surgeon who speaks a common language. However, these differences in providers clearly do not indicate objective differences in provider quality.

Key hurdles

The focus of this article has been on objective quality reports. First, an ideal data source must be identified (see Table 2). Second, a meaningful outcome measure must be selected for measurement, and the measurement process must be refined. Third, the hurdle of inadequate sample size may not ever be overcome when traditional outcome measures, like mortality, are used. Fourth, there is ongoing research to determine the most equitable method of risk adjustment. Fifth, the hurdle of timely reports is being compounded by the hurdles of obtaining timely data and timely risk adjustment. Last, the range of health literacy in the consumers of comparative reports makes choosing the right report format a challenging task.

Innovations

Video-based assessments. The increase in laparoscopic surgery makes direct monitoring and evaluating surgeon skill theoretically feasible. A group of bariatric surgeons in Michigan took advantage of this opportunity [27]. Operations were videotaped and submitted to the group. They were rated on a variety of measures by a cohort of blinded peers. The scores of each surgeon were then compared with his or her complication rate to identify any association. They found a broad range of technical skill and that greater skill was associated with fewer complications, reoperations, readmissions, and fewer Emergency Department visits. This association indicates not only that surgeon skill is correlated with outcomes but also that these skills can be measured in a reproducible manner. Next steps in this line of research include assessing interrater reliability to move toward an objective measure of surgeon skill rather than the current subjective measure; testing this strategy in other surgical specialties to assess the generalizability of the findings; and assessing the effect of the feedback generated to understand if this process improves surgeon skill and subsequent outcomes.

Patient-reported outcomes. Current research in comparative effectiveness is aimed at identifying what factors patients consider most important in choosing a physician [28]. It is hypothesized that patients will vary in their views, and therefore, surgeon choice will be influenced by the "best fit" rather than the absolute "best." This trend is especially important as the medical community becomes better at optimizing clinical outcomes (length of stay, morbidity, mortality), as the difference between providers becomes more difficult to measure and less clinically relevant, and as a patient becomes equally likely to have a good outcome across all surgeons. Patient-reported outcome measures are designed to measure those aspects of the medical encounter that are most important to patients and are likely to demonstrate differences among providers where clinical variation does not exist.

SUMMARY

For surgeon scorecards to be accurate, the data from which they are derived must be high quality, the risk adjustment must be validated, and the results must be presented in an easy-to-use format with methodologic transparency. In this article, the authors have discussed the different methods of data collection for quality assessments, explained the issue related to sample size, discussed structure, process, outcome measures, and the challenges of risk adjustment, and presented concerns regarding the potential adverse consequences when surgeon-specific data are publicly reported. Finally, the authors suggest some possibilities for future developments in this field. Public reporting of surgeon-specific outcome data has begun and continues to grow in popularity; thus, surgeons should understand how the available scorecards are developed and be able to explain the usefulness of such scorecards to their patients in an objective manner.

Acknowledgments

The authors would like to thank Kristen Ban for her work on this project.

References

[1] Young GJ, Burgess JF, White B. Pioneering pay-for-quality: lessons from the rewarding results demonstrations. Health Care Financ Rev 2007;29(1):59–70.

[2] Stundner O, Memtsoudis SG. Outcomes research in perioperative medicine. Adv Anesth 2014;2014:10.

[3] Zinman D. Heart surgeons rated. State reveals patient-mortality records. Newday 1991;34–7.

[4] Health NYSDO. Cardiovascular disease data and statistics. 2016. Available at: https://www.health.ny.gov/statistics/diseases/cardiovascular/. Accessed November 26, 2016.

[5] Wei S, Pierce O, Allen M. Surgeon scorecard. 2015. Available at: https://projects.propublica.org/surgeons/. Accessed July 29, 2016.

[6] Schneider EC, Epstein AM. Influence of cardiac-surgery performance reports on referral practices and access to care. A survey of cardiovascular specialists. N Engl J Med 1996;335(4):251–6.

[7] Chun J, Bafford AC. History and background of quality measurement. Clin Colon Rectal Surg 2014;27(1):5–9.

[8] Brand RA. Ernest Amory Codman, MD, 1869–1940. Clin Orthop Relat Res 2009;467(11): 2763–5.

[9] Institute of Medicine. Crossing the quality chasm: a new health system for the 21st century. Washington, DC: National Academy Press; 2001.

[10] Rajaram R, Barnard C, Bilimoria KY. Concerns about using the patient safety indicator-90 composite in pay-for-performance programs. JAMA 2015;313(9):897–8.

[11] Friedberg MW, Pronovost PJ, Shahian DM, et al. A methodological critique of the propublica surgeon scorecard. 2015. Available at: http://www.rand.org/pubs/perspectives/PE170.html. Accessed July 22, 2016.

[12] Pierce O, Allen M. Assessing surgeon-level risk of patient harm during elective surgery for public reporting. 2015. Available at: https://static.propublica.org/projects/patient-safety/methodology/surgeon-level-risk-methodology.pdf. Accessed July 29, 2016.

[13] Ban KA, Cohen ME, Ko CY, et al. Evaluation of the Propublica surgeon scorecard "adjusted complication rate" measure specifications. Ann Surg 2016;264(4):566–74.

[14] Donabedian A. Quality assurance. Structure, process and outcome. Nurs Stand 1992;7(11 Suppl QA):4–5.

[15] Stulberg JJ, Delaney CP, Neuhauser DV, et al. Adherence to surgical care improvement project measures and the association with postoperative infections. JAMA 2010;303(24): 2479–85.

[16] Hall BL, Huffman KM, Hamilton BH, et al. Profiling individual surgeon performance using information from a high-quality clinical registry: opportunities and limitations. J Am Coll Surg 2015;221(5):901–13.

[17] Jaffe TA, Hasday SJ, Dimick JB. Power outage—inadequate surgeon performance measures leave patients in the dark. JAMA Surg 2016;151(7):599–600.

[18] Cohen ME, Ko CY, Bilimoria KY, et al. Optimizing ACS NSQIP modeling for evaluation of surgical quality and risk: patient risk adjustment, procedure mix adjustment, shrinkage adjustment, and surgical focus. J Am Coll Surgeons 2013;217(2):336–46.e1.

[19] Krumholz HM, Brindis RG, Brush JE, et al. Standards for statistical models used for public reporting of health outcomes. Circulation 2006;113(3):456–62.

[20] Stulberg JJ, Quinn CM, Pavey ES, et al. Development of physician-level quality reports in the Illinois Surgical Quality Collaborative. San Diego (CA): Paper presented at the American College of Surgeons National Surgical Quality Improvement Project National Conference; July 16–19, 2016.

[21] Mad*Pow Insights. Available at: http://www.madpow.com/insights. Accessed May 11, 2016.

[22] Burns EM, Pettengell C, Athanasiou T, et al. Understanding the strengths and weaknesses of public reporting of surgeon-specific outcome data. Health Aff 2016;35(3):415–21.

[23] Burack JH, Impellizzeri P, Homel P, et al. Public reporting of surgical mortality: a survey of New York State cardiothoracic surgeons. Ann Thorac Surg 1999;68(4):1195–200 [discussion 1201–2].

[24] Radford PD, Derbyshire LF, Shalhoub J, et al. Publication of surgeon specific outcome data: a review of implementation, controversies and the potential impact on surgical training. Int J Surg 2015;13:211–6.

[25] Alderson D, Cromwell D. Publication of surgeon-specific outcomes. Br J Surg 2014;101(11):1335–7.

[26] Walker K, Neuburger J, Groene O, et al. Public reporting of surgeon outcomes: low numbers of procedures lead to false complacency. Lancet 2013;382(9905):1674–7.

[27] Birkmeyer JD, Finks JF, O'Reilly A, et al. Surgical skill and complication rates after bariatric surgery. N Engl J Med 2013;369(15):1434–42.

[28] Gabriel SE, Normand S-LT. Getting the methods right — the foundation of patient-centered outcomes research. N Engl J Med 2012;367(9):787–90.

[29] Healthgrades. 2016. Available at: https://www.healthgrades.com/. Accessed November 26, 2016.

[30] SurgeonRatings.org. 1996. Available at: http://www.checkbook.org/surgeonratings/. Accessed November 26, 2016.

[31] Top Doctors. 1992. Available at: http://castleconnolly.com/. Accessed November 26, 2016.

[32] Vitals. 2016. Available at: http://www.vitals.com/. Accessed November 26, 2016.

[33] Cohen ME, Bilimoria KY, Ko CY, et al. Development of an American College of Surgeons National Surgery Quality Improvement Program: morbidity and mortality risk calculator for colorectal surgery. J Am Coll Surg 2009;208(6):1009–16.

Advances in Surgery 52 (2018) 15–27

ADVANCES IN SURGERY

ELSEVIER
MOSBY

Laparoscopic Surgery for Small Bowel Obstruction: Is It Safe?

Ramy Behman, MD[a,b],
Avery B. Nathens, MD, MPH, PhD, FRCSC[a,c],
Paul J. Karanicolas, MD, PhD, FRCSC[a,d],*

[a]Division of General Surgery, University of Toronto, 600 University Avenue, Toronto, ON M5G 1X5, Canada; [b]Sunnybrook Health Sciences Centre, 2075 Bayview Avenue, Room K3W-11, Toronto, Ontario M4N 3M5, Canada; [c]Division of General Surgery, Sunnybrook Health Sciences Centre, 2075 Bayview Avenue, Room D574, Toronto, Ontario M4N 3M5, Canada; [d]Division of General Surgery, Sunnybrook Health Sciences Centre, 2075 Bayview Avenue, Room T2-16, Toronto, Ontario M4N 3M5, Canada

Keywords

- Small bowel obstruction • Adhesions • Adhesiolysis • Laparoscopy • Bowel injury
- Bowel resection

Key points

- Laparoscopic surgery for adhesive small bowel obstruction is becoming increasingly common.
- Existing evidence suggests that laparoscopic surgery for small bowel obstruction is associated with improved clinical outcomes.
- Laparoscopy in this patient population is associated with a higher risk of bowel injury than open surgery.
- Appropriate patient selection and techniques to mitigate the risks for bowel injury are necessary to make laparoscopy surgery a safe undertaking in this patient population.

 Video content accompanies this article at http://www. advancessurgery.com/.

Disclosure Statement: The authors have nothing to disclose.

*Corresponding author. Sunnybrook Health Sciences Centre, 2075 Bayview Avenue, Room T2-16, Toronto, Ontario M4N 3M5, Canada. E-mail address: paul.karanicolas@sunny-brook.ca

https://doi.org/10.1016/j.yasu.2018.03.001

INTRODUCTION

Small bowel obstruction (SBO) is among the most common reasons for admission to a surgical service in developed countries. Approximately 20% of all emergency admissions for acute abdomen are for SBO [1–3]. For approximately 20% to 30% of these admissions, surgical intervention is required, resulting in an estimated 350,000 operations performed annually in the United States. These operations are associated with 960,000 inpatient days and $2.3 billion in health care expenditures [4,5].

Over the last 2 decades, the use of minimally invasive techniques in surgery have proliferated. Across a wide range of surgical illnesses, laparoscopy reduces surgical site infections, serious complications, perioperative mortality, and postoperative duration of stay [6–15].

Among patients undergoing surgery for adhesive SBO (aSBO) in the province of Ontario, Canada, the use of laparoscopy increased from 4% to more than 14% between 2005 and 2014 [16]. However, a laparoscopic approach in patients with SBO has unique challenges. These challenges include trocar introduction into an abdomen filled with distended bowel and the manipulation of bowel using laparoscopic bowel graspers in the context of distended, potentially ischemic bowel. Some studies have suggested that a laparoscopic approach in this patient population may be associated with an increased risk of bowel injury [6,16–18].

The objective of this article is to summarize the existing literature regarding the safety of laparoscopic surgery for SBO. This article focuses on surgery for SBO caused by adhesions. Adhesions are responsible for approximately 70% to 75% of all admissions for SBO [19]. Other common etiologies of SBO, including hernias, intraluminal or extraluminal malignancy, volvulus, intussusception, and so on have considerably varying surgical approaches for which laparoscopy may or may not be appropriate.

SIGNIFICANCE

Bowel injuries and resections

Despite the potential advantages with regard to postoperative complications, mortality, and duration of stay, there are several challenges associated with laparoscopic procedures in patients with SBO. Adhesions that may secure loops of bowel to the anterior peritoneal surface as well as the limited intraabdominal space caused by distended bowel makes trocar introduction challenging. Additionally, the handling of heavy, fluid-filled bowel using laparoscopic graspers may result in injuries to the bowel wall. Together, these challenges place patients at risk for bowel injury and, potentially, resection. Bowel resections in patients with SBO are associated with increased risk of postoperative complications [20].

Limitations in the available data have made the study of bowel injuries in this patient population challenging. Many population-level datasets do not capture conversion from laparoscopy to open, and most datasets only record bowel resection, neglecting iatrogenic bowel injury. In the most commonly used database (the American College of Surgeons National Quality Improvement Program), bowel resections are recorded as laparoscopic if they are performed laparoscopically and as open if performed via laparotomy, regardless of how a case was initiated. In this database, there is no coding for conversion to an open procedure. Therefore, bowel injuries that occur laparoscopically and result in conversion to open with open bowel resections are misleadingly counted as bowel resections associated with open procedures. For example, a large study in 2013 that used data from the American College of Surgeons National Quality Improvement Program found a lower incidence of bowel resection with laparoscopic procedures (8.1% vs 31.5%). However, this dataset did not capture iatrogenic injuries or conversions and may have misclassified laparoscopic injuries as open bowel resections [7].

Our group recently examined a large cohort to compare the incidence of bowel injury between open and laparoscopic procedures for SBO. To mitigate limitations to the available data, we used validated operative billing codes, to define a composite outcome that included codes for "bowel resection," "bowel enterotomy," and "suture repair of intestine," which we called "bowel intervention." We also evaluated patients based on the approach by which their operation was initiated, in an intention-to-treat analysis. Therefore, bowel injuries during procedures that were initiated laparoscopically, which required conversion to an open procedure, were classified as laparoscopic-associated injuries. In our analysis, patients who underwent procedures that were initiated laparoscopically were more likely to require bowel intervention than those who underwent open procedures (53.5% vs 43.4%; $P<.0001$; Fig. 1). After adjusting for patient- and hospital-level covariates in a hierarchical multivariable regression model, laparoscopy was associated with an adjusted odds ratio (OR) for bowel intervention of 1.64 (95% confidence interval, 1.39–1.93) [16].

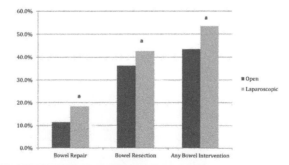

Fig. 1. Incidence of bowel injury and resection by surgical approach. Bowel repair is an enterotomy and/or suture of intestine. Any bowel intervention is bowel repair and/or bowel resection. [a] $P<.05$. (*From* Behman R, Nathens AB, Byrne JP, et al. Laparoscopic surgery for adhesives small bowel obstruction is associated with a higher risk of bowel injury: a population-based analysis of 8584 patients. Ann Surg 2017;266(3):492; with permission.)

The limitations to data sources have made the study of bowel injury with laparoscopic surgery challenging and likely contribute to discrepancy in findings. For example, in a systematic review by Sajid and colleagues [21], bowel resection and bowel injury were evaluated separately. The authors found that laparoscopy was associated lower risk of bowel resection (OR, 0.39; 95% confidence interval, 0.20–0.75), but a nonsignificantly higher risk of bowel injury (OR, 1.08; 95% confidence interval, 0.25–4.61). Among the 6 studies that evaluated bowel injury in this metaanalysis, the OR associated with a laparoscopic approach ranged from 0.09 to 8.55. The discrepancy in the existing literature may reflect the quality of the available data and the challenges to accurately evaluating intraoperative iatrogenic injuries. In another systematic review and metaanalysis, 2 studies were identified that compared the incidence of bowel injury between laparoscopic and open procedures. Laparoscopy was associated with an OR of 1.9 for bowel injury compared with open procedures, although the analysis was underpowered and did not yield statistical significance [22].

Bowel injuries and bowel resections in patients with aSBO are associated with increased postoperative morbidity and mortality [20]. In our population-based cohort study, we compared the incidence of serious complications and 30-day mortality between patients who underwent laparoscopic procedures that involved a bowel intervention and patients who had open procedures that did not involve a bowel intervention. The adjusted odds of experiencing a serious complication or of experiencing perioperative mortality were significantly higher in patients who had laparoscopic procedures that involved a bowel intervention compared with patients who had open procedures without bowel resection [16] (Fig. 2).

Our findings suggest that bowel intervention is a more significant driver of adverse outcomes than the morbidity associated with laparotomy. In cases

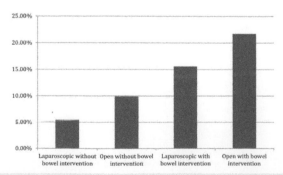

Fig. 2. Incidence of serious complications by surgical approach and bowel intervention. The χ^2 across all 4 groups: $P<.0001$; χ^2 between groups 2 and 3: $P = .013$. (*From* Behman R, Nathens AB, Byrne JP, et al. Laparoscopic surgery for adhesives small bowel obstruction is associated with a higher risk of bowel injury: a population-based analysis of 8584 patients. Ann Surg 2017;266(3):494; with permission.)

initiated laparoscopically in which the risk of bowel injury is high, conversion to an open procedure and avoiding a bowel injury is more important than completing a procedure laparoscopically and avoiding laparotomy.

Perioperative morbidity and mortality

Almost all studies that have compared laparoscopic and open approaches for SBO demonstrate a significant decrease in the incidence of perioperative complications and mortality associated with laparoscopic procedures. Table 1 contains a summary of the existing literature with a focus on large, population-based studies and metaanalyses. Laparoscopy is consistently associated with lower odds of superficial surgical site infections, lower odds of postoperative complications (both serious complications and overall complications), and lower odds of postoperative mortality.

A major limitation to the existing data with respect to evaluation of perioperative morbidity and mortality is in the inherent selection bias of retrospective data. Patients who undergo laparoscopic procedures are, in almost all studies, younger and have fewer comorbidities than patients who undergo open procedures [7,16,23]. A number of different statistical methods have been used in efforts to mitigate this selection bias. The results are reassuringly consistent across studies, with laparoscopy being associated with a lower risk of perioperative morbidity and mortality.

In summary, the existing literature suggests that laparoscopic adhesiolysis is safe with regards to the most clinically important perioperative outcomes: morbidity and mortality. The limitations of these studies should be noted and the findings should be considered in the context of appropriate patient selection.

Duration of stay

Almost 1 million days of inpatient care are attributed annually to patients undergoing surgical management for adhesive SBO in the United States alone. All large studies that we evaluated for this article identified a shorter length of stay associated with laparoscopic procedures compared with open procedures (see Table 1).

Given the volume of annual admissions for SBO and the high associated resource burden, the shorter duration of stay with laparoscopy is an important consideration from a health care use perspective. Moreover, shorter duration of hospital may reduce patients' exposure to potential nosocomial infections.

Although the existing evidence suggests that laparoscopic approaches in patients with SBO are associated with a shorter duration of stay, the limitations mentioned with regard to selection bias should be considered in evaluating the duration of stay.

PRESENT RELEVANCE AND FUTURE AVENUES

Surgery for SBO is a common undertaking in developed countries. The incidence of complications associated with surgery for aSBO is high, with rates that approach 25% in most large studies [7,21,23]. Moreover, these procedures are often performed in an emergent setting in patients who are malnourished, have high aspiration risk, and may have ischemic bowel or sepsis.

Table 1
Summary of results of studies comparing laparoscopic and open adhesiolysis

Authors	Setting/design	Cohort size	Timeframe	Findings
Behman et al [16], 2017	• Retrospective cohort study of Ontario administrative data • Multivariable logistic regression	8584	2005–2014	Laparoscopy associated with: • Greater odds of bowel intervention (OR, 1.64; 95% CI, 1.39 to 1.93) • Lower odds of serious complications (OR, 0.80; 95% CI, 0.61 to 1.04)[a] • Lower odds of 30-d mortality (OR, 0.63; 95% CI, 0.42 to 0.95) • Shorter duration of stay (7 d vs 10 d, P<.0001)
Kelly et al [7], 2014	• Retrospective cohort study of ACS-NSQIP • Multivariable logistic regression	9619	2005–2010	Laparoscopy associated with: • Lower odds of serious complications (OR, 0.70; 95% CI, 0.58 to 0.85) • Lower odds of incisional complications (OR, 0.22; 95% CI, 0.15 to 0.33) • Lower odds of 30-d mortality (OR, 0.55; 95% CI, 0.33 to 0.92) • Shorter duration of stay (4.7 d vs 9.9 d; P<.0001)

| Lombardo et al [23], 2014 | • Retrospective cohort study of ACS-NSQIP
• Propensity-matched analysis | 6762 (444 after matching) | 2005–2009 | Laparoscopy associated with:
• Lower odds of all complications (OR, 0.48; 95% CI, 0.30 to 0.77)
• Lower odds of incisional complications (OR, 0.17; 95% CI, 0.05 to 0.57)
• Lower odds of serious complications (OR, 0.56; 95% CI, 0.33 to 0.96)
• Shorter duration of stay (4 d vs 10 d; $P<.001$) |
| Sajid et al [21], 2016 | • Systematic review and metaanalysis | 38,C57 (14 studies) | 2003–2014 | Laparoscopy associated with:
• Lower odds of all complications (OR, 0.38; 95% CI, 0.13 to 0.65)
• Lower odds of postoperative mortality (OR, 0.31; 95% CI, 0.23 to 0.42)
• Shorter duration of stay (standard mean difference, −0.44; 95% CI, −0.65 to −0.22) |

Abbreviations: ACS-NSQIP, American College of Surgeons National Quality Improvement Program; CI, confidence interval; OR, odds ratio.

^aDid not reach statistical significance.

Based on the existing literature, a laparoscopic approach in patients with adhesive SBO is safe, with a duly cautious approach. Patients who undergo laparoscopic procedures have lower postoperative morbidity and mortality as well as shorter durations of stay. In multiple studies, these findings persist after adjusting for important patient and operative factors.

However, despite a lower incidence of serious complications and perioperative mortality, laparoscopic procedures are associated with a greater risk of bowel injury. Moreover, when bowel injury does occur, the associated morbidity is high. Patients who undergo open procedures without bowel intervention have lower adjusted morbidity than patients who undergo laparoscopic procedures with bowel intervention, suggesting that the morbidity associated with bowel injury or resection is greater than the morbidity associated with laparotomy.

Although a laparoscopic approach in this patient population may be safe, an understanding of the inherent challenges and risks of bowel injury is important. Given the volume of adhesiolysis procedures performed each year and the risks associated with these procedures, measures to optimize the safety of laparoscopy in this patient population are critical.

Patient selection

Patient selection is an important factor in optimizing the benefits of laparoscopy while minimizing the risks. In our previously published study, we used a hierarchical multivariable regression model to evaluate the impact of laparoscopy on bowel intervention. Our model identified 3 factors associated with increased odds of bowel intervention after adjusting for other patient- and hospital-level covariates, including laparoscopy. These factors were (1) older patient age, (2) female sex, and (3) undergoing an after-hours procedure, defined as procedures that were initiated between 5 PM and 7 AM on weekdays or on weekends [16].

Older patients undergoing surgery for SBO may have a more extensive prior surgical history as well as poorer vascular supply and friable tissue, which may explain the increased risk of bowel intervention. Female patients often have deep pelvic adhesions resulting from previous gynecologic procedures, which may be more challenging to lyse, particularly laparoscopically.

It is difficult to interpret the impact of after-hours procedures. It is unclear from our retrospective data if an after-hours procedure is a risk factor for bowel intervention or if patients who undergo after-hours procedures are inherently at greater risk of bowel interventions owing to clinical deterioration or signs of bowel ischemia necessitating emergent surgery.

Appropriate patient selection is important to mitigate the risks of laparoscopy in this patient population. Patient selection requires a thorough understanding of each patient's previous surgical history and abdominal wall anatomy—previous surgical scars and the presence of ventral hernias or abdominal wall mesh are important considerations for surgical planning. Careful evaluation of preoperative imaging can help to identify obstructions that may be amenable to laparoscopic adhesiolysis or may suggest dense, matted adhesions that may be better approached by laparotomy. Finally, our results suggest that older patients, female patients, and patients undergoing after-hours procedures may be at increased risk for bowel injuries.

Taken together, these factors should aid surgeons in identifying patients who are at elevated risk for bowel injury with a laparoscopic approach. In these patients, an open approach or early conversion to open should be considered.

Avoiding trocar injury

Safely establishing peritoneal access is challenging in patients with adhesive SBO (Video 1). Owing to distended bowel, patients with aSBO often have limited free space in the abdomen into which trocars may safely be introduced. Patients with a history of previous intraabdominal procedures often have midline adhesions to the anterior peritoneal surface, resulting in loops of bowel adherent to the anterior abdominal wall at the site of potential trocar insertion. Careful consideration of the patient's previous surgical history and preoperative imaging is necessary for safe trocar placement.

When establishing peritoneal access, care should be taken to avoid any previous surgical incisions, because these are likely to have associated adhesions. In cases of a previous midline incision, we recommend entry into the left or the right upper quadrant. When available, preoperative computed tomography scans should be inspected to determine which quadrant has fewer distended loops of bowel, while being mindful that bowel may have moved by the time of surgery. Previous reports have suggested improved safety with a Veress technique to establish pneumoperitoneum, followed by placement of optical trocars to visualize entry [10]. However, instances of bowel injury with optical trocar placement have been reported and surgeons should be wary of a false sense of security when using this technique. Ultimately, surgeon comfort should be considered and surgeons should only use an entry technique with which they are comfortable. Our approach is to use a Veress needle to establish access subcostally in the midclavicular line on either the left or the right side, depending on the computed tomography findings.

Once pneumoperitoneum is established and a laparoscopic camera has been introduced, inspection of the anterior peritoneal surface should be performed to identify safe entry points for additional trocars. A high-definition, 5-mm laparoscope with a 30° angle of view is critical to optimize visualization during this operation. After the introduction of a second port, abdominal wall adhesions may be carefully lysed to allow for additional working ports to be placed. The lysis of abdominal wall adhesions should use sharp dissection techniques where possible. In general, surgeons should minimize the use of energy devices in these patients, because the bowel-filled abdomen often has limited working space and compromised field of view, increasing the risk for collateral injury. Box 1 contains a summary of the steps required to safely establish peritoneal access.

Safe bowel handling

The manipulation of distended and potentially ischemic bowel using laparoscopic bowel graspers is another important hazard associated with a laparoscopic

Box 1: Steps for safely establishing peritoneal access

1. Evaluate preoperative imaging, inspect the abdomen and avoid previous surgical incisions.
2. Use the Veress technique in the RUQ or LUQ and optical trocars if comfortable doing so.
3. Inspect the anterior abdominal wall with the laparoscopic camera for additional safe entry points.
4. Take down anterior peritoneal adhesions to facilitate additional trocar entry.
5. Use sharp dissection of adhesions where possible and avoid energy use.

approach in this patient population (Video 2). Laparoscopic graspers may have a small contact area with the bowel, resulting in focal points of tension that are prone to tearing. Moreover, owing to the large diameter of distended bowel, it is often challenging to adequately grasp the bowel without the grasper sliding off. This situation results in small pieces of bowel wall captured in the grasper that are prone to tearing. Finally, the distended, fluid-filled bowel is often heavy, requiring more force to manipulate and adding to the risks of tearing.

Surgeons should avoid grasping dilated bowel altogether when possible. After establishing adequate port access, the terminal ileum should be identified, which should be collapsed in SBO. The small bowel can then be followed proximally from the terminal ileum until the obstruction-causing adhesion is found, with the surgeon only grasping collapsed bowel.

In situations where distended bowel must be manipulated, care should be taken to ensure that the bowel is grasped using the entire jaw of the grasper, with the aim of reaching across the entire width of the small bowel. Manipulation of the bowel should not be attempted until large, secure grasps of bowel have been secured. Where possible, distended bowel should be grasped using 2 graspers in 2 different points a few centimeters apart to maximize distribution of tension. Generous use of table tilt can help to mobilize heavy, distended bowel. Finally, the bowel should only be grasped on screen, where it can be clearly visualized. Box 2 contains a summary of techniques designed to mitigate the risks of injury during bowel manipulation.

Box 2: Safe bowel handling

1. Identify collapsed terminal ileum and run the bowel backward until obstructing adhesion is identified.
2. Avoid grasping distended bowel when possible.
3. If distended bowel must be grasped, ensure large bites that use the entire jaw of the grasper.
4. When possible, distended bowel should be grasped in 2 places.
5. Grasped bowel should only be held on screen.
6. Generous use of table tilt can be used to aid in mobilizing heavy bowel loops.

Converting to an open procedure

Another consideration is conversion from laparoscopy to laparotomy in patients with SBO. Approximately 30% of cases that are initiated laparoscopically for SBO are converted to an open procedure [6,17]. The majority of conversions are prompted by dense adhesions and bowel resections or injuries.

Surgeons should approach cases of laparoscopic lysis of adhesions with an understanding that approximately one-third of these procedures will require conversion to open. Conversion to open should not be perceived as a failure of a laparoscopic approach, but as a normal potential course of laparoscopic surgery of SBO.

There are several critical moments in which the decision to convert to an open procedure should be considered, to avoid or repair injured bowel (Box 3). These moments include at the time of trocar placement, during attempts to safely manipulate the bowel, upon inspecting the bowel if there are signs of ischemia, and in the event of bowel injury. Surgeon experience and comfort with laparoscopy should be considered, particularly when deciding whether to preform a bowel resection or bowel wall repair laparoscopically.

Future avenues

The body of existing literature has important limitations, and findings should be interpreted in the context of these limitations. Given the retrospective nature of all studies, selection bias and unmeasured confounding are invariably present. Future studies should aim to address these limitations.

Prospective collection of SBO-specific data will be critical to optimizing care in this large patient population. Although data collected in the American College of Surgeons National Quality Improvement Program are captured prospectively, this database is not specifically designed to study SBO and has important limitations. We have identified 6 areas for which data are largely unavailable in large, population-based databases. These areas include (1) findings of preoperative imaging, (2) type of adhesions (dense, matted vs bands), (3) previous surgical history (total number, previous procedures for SBO, presence of synthetic mesh), (4) surgeon training and/or experience with minimally invasive surgery, (5) whether there was conversion from laparoscopy to an open procedure, and (6) the incidence of iatrogenic bowel injury. An understanding of these perioperative findings and events is necessary to accurately evaluate interventions and to determine optimal care strategies.

Box 3: When to consider converting to an open procedure

1. If safe placement of adequate trocars is not possible.
2. If collapsed, distal bowel cannot be safely identified and grasped.
3. If the procedure cannot advance without significant manipulation of distended bowel.
4. If a bowel resection is necessary owing to ischemia.
5. If a bowel injury has occurred and requires repair.

SUMMARY

Laparoscopy for adhesive SBO is safe; however, appropriate patient selection, careful entry to the peritoneal cavity, gentle handling of the bowel, and early conversion to laparotomy are crucial to avoid undue injury to the bowel. Surgeons should be aware that laparoscopy is associated with an increased risk of bowel injury in this patient population and use techniques to mitigate this risk. The safe use of laparoscopy for SBO requires a balancing of the risks of bowel injury and the benefits of laparoscopy with the ultimate goal of improving outcomes in this common disease.

SUPPLEMENTARY DATA

Supplementary data related to this article can be found online at https://doi.org/ 10.1016/j.yasu.2018.03.001.

References

[1] Millet I, Ruyer A, Alili C, et al. Adhesive small-bowel obstruction: value of CT in identifying findings associated with the effectiveness of nonsurgical treatment. Radiology 2014;273(2): 425–32.

[2] Foster NM, McGory ML, Zingmond DS, et al. Small bowel obstruction: a population-based appraisal. J Am Coll Surg 2006;203(2):170–6.

[3] Irvin TT. Abdominal pain: a surgical audit of 1190 emergency admissions. Br J Surg 1989;76(11):1121–5.

[4] Sikirica V, Bapat B, Candrilli SD, et al. The inpatient burden of abdominal and gynecological adhesiolysis in the US. BMC Surg 2011;11(1):13.

[5] Ray NF, Denton WG, Thamer M, et al. Abdominal adhesiolysis: inpatient care and expenditures in the United States in 1994. J Am Coll Surg 1998;186(1):1–9.

[6] O'Connor DB, Winter DC. The role of laparoscopy in the management of acute small-bowel obstruction: a review of over 2,000 cases. Surg Endosc 2012;26(1):12–7.

[7] Kelly KN, Iannuzzi JC, Rickles AS, et al. Laparotomy for small-bowel obstruction: first choice or last resort for adhesiolysis? A laparoscopic approach for small-bowel obstruction reduces 30-day complications. Surg Endosc 2014;28(1):65–73.

[8] Garrett KA, Champagne BJ, Valerian BT, et al. A single training center's experience with 200 consecutive cases of diverticulitis: can all patients be approached laparoscopically? Surg Endosc 2008;22(11):2503–8.

[9] Saleh F, Ambrosini L, Jackson T, et al. Laparoscopic versus open surgical management of small bowel obstruction: an analysis of short-term outcomes. Surg Endosc 2014;28(8): 2381–6.

[10] Nagle A, Ujiki M, Denham W, et al. Laparoscopic adhesiolysis for small bowel obstruction. Am J Surg 2004;187(4):464–70.

[11] Agresta F, Piazza A, Michelet I, et al. Small bowel obstruction. Laparoscopic approach. Surg Endosc 2000;14(2):154–6.

[12] Agresta F, Ansaloni L, Baiocchi GL, et al. Laparoscopic approach to acute abdomen from the Consensus Development Conference of the Societa Italiana di Chirurgia Endoscopica e nuove tecnologie (SICE), Associazione Chirurghi Ospedalieri Italiani (ACOI), Societa Italiana di Chirurgia (SIC), Societa Italiana di Chirurgia d''Urgenza e del Trauma (SICUT), Societa Italiana di Chirurgia nell''Ospedalita Privata (SICOP), and the European Association for Endoscopic Surgery (EAES). Surg Endosc 2012;26(8): 2134–64.

[13] Winslow ER, Brunt LM. Perioperative outcomes of laparoscopic versus open splenectomy: a meta-analysis with an emphasis on complications. Surgery 2003;134(4):647–53 [discussion: 654–5].

[14] Nguyen NT, Neuhaus AM, Ho HS, et al. A prospective evaluation of intracorporeal laparo-scopic small bowel anastomosis during gastric bypass. Obes Surg 2001;11(2):196–9.

[15] Thaler K, Dinnewitzer A, Mascha E, et al. Long-term outcome and health-related quality of life after laparoscopic and open colectomy for benign disease. Surg Endosc 2003;17(9): 1404–8.

[16] Behman R, Nathens AB, Byrne JP, et al. Laparoscopic surgery for adhesive small bowel obstruction is associated with a higher risk of bowel injury: a population-based analysis of 8584 patients. Ann Surg 2017;266(3):489–98.

[17] Ghosheh B, Salameh JR. Laparoscopic approach to acute small bowel obstruction: review of 1061 cases. Surg Endosc 2007;21(11):1945–9.

[18] Halling A, Fridh G, Ovhed I. Validating the Johns Hopkins ACG case-mix system of the elderly in Swedish primary health care. BMC Public Health 2006;6(1):171.

[19] Mullan CP, Siewert B, Eisenberg RL. Small bowel obstruction. AJR Am J Roentgenol 2012;198(2):W105–17.

[20] Margenthaler JA, Longo WE, Virgo KS, et al. Risk factors for adverse outcomes following surgery for small bowel obstruction. Ann Surg 2006;243(4):456–64.

[21] Sajid MS, Khawaja AH, Sains P, et al. A systematic review comparing laparoscopic vs open adhesiolysis in patients with adhesional small bowel obstruction. Am J Surg 2016;212(1): 138–50.

[22] Li M-Z, Lian L, Xiao L-B, et al. Laparoscopic versus open adhesiolysis in patients with adhesive small bowel obstruction: a systematic review and meta-analysis. Am J Surg 2012;204(5):779–86.

[23] Lombardo S, Baum K, Filho JD, et al. Should adhesive small bowel obstruction be managed laparoscopically? A National Surgical Quality Improvement Program propensity score analysis. J Trauma Acute Care Surg 2014;76(3):696–703.

Advances in Surgery 52 (2018) 29–42

ADVANCES IN SURGERY

ELSEVIER
MOSBY

Prevention and Treatment of *Clostridium difficile* Enterocolitis

Lisa M. Kodadek, MD[a,*], Pamela A. Lipsett, MD, MHPE[a,b]

[a]Department of Surgery, Johns Hopkins University School of Medicine, 600 North Wolfe Street, Tower 110, Baltimore, MD 21287, USA; [b]Anesthesiology and Critical Care Medicine, Johns Hopkins University School of Medicine, 600 North Wolfe Street, Osler 603, Baltimore, MD 21287, USA

Keywords

- *Clostridium difficile* • Enterocolitis • Infection

Key points

- *Clostridium difficile* infection is a major cause of nosocomial infection and is increasing in incidence and severity.
- Metronidazole and vancomycin are considered first-line medical therapies.
- Surgical management is subtotal colectomy with preservation of the rectum and end ileostomy.
- Diverting loop ileostomy with colonic lavage and installation of antibiotics via the ileostomy may be appropriate for selected patients.

INTRODUCTION

Clostridium difficile infection (CDI) is a symptomatic disease caused by the spore-forming and toxin-producing anaerobic bacterium *C difficile*. CDI is the most common cause of pseudomembranous colitis and remains a major cause of nosocomial infection and antibiotic-associated diarrhea. Surgical patient populations, especially patients undergoing colorectal procedures and those with inflammatory bowel disease, are susceptible. Rates of CDI are increasing in incidence in the United States, and associated morbidity and mortality are high. Antibiotic stewardship, hand hygiene, and environmental control are critical to help prevent spread of this transmissible disease. Most cases will respond to medical management, but early operative consultation is recommended. The mainstay of surgical management is subtotal colectomy with preservation of the rectum and end ileostomy. Some patients may be appropriate for a newer

Disclosure: The authors have nothing to disclose.

*Corresponding author. E-mail address: lkodadek@jhmi.edu

approach using diverting loop ileostomy with colonic lavage and installation of antibiotics via the efferent limb of the ileostomy.

HISTORY

The first reported case of pseudomembranous colitis was published in 1893 by JM.T. Finney at The Johns Hopkins Hospital [1]. A 22-year-old woman developed bloody diarrhea on the tenth postoperative day after uncomplicated peptic ulcer surgery and died on postoperative day 15. The autopsy report described pseudomembranous changes of the colon: "...appearing gray in contrast with the haemorrhagic mucous membrane about it, and a coating of what is apparently fibrin (and blood) can be scraped from the surface." Although the *C difficile* organism would not be identified until more than 40 years later, this case has been cited as the first report of a *C difficile*–associated diseaselike process [2,3]. Pseudomembranous colitis became a commonly recognized complication of antibiotic use in the early 1950s. Surgeons reported rates as high as 14% to 27% among postoperative patients [4]. An early study used routine endoscopy and reported high rates of pseudomembranous colitis (21%) among patients receiving the antibiotic clindamycin [5]. Further efforts were directed at identifying the cause of "clindamycin colitis." By the late 1970s, *C difficile* was isolated from the stool of patients with pseudomembranous colitis [6,7].

SIGNIFICANCE AND EPIDEMIOLOGY

CDI is common and remains the most frequently reported health care–associated pathogen in the United States [8]. CDI is an independent predictor of increased length of stay in the intensive care unit, increased hospital length of stay, and higher total hospital charges [3]. A major burden for both patients and hospitals, CDI has demonstrated increasing incidence and greater severity of disease since the year 2000 [9–11]. Currently, at least 500,000 cases are reported each year in the United States, and mortality may be as high as 5% to 10% [11,12]. The economic burden of CDI on the US health care system is estimated at more than $1.5 to $2 billion per year [9,11].

Although most CDI cases are acquired in the hospital, a growing number of individuals without traditional risk factors have acquired the infection in the community [13]. Community-acquired CDI may account for more than one-third of *C difficile*–associated diarrhea. Specifically, nursing home–acquired CDI represents nearly one-quarter of all cases in the United States with a 19% recurrence and 8% 30-day mortality [14]. Although community-acquired cases are usually associated with lower mortality than hospital-acquired cases, rates of hospitalization, morbidity, and mortality remain high.

PATHOGENESIS

C difficile is present within the normal microbial population of the gut in as many as 5% to 15% of healthy adults and 40% to 60% of neonates [15,16]. Asymptomatic colonization is not a risk factor for symptomatic CDI and may in fact protect against development of the disease [17]. Healthy carriers are thought to be protected by their normal intestinal flora as well as the formation of immunoglobulin G antibody to the toxins produced by *C difficile* [18]. Individuals colonized with *C difficile* likely develop immune memory, which confers a protective effect through the sixth or seventh decade but then wanes [3]. Waning immune memory may account for the increased incidence of CDI among older patients.

CDI requires both the presence of the bacterium and disruption of intestinal flora. The bacterium itself is not invasive, but *C difficile* can produce several toxins, including toxin A and toxin B, which are thought to contribute to its pathogenesis. Although toxin A and toxin B are necessary to cause CDI, they are not sufficient [19]. The toxins disrupt epithelial integrity by glycosylation of cytoskeletal proteins, which cause loss of cell-cell tight junctions and subsequent release of inflammatory mediators. An inflammatory infiltrate may develop in the colonic mucosa, which further leads to fluid shifts responsible for diarrhea and epithelial necrosis [20].

A new strain of *C difficile* (B1/NAP1/027, also known as ribotype 027) is proving to be more virulent with higher production of toxin A and toxin B. This strain has been associated with several outbreaks of infection in the United States and worldwide [21]. As many as 28.1% of CDI may be caused by this new strain, and reports indicate that it is the most common strain currently found in health care facilities in the United States [22]. Reduced susceptibility to vancomycin has been noted in 39.1% of ribotype 027 isolates, and metronidazole may be a superior antibiotic regimen in these cases [22,23]. In patients infected with ribotype 027, mortality at 6 months has been shown to be higher than those with non–ribotype 27 strains [24].

RISK FACTORS
The most important risk factors for the development of both initial and recurrent CDI are exposure to antibiotics and exposure to *C difficile* [3,19]. Classically, antibiotics such as clindamycin or fluoroquinolones have been implicated in the pathogenesis of this disease, but any antibiotic can cause CDI. A single dose of antibiotics may serve as a risk factor, although rate of CDI following administration of perioperative antibiotics is low. One study has shown that the risk of developing subsequent CDI from a single dose of perioperative ertapenem is 1.7% among patients undergoing colorectal surgery [25]. Extended duration and repeated doses of antibiotics confer higher risk. Among community-acquired cases of CDI, however, 43% of patients had no known antibiotic exposure [26].

Other important risk factors for CDI are common among surgical patients: gastrointestinal surgery (especially colectomy), emergency surgery, solid organ transplant, inflammatory bowel disease, and nasogastric tube use. Advanced age, immunodeficiency, and prolonged or recent stay in a hospital or long-term care facility may also increase risk of infection. Administration of proton pump inhibitors (PPI) has been associated with increased risk of CDI. Histamine-2 receptor antagonists are less commonly associated with CDI than PPIs [27].

PREVENTION

Prevention of CDI is a multidisciplinary effort. Antibiotic stewardship aims to limit the development of antibiotic-resistant microorganisms through directed use of antibiotics. Tactics include limiting duration of empiric antibiotic treatment, selecting the most appropriate narrow-spectrum antibiotic based on culture data, and ensuring appropriate dosing and duration of antibiotic therapy [28]. Environmental control includes use of disposable medical supplies, personal protective equipment (contact precautions), private or separated rooms, and terminal room cleaning. Although glove use has been shown to reduce the incidence of CDI, the efficacy of gown use for disease prevention has not been studied [29,30]. The cost-benefit ratio of disposable gown use has also not been established. Terminal room cleaning with bleach is recommend by the Centers for Disease Control and Prevention after a patient has been discharged or transferred; hydrogen peroxide vapor or pulsed xenon ultraviolet light may also be used for terminal cleaning [31]. *C difficile* spores are not eradicated by typical alcohol-based approaches to hand hygiene; providers must be diligent about washing their hands with soap and water or 4% chlorhexidine to prevent transmission of infectious spores [32].

DIAGNOSIS

Diagnosis of CDI requires the presence of diarrhea (3 or more unformed stools in 24 hours) or radiographic evidence of ileus or toxic megacolon, *and* a positive stool test for toxigenic *C difficile* or its toxins or evidence of pseudomembranous colitis (by colonoscopic or histopathologic findings) [9]. Simple stool cultures for *C difficile* are not useful because strains that do not produce toxins are not clinically relevant, and as many as 20% to 46% of *C difficile* isolates are nontoxigenic [3]. Laboratory testing is unable to distinguish between colonization and symptomatic infection with *C difficile*. Testing should be limited to those patients with diarrhea, unless ileus from CDI is suspected [33]. Testing should not be repeated within 7 days because this will increase the rate of false positive results [19]. It is not appropriate to complete testing after treatment of known CDI to establish cure. Patients may continue to have a positive test for several months even after resolution of symptoms [34].

A variety of methods are currently available for diagnosis of toxigenic *C difficile* (Table 1) [35–38]. Toxigenic culture and cell cytotoxicity assays are generally considered the gold standards for diagnosis, but they are too time-consuming and resource intensive for practical clinical use. A 2-step method uses glutamate dehydrogenase (GDH) enzyme immunoassay (EIA) with subsequent EIA to detect toxins A and B. GDH is produced by both toxigenic and nontoxigenic strains of *C difficile* so confirmatory testing for toxins is critical to establish the diagnosis. Nucleic acid amplification test (NAAT), also known as real-time polymerase chain reaction (PCR), allows for detection of *C difficile* toxin genes in a single step. NAAT is now more commonly used in clinical practice because it is a rapid test with high sensitivity and specificity. The

Table 1

Laboratory tests for the diagnosis of *Clostridium difficile* infection

Assay	Methodology/assay target	Sensitivity and specificity	Assay turnaround time	Availability of assay	Notes
Toxigenic culture	Detects toxigenic *C difficile*	High	24–43 h+	Limited availability and resource intensive	Reference standard
Cell cytotoxicity assay	Detects toxins A or B	High	24–48 h+	Limited availability and resource intensive	Reference standard
EIA	Detects GDH	GDH: high sensitivity with low specificity	Rapid, 15 min to 1 h	Widely available	GDH detection is nonspecific because GDH is produced by both toxigenic and nontoxigenic *C difficile* strains. When GDH EIA is used, a confirmatory EIA for toxins A and B must be performed
	Detects toxins A or B	Toxins A or B: low sensitivity with high specificity			
NAAT	PCR to detect *tcdB* or *tcdC* genes	High	Rapid, 45–180 min	Widely available	More expensive than other methods

Data from Refs. [35–38].

sensitivity of EIA testing may vary with *C difficile* strain, but NAAT is less variable. Although false positive results have been reported using NAAT, these false positives are usually seen in patients who are asymptomatic and for whom testing is not recommended [15,39].

Computed tomographic (CT) imaging may be used as an adjunct to diagnosis of *C difficile*–associated pathology, including fulminant colitis and toxic megacolon [40,41]. In the case of fulminant colitis, the colon wall may appear edematous and thickened with characteristic "thumb-printing." Pneumatosis intestinalis, mesenteric stranding, and ascites may also be noted. CT features that distinguish toxic megacolon from severe acute colitis include colonic dilatation or colonic wall thinning with intraluminal air and/or fluid with a distorted colonic contour or an ahaustral pattern and air-filled colonic distension greater than 6 cm. Diffuse colonic wall thickening and submucosal edema are more often present in cases of uncomplicated severe acute colitis (Fig. 1). However, some cases of CDI may manifest with diffuse colonic and rectal wall thickening with associated fat stranding (Fig. 2).

Endoscopy may be useful for diagnosis of CDI in cases whereby a false negative laboratory result is suspected, when a stool sample is not available for laboratory testing secondary to ileus, or when the differential diagnosis is broad and includes other colonic pathology [42]. Yellow plaques adherent to colonic mucosa or pseudomembranes are highly suggestive of CDI and warrant empiric treatment.

CLINICAL MANIFESTATION AND DISEASE SEVERITY

CDI is a spectrum of disease, and the clinical presentation is highly variable, ranging from mild diarrhea to toxic megacolon. Some patients with infection may not have diarrhea at all, but instead may demonstrate a distended abdomen, obstipation, and signs of systemic illness. Small bowel enteritis may also result from *C difficile*.

CDI is generally divided into categories and treated based on disease severity (Table 2). Clinical practice guidelines delineate criteria for mild to moderate disease, severe disease, complicated disease, and recurrent disease [33]. Mild to moderate disease is marked by a white blood cell count less than 15,000/mL and serum creatinine less than 1.5 times premorbid level. Severe disease is marked by a white blood cell count of at least 15,000/mL or serum creatinine of at least 1.5 times premorbid level. Severe/complicated disease manifests as systemic signs of infection plus hypotension or shock, ileus, or toxic megacolon. Recurrent disease is defined as recurrence of infection within 8 weeks of successful treatment of CDI [43]. As many as 15% to 35% of patients with CDI may experience recurrence [3].

Mild to moderate *C difficile* colitis may cause diarrhea and abdominal pain and usually appears as a diffuse or patchy erythematous colitis on colonoscopy. Pseudomembranous colonic changes are usually not seen in mild to moderate cases. However, in severe or complicated cases, systemic systems are apparent and pseudomembranes are usually visualized during colonoscopy.

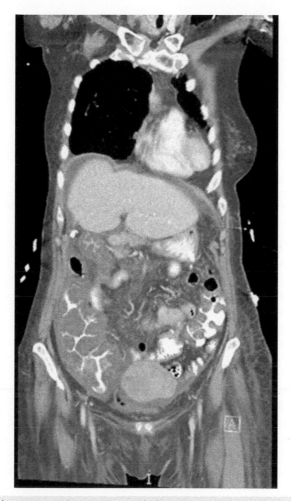

Fig. 1. Pancolitis on coronal CT imaging with disease present throughout colon but worse in the cecum and ascending colon.

Pseudomembranes, however, are not specific for *C difficile* colitis and may be seen in other types of infectious colitis.

Rarely, in less than 5% of cases, *C difficile* colitis may present as toxic megacolon [19]. Patients will have evidence of colonic dilation such as a distended abdomen or a radiologic finding of segmental or total colonic distension. The patient will also exhibit signs of systemic toxicity, such as fever, tachycardia, leukocytosis, or anemia. Typically, mental status changes, electrolyte disturbance, and/or hypotension are present [44]. One series examined cause of toxic megacolon among patients requiring operative intervention, and 34% of cases were caused by infectious colitis, second only to ulcerative colitis [45].

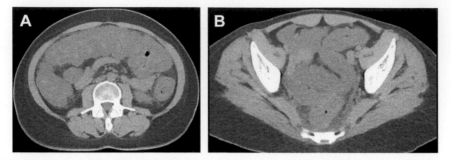

Fig. 2. CDI may manifest with diffuse colonic (A) and rectal wall (B) thickening with associated fat stranding.

MEDICAL TREATMENT

CDI often develops in the setting of treatment with antibiotics, especially clindamycin, fluoroquinolones, and third-generation cephalosporins [46–48]. When possible, the offending antibiotic should be discontinued if CDI is suspected or confirmed.

Metronidazole and vancomycin are considered first-line medical therapies for most patients with CDI. In cases of high clinical suspicion, antibiotic therapy may be started before laboratory confirmation of CDI. Metronidazole is appropriate for mild disease but has been associated with medical treatment failure in severe or complicated cases [49,50]. For mild to moderate CDI, a standard treatment regimen is 500 mg oral metronidazole 3 times daily for 10 to 14 days. If a patient is unable to take oral medications, metronidazole may be given by intravenous route at the same dose, but such a regimen should not be given as monotherapy [33,43]. Oral vancomycin may be indicated for treatment of mild to moderate infection when there is intolerance, contraindication, or lack of response to metronidazole.

Vancomycin is the preferred therapy in severe or complicated cases of CDI and may be combined with other adjunctive therapies. Available data show a clinical success rate of 66.3% for metronidazole versus 78.5% for vancomycin for severe CDI [9]. A typical regimen is 125 mg oral vancomycin 4 times daily for 10 to 14 days. Experts recommend higher doses of vancomycin (eg, 500 mg orally 4 times daily) in severe or complicated cases [33,43]. Rectal administration of vancomycin may be used as an adjunct therapy, but is not used as monotherapy. Intravenous metronidazole may be used as an adjunct in cases of severe or complicated CDI.

Recurrent CDI is increasing in incidence. Oral metronidazole or vancomycin may be used for the first recurrence of mild to moderate infection. Vancomycin is appropriate for patients who have had 2 or more recurrences of CDI. Fidaxomicin, a new macrocycle antibiotic approved for use in 2011, has been shown to be noninferior to vancomycin and may be beneficial for patients with recurrent CDI or those patients at high risk of recurrence. Lower recurrence rates

Table 2
Clostridium difficile infection disease severity and treatment

Disease severity category	Symptoms and signs	Treatment
Mild to moderate	Diarrhea White blood cell count <15,000/mL Serum creatinine <1.5 times baseline	Oral metronidazole 500 mg, 3 times daily, for 10–14 d OR Oral vancomycin 125 mg, 4 times daily, 10–14 d (if intolerance, contraindication, or lack of response to metronidazole) OR Oral fidaxomicin 200 mg, 2 times daily, for 10 d
Severe	Systemic signs of infection White blood cell count ≥15,000/mL Serum creatinine ≥1.5 times baseline	Oral vancomycin 125 mg, 4 times daily, 10–14 d OR Oral fidaxomicin 200 mg, 2 times daily, for 10 d (if significant risk of recurrence)
Severe, complicated	Systemic signs of infection Hypotension, ileus, or megacolon	Oral vancomycin 125–500 mg, 4 times daily, duration varies AND/OR Vancomycin per rectum, 500 mg/500 mL saline, 4 times daily AND Metronidazole, 500 mg intravenous, every 8 h AND Surgical consultation
Recurrent	Recurrence within 8 wk of successful completion of treatment	First recurrence: Repeat initial therapy OR Oral fidaxomicin 200 mg, 2 times daily, for 10 d Two or more recurrences: Oral fidaxomicin 200 mg, 2 times daily, for 10 d OR Vancomycin oral taper

Adapted from Cohen SH, Gerding DN, Johnson S, et al. Clinical practice guidelines for Clostridium difficile infection in adults: 2010 update by the Society for Healthcare Epidemiology of America (SHEA) and the Infectious Diseases Society of America (IDSA). Infect Control Hosp Epidemiol 2010;31(5):447; with permission.

have been shown with use of fidaxomicin (15.4%) as compared with vancomycin (25.3%) [51]. Fecal microbiota transfer (FMT) has an established role for treatment of recurrent CDI and may have response rates as high as 83% to 94% [9]. This procedure entails instillation of donor stool into the gastrointestinal tract of the patient via enema, upper or lower endoscopy, or nasojejunal tube. A randomized controlled trial published in 2013 demonstrated a 94% rate of symptom resolution with vancomycin followed by FMT (1 or 2 treatments) as compared with a 31% rate of resolution with vancomycin alone or a 23% rate of resolution with vancomycin plus bowel lavage. The trial was stopped early after interim analysis showed the clear benefit of FMT [52]. Regulation and standardization of FMT as well as further studies are needed to understand the impact of this therapy.

A role for immunotherapy in the treatment of CDI is emerging. An early study demonstrated that use of monoclonal antibodies against *C difficile* toxins A and B combined with standard therapy demonstrated a lower recurrence rate (7% vs 25%) [53]. A recent study demonstrated that among patients receiving standard treatment of primary or recurrent CDI, treatment with a human monoclonal antibody against *C difficile* toxin B (bezlotoxumab) was associated with a substantially lower rate of recurrent infection [54]. An anti–*C difficile* toxoid vaccine has also been developed that contains formalin-inactivated partially purified *C difficile* toxins A and B [55]. Clinical trials have shown the vaccines to be relatively safe, but further research is needed to understand the clinical benefits of *C difficile* vaccination [56,57]. A phase 3 clinical trial (Cdiffense) is underway that is enrolling at-risk patients [58].

SURGICAL TREATMENT
Early surgical consultation is critical for timely and optimal management of CDI, especially in cases of severe, complicated disease. Operative management is clearly necessary in rare cases of toxic megacolon, perforation, or peritonitis. It may be difficult to determine which patients will fail medical management and require surgical intervention. Some patients may not manifest signs of severe infection, but a low threshold for operative intervention should be maintained in patients aged 60 and older and/or those with baseline coagulopathy, baseline pulmonary or renal insufficiency, peripheral vascular disease, or congestive heart failure. These patients have worse outcomes and may benefit from earlier surgical management [59,60]. Patients with CDI cared for by a surgical team may benefit from shorter time to operative intervention, more frequent operative intervention, and lower mortality [61].

The mortality for total colectomy in patients with severe, complicated CDI may be as high as 30% to 50% [60]. Predictors of mortality in patients with *C difficile* colitis include higher APACHE II score, higher ASA class, baseline pulmonary or renal disease, steroid use, leukocytosis with white blood cell count greater than 20,000/mL, presence of toxic megacolon, and clinical signs of organ dysfunction. Predictors of postoperative mortality include preoperative shock requiring vasopressors, respiratory failure requiring mechanical ventilation, acute renal failure, and multiorgan failure [59]. In general, one should operate for *C difficile* colitis before a patient develops organ dysfunction or failure and before vasopressors are needed for management of shock, because this results in the highest survival and best outcomes [19].

The definitive surgical treatment remains subtotal colectomy with end ileostomy and preservation of the rectum. An open approach is preferred over a laparoscopic approach given the shorter duration of surgery, technical ease, and lower risk for compartment syndrome. It is important to remember that the external colon may appear deceptively normal at the time of operation [2]. The surgeon should not be tempted to perform a limited resection.

An alternative to colectomy in selected patients may be an approach developed and published by the University of Pittsburgh group [62]. This approach uses loop ileostomy and intraoperative colonic lavage with warmed polyethylene glycol solution and postoperative intravenous metronidazole and antegrade vancomycin flushes via the efferent limb of the ileostomy. This protocol was completed in most patients with a laparoscopic approach, and these patients were compared with historical controls, who underwent open subtotal colectomy and end ileostomy. This novel surgical approach was associated with lower mortality (19%) than the historical open approach (50%). Most patients (39/42) were able to be successfully treated without colon resection. Three patients underwent total abdominal colectomy for ongoing sepsis or compartment syndrome. This study was limited by a selection bias because the patients enrolled were not randomized. The patients undergoing formation of a loop ileostomy were generally healthier than those historical controls undergoing colectomy. This study is innovative, and the results are important, but should be considered and applied with caution [10].

SUMMARY

C difficile remains a major cause of nosocomial infection, and surgical patient populations are especially susceptible. Most cases will respond to medical management, but surgical consultation should be sought early in cases of severe, complicated disease. Surgical management is subtotal colectomy with preservation of the rectum and end ileostomy. Some patients may be appropriate for diverting loop ileostomy with colonic lavage and installation of antibiotics via the efferent limb of the ileostomy. Vaccines, monoclonal antibodies, and FMT may offer protection and benefit to patients. Further research is needed to understand the clinical implications of these newer therapies.

References

[1] Finney JMT. Gastro-enterostomy for cicatrizing ulcer of the pylorus. Dis Colon Rectum 1893;29:218–21.

[2] Lipsett PA, Samantaray DK, Tam ML, et al. Pseudomembranous colitis: a surgical disease? Surgery 1994;116:491–6.

[3] Napolitano LM, Edmiston CE. Clostridium difficile disease: diagnosis, pathogenesis, and treatment update. Surgery 2017;162:325–48.

[4] Bartlett JG. Historical perspectives on studies of Clostridium difficile and C. difficile infection. Clin Infect Dis 2008;46:S4–11.

[5] Tedesco FJ, Barton RW, Alpers DH. Clindamycin-associated colitis: a prospective study. Ann Intern Med 1974;81:429–33.

[6] Bartlett JG, Chang CW, Gurwith M, et al. Antibiotic-associated pseudomembranous colitis due to toxin-producing clostridia. N Engl J Med 1978;298:531–4.

[7] George WL, Sutter VL, Goldstein EJ, et al. Aetiology of antimicrobial-agent-associated colitis. Lancet 1978;1:802–3.

[8] Leffler DA, Lamont JT. Clostridium difficile infection. N Engl J Med 2015;372:1539–48.

[9] Bagdasarian N, Rao K, Malani PN. Diagnosis and treatment of Clostridium difficile in adults: a systematic review. JAMA 2015;313:398–408.

[10] Steele SR, McCormick J, Melton GB, et al. Practice parameters for the management of Clostridium difficile infection. Dis Colon Rectum 2015;58:10–24.

[11] Honda H, Dubberke ER. Overview and changing epidemiology of Clostridium difficile infection. Curr Opin Gastroenterol 2014;30:54–62.

[12] Kuehn BM. Scientists seek strategies to prevent Clostridium difficile infections. JAMA 2011;306:1849–50.

[13] Leffler DA, Lamont JT. Editorial: not so nosocomial anymore: the growing threat of community-acquired Clostridium difficile. Am J Gastroenterol 2012;107(1):96–8.

[14] Hunter JC, Mu Y, Dumyati GK, et al. Burden of nursing home-onset Clostridium difficile infection in the United States: estimates of incidence and patient outcomes. Open Forum Infect Dis 2016;3:ofv196.

[15] Galdys AL, Curry SR, Harrison LH. Asymptomatic Clostridium difficile colonization as a reservoir for Clostridium difficile infection. Expert Rev Anti Infect Ther 2014;12(8):967–80.

[16] McFarland LV, Brandmarker SA, Guandalini S. Pediatric Clostridium difficile: a phantom menace or clinical reality? J Pediatr Gastroenterol Nutr 2000;31:220–31.

[17] Shim JK, Johnson S, Samore MH, et al. Primary symptomless colonisation by Clostridium difficile and decreased risk of subsequent diarrhoea. Lancet 1998;351(9103):633–6.

[18] Blondeau JM. What have we learned about antimicrobial use and the risk of Clostridium difficile-associated diarrhea? J Antimicrob Chemother 2009;63:238–42.

[19] Kaiser AM, Hogen R, Bordeianou L, et al. Clostridium difficile infection from a surgical perspective. J Gastrointest Surg 2015;19:1363–77.

[20] Pothoulakis C. Effects of Clostridium difficile toxins on epithelial cell barrier. Ann N Y Acad Sci 2000;915:347–56.

[21] McDonald LC, Killgore GE, Thompson A, et al. An epidemic, toxin gene-variant strain of Clostridium difficile. N Engl J Med 2005;353:2433–41.

[22] Tickler IA, Goering RV, Whitmore JD, et al, Healthcare Associated Infection Consortium. Strain types and antimicrobial resistance patterns of Clostridium difficile isolates from the United States, 2011 to 2013. Antimicrob Agents Chemother 2014;58(7):4214–8.

[23] Pépin J, Valiquette L, Gagnon S, et al. Outcomes of Clostridium difficile-associated disease treated with metronidazole or vancomycin before and after the emergence of NAP1/027. Am J Gastroenterol 2007;102:2781–8.

[24] Archbald-Pannone LR, Boone JH, Carman RJ, et al. Clostridium difficile ribotype 027 is most prevalent among inpatients admitted from long-term care facilities. J Hosp Infect 2014;88:218–21.

[25] Itani KM, Wilson SE, Awad SS, et al. Ertapenem versus cefotetan prophylaxis in elective colorectal surgery. N Engl J Med 2006;355:2640–51.

[26] Collins CE, Ayturk MD, Flahive JM, et al. Epidemiology and outcomes of community-acquired Clostridium difficile infections in medicare beneficiaries. J Am Coll Surg 2014;218:1141–7.e1.

[27] Marik PE, Vasu T, Hirani A, et al. Stress ulcer prophylaxis in the new millennium: a systematic review and meta-analysis. Crit Care Med 2010;38:2222–8.

[28] Rebmann T, Carrico RM, Association for Professionals in Infection Control and Epidemiology. Preventing Clostridium difficile infections: an executive summary of the Association for Professionals in Infection Control and Epidemiology's elimination guide. Am J Infect Control 2011;39:239–42.

[29] Johnson S, Gerding DN, Olson MM, et al. Prospective, controlled study of vinyl glove use to interrupt Clostridium difficile nosocomial transmission. Am J Med 1990;88:137–40.

[30] Surawicz CM, Brandt LJ, Binion DG, et al. Guidelines for diagnosis, treatment, and prevention of Clostridium difficile infections. Am J Gastroenterol 2013;108:478–98 [quiz: 499].

[31] Loo VG. Environmental interventions to control Clostridium difficile. Infect Dis Clin North Am 2015;29:83–91.

[32] Bettin K, Clabots C, Mathie P, et al. Effectiveness of liquid soap vs. chlorhexidine gluconate for the removal of Clostridium difficile from bare hands and gloved hands. Infect Control Hosp Epidemiol 1994;15:697–702.

[33] Cohen SH, Gerding DN, Johnson S, et al. Clinical practice guidelines for Clostridium difficile infection in adults: 2010 update by the Society for Healthcare Epidemiology of America (SHEA) and the Infectious Diseases Society of America (IDSA). Infect Control Hosp Epidemiol 2010;31(5):431–55.

[34] Fekety R, Silva J, Kauffman C, et al. Treatment of antibiotic-associated Clostridium difficile colitis with oral vancomycin. Am J Med 1989;86(1):15–9.

[35] Chapin KC, Dickenson RA, Wu F, et al. Comparison of five assays for detection of Clostridium difficile toxin. J Mol Diagn 2011;13(4):395–400.

[36] Naaber P, Stsepetova J, Smidt I, et al. Quantification of Clostridium difficile in antibiotic-associated-diarrhea patients. J Clin Microbiol 2011;49(10):3656–8.

[37] Tenover FC, Baron EJ, Peterson LR, et al. Laboratory diagnosis of Clostridium difficile infection can molecular amplification methods move us out of uncertainty? J Mol Diagn 2011;13(6):573–82.

[38] Kvach EJ, Ferguson D, Riska PF, et al. Comparison of BD GeneOhm Cdiff real-time PCR assay with a two-step algorithm and a toxin A/B enzyme-linked immunosorbent assay for diagnosis of toxigenic Clostridium difficile infection. J Clin Microbiol 2010;48(1):109–14.

[39] Carroll KC. Tests for the diagnosis of Clostridium difficile infection: the next generation. Anaerobe 2011;17:170–4.

[40] Imbriaco M, Balthazar EJ. Toxic megacolon: role of CT in evaluation and detection of complications. Clin Imaging 2001;25:349–54.

[41] Moulin V, Dellon P, Laurent O, et al. Toxic megacolon in patients with severe acute colitis: computed tomographic features. Clin Imaging 2011;35:431–6.

[42] Fekety R. Guidelines for the diagnosis and management of Clostridium difficile-associated diarrhea and colitis. American College of Gastroenterology, Practice Parameters Committee. Am J Gastroenterol 1997;92:739–50.

[43] Debast SB, Bauer MP, Kuijper EJ. European Society of Clinical Microbiology and Infectious Diseases: update of the treatment guidance document for Clostridium difficile infection. Clin Microbiol Infect 2014;20(suppl 2):1–26.

[44] Jalan K, Sircus W, Card WI, et al. An experience of ulcerative colitis. I. Toxic dilation in 55 cases. Gastroenterology 1969;57:68–82.

[45] Ausch C, Madoff D, Gnant M, et al. Aetiology and surgical management of toxic megacolon. Colorectal Dis 2005;8:195–201.

[46] Slimings C, Riley TV. Antibiotics and hospital-acquired Clostridium difficile infection: update of systematic review and meta-analysis. J Antimicrob Chemother 2014;69(4):881–91.

[47] Thomas C, Stevenson M, Riley TV. Antibiotics and hospital-acquired Clostridium difficile-associated diarrhoea. J Antimicrob Chemother 2003;51(6):1339–50.

[48] Owens RC Jr, Donskey CJ, Gaynes RP, et al. Antimicrobial-associated risk factors for Clostridium difficile infection. Clin Infect Dis 2008;46(suppl 1):S19–31.

[49] Belmares J, Gerding DN, Parada JP, et al. Outcome of metronidazole therapy for Clostridium difficile disease and correlation with a scoring system. J Infect 2007;55(6):495–501.

[50] Johnson S, Louie TJ, Gerding DN, et al. Vancomycin, metronidazole, or tolevamer for Clostridium difficile infection: results from two multinational, randomized, controlled trials. Clin Infect Dis 2014;59(3):345–54.

[51] Louie TJ, Miller MA, Mullane KM, et al, OPT-80-003 Clinical Study Group. Fidaxomicin versus vancomycin for Clostridium difficile infection. N Engl J Med 2011;364:422–31.

[52] van Nood E, Vrieze A, Nieuwdorp M, et al. Duodenal infusion of donor feces for recurrent Clostridium difficile. N Engl J Med 2013;368(5):407–15.

[53] Lowy I, Molrine DC, Leav BA, et al. Treatment with monoclonal antibodies against Clostridium difficile toxins. N Engl J Med 2010;362:197–205.

[54] Wilcox MH, Gerding DN, Poxton IR, et al, MODIFY I and MODIFY II Investigators. Bezlo-
    toxumab for prevention of recurrent Clostridium difficile infection. N Engl J Med
    2017;376(4):305–17.
[55] Sougioultzis S, Kyne L, Drudy D, et al. Clostridium difficile toxoid vaccine in recurrent C.
    difficile associated diarrhea. Gastroenterology 2005;128:764–70.
[56] Gerding DN. Clostridium difficile infection prevention. Discov Med 2012;13(68):75–83.
[57] Henderson M, Bragg A, Fahim G, et al. A review of the safety and efficacy of vaccines as
    prophylaxis for Clostridium difficile infections. Vaccines (Basel) 2017;25(3) [pii:E25].
[58] Clostridium difficile vaccine trial. Paris: Sanofi; 2013. Available at: http://www.cdiffen-
    se.org/home. Accessed September 11, 2017.
[59] Bhangu A, Nepogodiev D, Gupta A, et al, Collaborative WMR. Systematic review and
    meta-analysis of outcomes following emergency surgery for Clostridium difficile colitis. Br
    J Surg 2012;99:1501–13.
[60] Dudukgian H, Sie E, Gonzalez-Ruiz C, et al. C. difficile colitis–predictors of fatal outcome.
    J Gastrointest Surg 2010;14:315–22.
[61] Sailhamer EA, Carson K, Chang Y, et al. Fulminant Clostridium difficile colitis: patterns of
    care and predictors of mortality. Arch Surg 2009;144:433–9 [discussion: 439–40].
[62] Neal MD, Alverdy JC, Hall DE, et al. Diverting loop ileostomy and colonic lavage: an alter-
    native to total abdominal colectomy for the treatment of severe, complicated Clostridium
    difficile-associated disease. Ann Surg 2011;254:423–7 [discussion: 427–9].

Advances in Surgery 52 (2018) 43–56

ADVANCES IN SURGERY

ELSEVIER
MOSBY

The Management of Venous Thromboembolic Disease
New Trends in Anticoagulant Therapy

Andrea Obi, MD[a],*, Thomas Wakefield, MD[b]

[a]Section of Vascular Surgery, Department of Surgery, University of Michigan, 5372 Cardiovascular Center, 1500 East Medical Center Drive, Ann Arbor, MI 48109-5867, USA; [b]Section of Vascular Surgery, Department of Surgery, University of Michigan, 5463 Cardiovascular Center, 1500 East Medical Center Drive, Ann Arbor, MI 48109-5867, USA

Keywords
• Deep vein thrombosis • Anticoagulation • Extended treatment • Iliofemoral DVT
• Femoropopliteal DVT • Distal (calf) DVT

Key points

• Based on ease of dosing and large noninferiority trials, direct oral anticoagulants (DOACs) should be considered first-line therapy for treatment of venous thromboembolism (VTE)

• New strategies for treatment (besides long-term anticoagulation) of unprovoked (idiopathic) VTE now exist: prophylactic dose rivaroxaban or apixaban, aspirin, and use of HERDOO2 scoring rule to identify women at low risk of VTE recurrence.

• Aggressive pharmacomechanical thrombolysis appears indicated for iliofemoral deep vein thrombosis (DVT) to decrease immediate symptoms.

• Controversy still exists on the role of anticoagulation after calf vein thrombosis.

INTRODUCTION

In the past several years, the Food and Drug Administration (FDA) has approved 5 new direct oral anticoagulant (DOAC) agents. In the 2012 American College of Chest Physicians (ACCP) recommendations, vitamin K antagonists (VKAs) remained the central mainstay of therapy for treatment of acute VTE [1]. In the 2016 ACCP guidelines, DOACs gained preference over VKAs

Disclosure: None of the authors report conflicts of interest.

*Corresponding author. E-mail address: easta@med.umich.edu

https://doi.org/10.1016/j.yasu.2018.03.005

as first-line therapy for the treatment of venous thromboembolism (VTE). With these new agents, an explosion of clinical studies is occurring to determine the utility of each medication for several different indications. This article discusses how to choose the best anticoagulant for VTE treatment and when extended anticoagulation for prevention of recurrent VTE should be used, and specific discussions are provided on calf vein DVT and iliofemoral DVT.

SIGNIFICANCE
Anticoagulant choice for venous thromboembolism
Approved in 1954, VKAs (warfarin [Coumadin]) have been the mainstay of therapy for thrombotic diseases for greater than a half century. Given the established safety profile of VKAs and their efficacy in reducing the risk for recurrent thrombosis and fatal pulmonary embolism (PE), they represent the gold standard against which every new agent is compared. There are several shortcomings associated with VKAs, not the least of which is that they have a defined bleeding risk of 5% to 6% per year [2], which cannot be mitigated by targeting a lower International Normalized Ratio (INR) [3,4]. Other shortcomings include that they require monitoring and that the metabolism of the drug is affected by diet and many commonly prescribed medications. Until recently, few alternatives existed other than low-molecular-weight heparins (LMWHs). Despite the downside of subcutaneous administration with the need for daily or twice-daily home injections, the LMWHs hold several advantages: predictable weight-based dosing, routine laboratory monitoring not necessary in most circumstances, and efficacy similar to VKAs. In a pooled analysis of the treatment of VTE involving LMWH and VKAs, the rate of fatal PE during treatment of DVT was 0.4% and of all PE was 1.5%, with the rates similarly low after cessation of anticoagulation [5]. In several circumstances, LMWHs are superior to VKAs. For example, in patients with malignancy, treatment with LMWH decreased the risk of recurrent VTE by approximately 50% at 6 months to 1 year compared with warfarin without an increase in bleeding [6]. In the Home-LITE (Home therapy of venous thrombosis with long-term LMWH versus usual care: patient satisfaction and post-thrombotic syndrome) trial, tinazparin (a LMWH), was superior to warfarin for prevention of post-thrombotic syndrome (PTS), development of leg ulcers, and treatment satisfaction after significant DVT [7].

Although VKAs and LMWH remain important agents for the treatment of VTE, there has been rapid development of evidence supporting the use of DOACs. The 2 categories of DOACs are the direct thrombin inhibitors and factor Xa inhibitors. Currently, of the direct Xa inhibitors, apixaban, rivaroxaban, and edoxaban have all been FDA approved for the treatment of VTE, whereas dabigatran is the approved direct thrombin inhibitor. The DOACs are appealing because they are all administered orally, do not need monitoring, and have fixed doses that do not need to be weight based adjusted. Two major initial clinical concerns regarding these agents is their efficacy/safety and reversibility in the event of major bleeding. In the past 10 years, all the DOACs each have had at least 1 large randomized controlled trial demonstrating noninferiority in the treatment of VTE compared with VKAs [8–11]. Apixaban is the only one to show a superior reduction in bleeding, major bleeding, and clinically relevant nonmajor bleeding compared with VKAs.

One of the appealing aspects of VKAs (and to a lower extent LMWH) is the ability to be quickly reversed. For heparin and to a lesser degree LMWH, reversal is by protamine, whereas for VKAs, reversal by achieved by fresh frozen plasma or prothrombin complex concentrate. In addition, the reversal can be monitored (international normalized ratio for VKAs and anti-Xa level for heparin and LMWH). Historically, for the DOACs, reversal has been limited to supportive measures, prothrombin complex concentrate, or selective dialysis for dabigatran [12]. Although the issue of reversibility has not been fully resolved, progress occurred when the FDA approved idarucizumab (Praxbind) in October 2015, a monoclonal antibody that binds dabigatran to rapidly reverse its anticoagulant effects [13]. Two other agents currently in development include andexanet alfa and aripazine. Andexanet alfa is recombinant factor Xa decoy for all factor Xa inhibitors, including DOACs, LMWHs, and fondaparinux. [14], whereas aripazine is a small molecule inhibitor of all anticoagulants. Clinical trials have shown the andexanet alfa can effectively reverse DOACs anticoagulant effect without any known thrombotic events in healthy patients [15]. Currently, ANNEXA-4 (Andexanet alfa, a novel antidote to the anticoagulation effects of FXa inhibitors [NCT02329327]) is a phase III open-label study to evaluate the use of the medication in patients with ongoing major bleeding, with an estimated completion in 2022. The FDA has recently (May, 2018) approved AndexXa® for reversal of Factor Xa inhibitors. The final reversal agent progressing in development with FDA fast-track designation for hemorrhage is Aripazine (ciraparantag [PER977], Perosphere Pharmaceuticals, Danbury, CT), a water-soluble, catatonic molecule available in intravenous formulation that noncovalently binds to and reverses the anticoagulation of all anticoagulation agents (LMWH, UFH, FXa inhibitors, and dabigatran) in animal models and healthy volunteers [15]. At least 5 phase I/II trials have been completed or are ongoing to evaluate aripazine for anticoagulant reversal.

In 2016, the ACCP recommended DOACs as first-line treatment of acute VTE over VKAs in patients whom do not have an associated cancer (grade 2B) [1]. In patients with cancer who develop acute VTE, LMWH remains the recommended first-line treatment. This is not because they are not effective, but because in most studies, there are not enough patients with cancer to evaluate the DOACs in these patients. The SELECT-d trial is an open-label multicenter prospective blinded study currently evaluating LMWH (dalteparin) versus rivaroxaban in patients with cancer and VTE. Preliminary results from this study demonstrate a lower risk of recurrence in the rivaroxaban arm (4% vs 11% for dalteparin) but at the expense of an increase in major and clinically relevant nonmajor bleeding (17% vs 5%). Although guidelines recommend DOACs over VKA in non–malignancy-related VTE, there are several clinical situations in which DOACs should not be used. For example, DOACs should not be used in patients with impaired renal function or mechanical heart valves or for patients who cannot afford the medication. Given that all of the comparison studies have shown noninferiority, in many cases either a DOAC or a VKA is acceptable. Recent work has shown, however, that certain patients are at much higher risk of treatment failure with VKAs than others [16], using a clinical scoring system, SAMe-TT$_2$R$_2$ (Sex, age, medical history, treatment, tobacco use, race) (Fig. 1). As the anticoagulation field continues to expand with increased agents and changing guidelines, providers need to decide which anticoagulation treatment is best for each individual patient (Table 1) based on the risks and benefits of each medication as they align to patients' comorbidities and preferences.

Extended anticoagulation treatment to reduce the risk of recurrent venous thromboembolism

For the treatment of provoked proximal and symptomatic distal DVT and PE (VTE), the recommended duration of anticoagulation is 3 months (grade 1B). Extended therapy traditionally is considered under the following circumstances: previous VTE, thrombophilia associated with a high a risk of recurrence, and unprovoked (idiopathic) VTE. Virtually all investigators agree that for a second idiopathic VTE, anticoagulant therapy should be continued due to the high recurrence risk well past 3 months in those patients with low and moderate

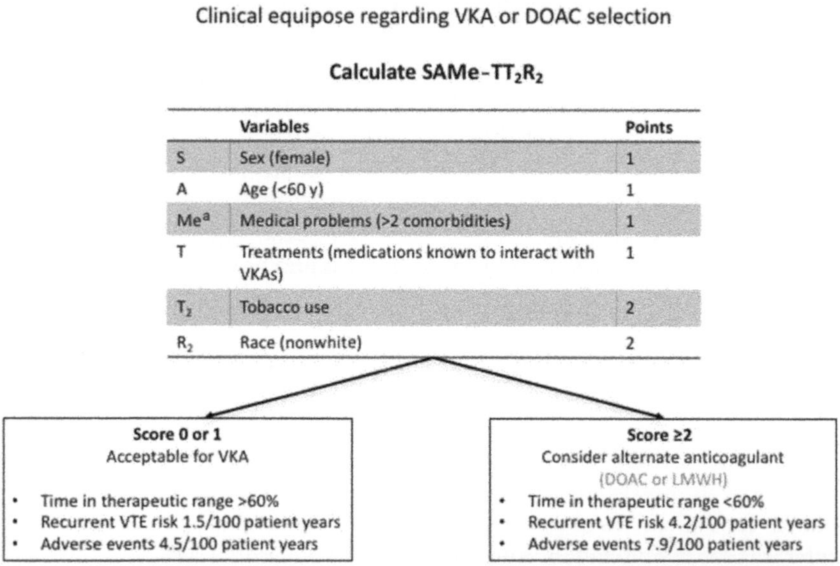

Clinical equipose regarding VKA or DOAC selection

Calculate SAMe-TT$_2$R$_2$

	Variables	Points
S	Sex (female)	1
A	Age (<60 y)	1
Me[a]	Medical problems (>2 comorbidities)	1
T	Treatments (medications known to interact with VKAs)	1
T$_2$	Tobacco use	2
R$_2$	Race (nonwhite)	2

Score 0 or 1
Acceptable for VKA
- Time in therapeutic range >60%
- Recurrent VTE risk 1.5/100 patient years
- Adverse events 4.5/100 patient years

Score ≥2
Consider alternate anticoagulant (DOAC or LMWH)
- Time in therapeutic range <60%
- Recurrent VTE risk 4.2/100 patient years
- Adverse events 7.9/100 patient years

Fig. 1. In the event of clinical equipoise regarding selection of VKAs or DOACs for the treatment of VTE, the SAMe-TT$_2$R$_2$ score can be used to predict individuals likely to have adverse events, VTE recurrence and poor time in therapeutic range with VKA treatment. [a] Medical comorbidities include diabetes, hypertension, renal disease, hepatic disease, pulmonary disease, congestive heart failure, coronary artery disease, peripheral vascular disease, and previous stroke. (*From* Smith M, Wakam G, Wakefield T, et al. New trends in anticoagulation therapy. Surg Clin N Am 2018;98(2):222; with permission.)

Table 1
Dosing and considerations for various anticoagulant choices

	Dosing	Half-life	Considerations
Apixaban	10 mg BID × 7 days Then 5-mg BID (2.5 mg BID for long-term therapy)	7–11 h	Superior to standard therapy with no increase in bleeding Twice-daily dosing No renal adjustment
Rivaroxaban	15-mg BID × 3 wk Then 20 mg daily	12 h	Once-daily regimen May need to be renal adjusted Increase in GI bleeding compared with warfarin
Dabigatran	LMWH for 5–10 d 150 mg BID	8–15 h	Poor choice in renal dysfunction Requires heparin bridge Increase in GI bleeding compared with warfarin Up to 10% have dyspepsia Avoid in patients with significant CAD
Edoxaban	LMWH for 5–10 d 60 mg daily 30 mg daily ≤60 kg or CrCl 15–50	10–14 h	Once daily dosing Requires heparin bridge Needs to be renal adjusted Increase in GI bleeding compared with warfarin
Warfarin	Variable dosing titrate to goal INR	~40 h	Reliable and predictable reversal Can use SAMe-TT$_2$R$_2$ to predict poor candidates Requires bridging Requires frequent monitoring Has many interactions with food and other medications

Abbreviations: CAD, coronary artery disease; CrCl, creatinine clearance; GI, gastrointestinal.
From Smith M, Wakam G, Wakefield T, et al. New trends in anticoagulation therapy. Surg Clin N Am 2018;98(2):223; with permission.

bleeding risks [1]. Even for patients with high bleeding risks, extended anticoagulation may still be recommended. For patients with thrombophilias, those that are associated with a higher risk of VTE recurrence, including protein C or protein S deficiency (especially with a family history), antithrombin deficiency, homozygous factor V Leiden and homozygous prothrombin 20,210 gene mutation, and multiple thrombophilic states in the same patient. The most common state, factor V Leiden heterozygous mutation alone, does not confer an increased risk of recurrence for patients. When combined with prothrombin 20210 gene mutation, however, recurrence is increased and prolonged anticoagulant therapy is usually recommended. Among acquired thrombophilias, the presence of antiphospholipid antibodies and active cancer mandate extended therapy, because these are severe thrombotic states [17].

For idiopathic first-time VTE, the practitioner must balance the competing risks and implications of recurrent VTE and major bleeding. D-dimer and repeat duplex testing have both been suggested to be useful tests to determine risk of recurrence with cessation of anticoagulation. D-dimer is measured approximately 1 month after stopping oral anticoagulation. If elevated, this suggests that active thrombosis is occurring somewhere in the circulation and the rate of recurrence in patients with a positive D-dimer is 15% compared with 6.2% with a normal D-dimer. This risk can be reduced with resumption of anticoagulation, which reduces the VTE rate to 2.9% [1,18]. The use of repeat serial lower-extremity ultrasound to determine the state of the thrombosed veins has also been suggested, with the belief that if the veins are occluded with fibrotic scar tissue, flow will be sluggish and the risk of recurrent VTE elevated. The usefulness of this test is less certain, because this approach used a complicated quantification scheme, which is difficult to reproduce in day-to-day clinical practice in most clinical vascular laboratories.

Two major new advances that have come about in recent years include the validation of the HERDOO2 score and low-dose anticoagulant/antiplatelet therapies for the prevention of recurrent VTE. The HERDOO2 (hyperpigmentation, edema, or redness in either leg; D-dimer level > 250 µg/ml; obesity with body mass index $\geq$ 30; or older age $\geq$ 65 years) score identified women at low risk of VTE recurrence after unprovoked VTE who may safely discontinue anticoagulants after short-term treatment. Points are assigned for (1) hyperpigmentation, edema, or redness in either leg; (2) VIDAS (VIDAS®, Biomerieux, USA) D-dimer greater than or equal to 250 µg/L; (3) obesity (body mass index [BMI] $\geq$30); and (4) older age ($\geq$65 years). Patients with 0 or 1 point are considered low risk for recurrent VTE and long-term anticoagulation therapy was discontinued (Fig. 2). Women defined as low risk with discontinued therapy had a 3.0% per patient year risk of recurrent VTE compared with an 8.1% per patient-year risk in high-risk women who discontinued anticoagulants (see Fig. 2) [19]. This scoring system was derived from a cohort of 646 men and women with first-time unprovoked VTE and validated in a multinational study of 2785 patients. No reliable predictors were noted for male patients [20].

Another approach is the use of low-dose anticoagulation for the prevention of recurrent thrombosis to improve the risk-benefit profile by decreasing the

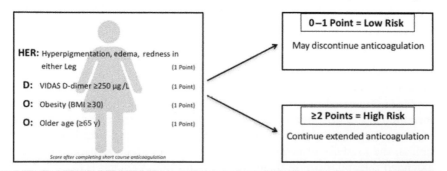

Fig. 2. In women with first time unprovoked VTE, the HERDOO2 score can identify those that are at low risk of recurrent VTE after initial standard anticoagulant therapy and can safely stop anticoagulation. (*From* Smith M, Wakam G, Wakefield T, et al. New trends in anticoagulation therapy. Surg Clin N Am 2018;98(2):224; with permission.)

bleeding risks associated with anticoagulant therapy. Previous studies with low-dose VKAs failed to demonstrate an improvement in bleeding profile and have been largely abandoned in clinical practice [21]. Aspirin has been suggested as an alternative to lower bleeding risk while still providing some benefit in decreasing VTE recurrence. Several studies, including the INSPIRE (International collaboration of aspirin trials for recurrent venous thromboembolism) trial, a collaboration of the WARFASA (Warfarin and Aspirin Study) and ASPIRE (Aspirin to prevent recurrent venous thromboembolism) trials, have shown that it is possible to reduce the risk of recurrent VTE by more than 30% in patients treated with aspirin compared with placebo [22,23]. More recently, both rivaroxaban and apixaban have been shown significantly more effective in prevention of VTE recurrence with no increased risk of bleeding compared with placebo and aspirin [24,25]. Although evidence exists that lower-dose anticoagulants may reduce VTE recurrence, the most effective therapy with the safest treatment profile and lowest cost is still not yet determined.

Proximal (iliofemoral and femoropopliteal) deep vein thrombosis

Proximal DVT (popliteal vein or more rostral) is usually manifested by unilateral leg swelling, pitting edema, and pain of the affected leg. Proximal DVT includes thrombosis of the iliac, common femoral, femoral, and popliteal vein segments. For severe obstructive iliofemoral DVT, symptoms may consist of severe swelling and pain. In all cases, the mainstay of therapy involves prompt initiation of anticoagulation, compression, and elevation. If an absolute contraindication to anticoagulation exists, consideration should be given for inferior vena cava filter placement to prevent PEs.

The gold standard for diagnosis is duplex ultrasound imaging. If iliofemoral venous thrombosis is suspected but not confirmed, using standard diagnostic modalities, such as venous duplex ultrasound imaging, the use of other imaging modalities, including CT venography (CTV) or magnetic resonance venography (MRV), to characterize the most proximal extent is recommended [26,27]. CTV and MRV evaluate the inferior vena cava and veins of the pelvis better than ultrasound or contrast venography. Studies comparing CTV to ultrasound or venography demonstrate a sensitivity/specificity greater than 95% [28]. MRV has also been found to be accurate in the diagnosis of DVT. In a large meta-analysis, when compared with venography or ultrasound imaging, MRV was found to have a sensitivity and specificity of 92% (94% for proximal DVT) and 95% [29]. Additionally, MRV is accurate and useful in the diagnosis of pelvic vein thrombosis [30].

For proximal DVT treatment, the goals are 3-fold: (1) to prevent extension or recurrence of DVT, (2) to prevent PE, and (3) to minimize the late sequelae of thrombosis, namely chronic venous insufficiency and PTS. Standard anticoagulants accomplish the first 2 goals but do not always accomplish the third goal. Pain and swelling after DVT occurs in up to 30% of patients after DVT, and that number is even higher in patients with iliofemoral DVT or ipsilateral recurrent DVT [31]. In select ambulatory patients with reasonable life expectancy and a good risk profile, more aggressive therapies for extensive thrombosis may be indicated. Experimentally, the thrombosis initiates an inflammatory response in the vein wall that leads to vein wall fibrosis and valvular dysfunction. Prolonged contact of the thrombus with the vein wall increases damage [32]. Thus, removing the thrombus may be an excellent solution to decrease this interaction, although it may not eliminate the pathophysiology depending on the timing of its initiation. The longer a thrombus is in contact with a vein valve, the more chance that valve will no longer function and the vein wall will become fibrotic [33]. For DVT limited to the femoropopliteal region, without extension into the iliac system, anticoagulation alone is recommended. Patients with femoropopliteal DVT show a lower risk of thrombosis recurrence [34], a lower risk of the development of PTS [35], and inferior outcomes with thrombolysis.

The 2016 ACCP guidelines emphasize anticoagulation over catheter-directed thrombolysis (CDT) except in patients who attach a high value to the prevention of PTS and a lower value to the initial complexity, cost, and risk of bleeding of aggressive therapies compared with anticoagulation alone [1]. Early thrombus removal may be performed [26,36–42] for patients with all of the following: (1) first episode of acute iliofemoral DVT, (2) symptoms less than 14 days in duration (although may be considered up to 28 days), (3) low risk of bleeding, (4) ambulatory with a good functional capacity and acceptable life expectancy, and (5) moderate to severe symptoms (as assessed by Villalta score ≥ 10 after a trial of anticoagulation).

An older technique, venous thrombectomy, which is removal of thrombus with a catheter under direct operative vision, has proved superior to anticoagulation over 6 months to 10 years, as measured by prevention of venous reflux and venous patency [43]. CDT has been used in many nonrandomized studies and in small, randomized trials was more effective than standard therapy in improving quality of life. Results are optimized further by combining CDT with mechanical devices, so-called pharmacomechanical thrombolysis [37,42]. These various devices hasten thrombolysis and decrease the amount of thrombolytic agent needed, potentially decreasing bleeding potential. CDT, although not currently endorsed by major society guidelines, decreases symptoms of pain and swelling at 30 days and may decrease PTS in highly select groups of patients (acute iliofemoral DVT, Villalta score ≥ 10 after a trial of anticoagulation). This should be performed ideally within 2 weeks but may be effective up to 4 weeks after initial symptoms. The preliminary data from the ATTRACT trial suggest that CDT is effective primarily for iliofemoral DVT with significant symptoms. Additionally, the use of venous stents for iliac venous obstruction has been shown to decrease the incidence of PTS and chronic venous insufficiency and to be important in conjunction with CDT [44].

Phlegmasia (alba or cerulea dolens) and venous gangrene are rare clinical events that can place the affected limb at risk of ischemia. Phlegmasia cerulea dolens is defined as an uncommon form of DVT characterized by severe pain, swelling, cyanosis, and edema; this is usually preceded by phlegmasia alba dolens, characterized by the same clinical signs except the limb is pale and white due to early ischemia. Venous gangrene is defined as skin necrosis, discoloration, and documented VTE. Treatment is the same as for proximal DVT with an emphasis on immediate anticoagulation. Procedural interventions include CDT or surgical embolectomy.

In summary, all patients with iliofemoral DVT should undergo standard anticoagulation. For selected patients with iliofemoral DVT or with limb-threatening venous ischemia, early thrombus removal is the treatment of choice with or without associated femoropopliteal venous thrombosis [26,45,46]. For DVT limited to the femoropopliteal region, without extension into the iliac system, anticoagulation alone is recommended.

Distal (calf) deep vein thrombosis

The need for treatment of distal DVT is controversial, with recommendations for anticoagulation and against anticoagulant treatment (Table 2). [47,48] The magnitude of the problem is demonstrated by studies reporting that the proportion of all DVTs that are "distal" is as much as 60% to 70% [48,49]. Calf DVT is commonly associated with transient risk factors and carries a lower mortality than proximal DVT (4.4% vs 8.0%, $P<.01$) [50]. Consequences of calf DVT include proximal extension, recurrence, PE, and PTS. These complications, including PE and PTS, are decreased compared with proximal DVT, although the rates still remain somewhat high [51]. Because studies are highly heterogeneous, rates do vary considerably between older and more modern studies. Compression ultrasonography is the first-line imaging modality for the diagnosis of distal DVT. The performance of the D-dimer to evaluate symptomatic distal DVT is controversial, with not all assays found reliable for this purpose [52]. Therefore, their use is not recommended for distal DVT.

Table 2
Distal (calf) deep vein thrombosis

When anticoagulation can be considered	When serial compression ultrasound is recommended
Patient has 1 or more of the following: • Thrombosis not provoked[a] • History of prior VTE • Significant calf pain • Patient immobility • Active cancer	Patient has none of the factors listed for "When anticoagulation can be considered."
If anticoagulation was initially withheld, but thrombus extension occurs, particularly into a proximal deep vein	High bleeding risk from anticoagulation
Patient preference to avoid DVT extension, PE, and DVT recurrence more than the risk of bleeding	Patient preference to avoid bleeding risk more than the risk of DVT extension, PE, and DVT recurrence

[a]Examples of provoked VTE include: postoperative status, active cancer, immobility, exposure to oral contraceptives/hormone replacement therapy, pregnancy, presence of central venous catheters, current/recent hospitalization, and diagnosis of severe thrombophilia.

Because there is clinical equipoise regarding treatment and surveillance for distal DVT, there are 2 recommended options for the management of distal (calf) DVT. These include either (1) anticoagulation therapy using the same schedule as for patients with acute proximal DVT or (2) weekly serial compression ultrasound for 2 weeks to assess for clot propagation and using anticoagulation only if there is propagation. Most calf-level DVTs (gastrocnemius and soleus veins) do not require anticoagulation but should still be followed by serial compression ultrasound surveillance.

The CALTHRO (Natural history of isolated deep vein thrombosis of the calf) study assessed the consequence of untreated calf DVT in 431 symptomatic outpatients with an abnormal D-dimer and an initial negative ultrasound for proximal vein DVT [53]. With a 3 month follow-up, adverse outcomes occurred in only 3 patients, including 1 patient with proximal vein extension, 1 patient with PE, and 1 patient with worsening symptoms [53]. In contrast, however, limited randomized studies have shown recurrent thrombotic events in up to 29% of patients with inadequately treated calf vein thrombosis [54]. In prospective cohorts of patients with isolated calf-level DVT largely treated with anticoagulation, VTE recurrence rates at 3 months were 2% to 2.2%, including 0.7% to 1.1% rates of PE [50,55].

Widely accepted management studies suggest that it is safe to withhold anticoagulation in outpatients with suspected DVT if serial compression ultrasound is negative for proximal DVT at baseline and at 1 week [56–61]. The pooled estimate of the 3-month thromboembolic risk in untreated patients in studies using only serial proximal vein ultrasound is 0.6% (95% CI, 0.4%–0.9%) [47]. The most recent randomized controlled trial, the CACTUS (Anticoagulant therapy for symptomatic calf deep vein thrombosis) trial, found no advantage for LMWH in reducing the risk of proximal extension or venous thromboembolic events in low-risk outpatients with symptomatic calf DVT (5.4% vs 3.3%; $P = .054$). There was an increase, however, in the risk of bleeding (0% vs 4%) [62]. This study, however, was underpowered for its endpoints, enrolling 259 patients when the calculated power required 572 patients.

Regarding PTS, in a prospective cohort of patients with acute DVT, PTS symptoms occurred in 23% of limbs with calf DVT at 12 months versus 54% with proximal DVT [63]. In studies, the proportion of patients treated with anticoagulation has varied from 51% to 72%, and there has been variation in the length of time of anticoagulation as well [64–66].

The 2016 ACCP guidelines recommend that patients with isolated distal DVT of the leg receive weekly serial imaging of the deep veins for 2 weeks over anticoagulation if they do not have severe symptoms or risk factors for extension. Conversely, if significant calf pain or risk factors for extension are present, 3 months of anticoagulation is recommended [1].

In patients with acute isolated distal DVT who are managed with anticoagulation, the treatment is the same as for patients with acute proximal DVT. Anticoagulation options include a DOAC or warfarin. In patients with an acute isolated distal DVT who are managed with serial imaging, switching to anticoagulation is recommended if the thrombus extends but remains confined to the distal veins or extends into a proximal vein. A patient's bleeding risk may influence the decision to prescribe anticoagulation versus prescribe serial compression ultrasonography for patients with distal DVT. Furthermore, in addition, patient preferences in regard to proximal DVT or PE risk versus bleeding risk need to be taken into consideration in cases where 2 different options are available for treatment and may be a guide to which treatment is recommended for a particular patient.

FUTURE DIRECTIONS

Despite all the trials and drug development over the past decade, there remain many unanswered questions and studies to be done. For instance, there are as yet no strong data on the use of DOACs in cancer patients, relegating a large group of individuals to daily or twice-daily injections with LMWH. Much of decision making regarding anticoagulation therapy centers around risk and benefit; the ideal agent that inhibits thrombus without bleeding does not yet exist. Such an agent is sorely needed and will be a valued addition to the anticoagulation arsenal. Until such an ideal agent is discovered, scoring systems to determine anticoagulation length of treatment will likely become more common. Finally, as newer expensive anticoagulants paired with their reversal agents enter the market, cost-effectiveness must be taken into consideration.

SUMMARY

After a half a decade of incremental gains, and in some areas, stagnation of forward progress, anticoagulation pharmacology has abruptly become a rapidly developing, expansive and progressive field. The standard of care is quickly evolving (see the difference between the 2012 and the 2016 ACCP guidelines) and even for an experienced clinician, the onslaught of newly approved medications and studies is difficult to interpret and implement in the context of practice. This article identifies the most recent trends in anticoagulation in the context of current standard of care. It is the authors' hope that this may serve as a practical guide to their usage.

References

[1] Kearon C, Akl EA, Ornelas J, et al. Antithrombotic therapy for VTE disease: CHEST guideline and expert panel report. Chest 2016;149(2):315–52.

[2] Schulman S, Rhedin AS, Lindmarker P, et al. A comparison of six weeks with six months of oral anticoagulant therapy after a first episode of venous thromboembolism. Duration of Anticoagulation Trial Study Group. N Engl J Med 1995;332(25):1661–5.

[3] Ridker PM, Goldhaber SZ, Glynn RJ. Low-intensity versus conventional-intensity warfarin for prevention of recurrent venous thromboembolism. N Engl J Med 2003;349(22):2164–7 [author reply: 2164–7].

[4] Kearon C, Ginsberg JS, Kovacs MJ, et al. Comparison of low-intensity warfarin therapy with conventional-intensity warfarin therapy for long-term prevention of recurrent venous thromboembolism. N Engl J Med 2003;349(7):631–9.

[5] Douketis JD, Kearon C, Bates S, et al. Risk of fatal pulmonary embolism in patients with treated venous thromboembolism. JAMA 1998;279(6):458–62.

[6] Lee AY, Levine MN, Baker RI, et al. Low-molecular-weight heparin versus a coumarin for the prevention of recurrent venous thromboembolism in patients with cancer. N Engl J Med 2003;349(2):146–53.

[7] Hull RD, Pineo GF, Brant R, et al. Home therapy of venous thrombosis with long-term LMWH versus usual care: patient satisfaction and post-thrombotic syndrome. Am J Med 2009;122(8):762–9.e3.

[8] EINSTEIN Investigators, Bauersachs R, Berkowitz SD, Brenner B, et al. Oral rivaroxaban for symptomatic venous thromboembolism. N Engl J Med 2010;363(26):2499–510.

[9] Schulman S, Kearon C, Kakkar AK, et al. Dabigatran versus warfarin in the treatment of acute venous thromboembolism. N Engl J Med 2009;361(24):2342–52.

[10] Hokusai-VTE Investigators, Büller HR, Décousus H, Grosso MA, et al. Edoxaban versus warfarin for the treatment of symptomatic venous thromboembolism. N Engl J Med 2013;369(15):1406–15.

[11] Agnelli G, Buller HR, Cohen A, et al. Oral apixaban for the treatment of acute venous thromboembolism. N Engl J Med 2013;369(9):799–808.

[12] Knepper J, Horne D, Obi A, et al. A systematic update on the state of novel anticoagulants and a primer on reversal and bridging. J Vasc Surg Venous Lymphat Disord 2013;1(4):418–26.

[13] Pollack CV Jr, Reilly PA, Eikelboom J, et al. Idarucizumab for dabigatran reversal. N Engl J Med 2015;373(6):511–20.

[14] Siegal DM, Curnutte JT, Connolly SJ, et al. Andexanet alfa for the reversal of Factor Xa inhibitor activity. N Engl J Med 2015;373(25):2413–24.

[15] Crowther M, Crowther MA. Antidotes for novel oral anticoagulants: current status and future potential. Arterioscler Thromb Vasc Biol 2015;35(8):1736–45.

[16] Kataruka A, Kong X, Haymart B, et al. SAMe-TT2R2 predicts quality of anticoagulation in patients with acute venous thromboembolism: the MAQI2 experience. Vasc Med 2017;22(3):197–203.

[17] Gabriel F, Portolés O, Labiós M, et al. Usefulness of thrombophilia testing in venous thromboembolic disease: findings from the RIETE registry. Clin Appl Thromb Hemost 2013;19(1):42–7.

[18] Palareti G, Cosmi B, Legnani C, et al. D-dimer testing to determine the duration of anticoagulation therapy. N Engl J Med 2006;355(17):1780–9.

[19] Rodger MA, Le Gal G, Anderson DR, et al. Validating the HERDOO2 rule to guide treatment duration for women with unprovoked venous thrombosis: multinational prospective cohort management study. BMJ 2017;356:j1065.

[20] Rodger MA, Kahn SR, Wells PS, et al. Identifying unprovoked thromboembolism patients at low risk for recurrence who can discontinue anticoagulant therapy. CMAJ 2008;179(5):417–26.

[21] Kearon C, Gent M, Hirsh J, et al. A comparison of three months of anticoagulation with extended anticoagulation for a first episode of idiopathic venous thromboembolism. N Engl J Med 1999;340(12):901–7.

[22] Simes J, Becattini C, Agnelli G, et al. Aspirin for the prevention of recurrent venous thromboembolism: the INSPIRE collaboration. Circulation 2014;130(13):1062–71.

[23] Becattini C, Agnelli G, Schenone A, et al. Aspirin for preventing the recurrence of venous thromboembolism. N Engl J Med 2012;366(21):1959–67.

[24] Weitz JI, Lensing AWA, Prins MH, et al. Rivaroxaban or aspirin for extended treatment of venous thromboembolism. N Engl J Med 2017;376(13):1211–22.

[25] Agnelli G, Buller HR, Cohen A, et al. Apixaban for extended treatment of venous thromboembolism. N Engl J Med 2013;368(8):699–708.

[26] Meissner MH, Gloviczki P, Comerota AJ, et al. Early thrombus removal strategies for acute deep venous thrombosis: clinical practice guidelines of the Society for Vascular Surgery and the American Venous Forum. J Vasc Surg 2012;55(5):1449–62.

[27] Bates SM, Jaeschke R, Stevens SM, et al. Diagnosis of DVT: antithrombotic therapy and prevention of thrombosis, 9th ed: American College of Chest Physicians evidence-based clinical practice guidelines. Chest 2012;141(2 Suppl):e351S–418S.

[28] Thomas SM, Goodacre SW, Sampson FC, et al. Diagnostic value of CT for deep vein thrombosis: results of a systematic review and meta-analysis. Clin Radiol 2008;63(3):299–304.

[29] Sampson FC, Goodacre SW, Thomas SM, et al. The accuracy of MRI in diagnosis of suspected deep vein thrombosis: systematic review and meta-analysis. Eur Radiol 2007;17(1):175–81.

[30] Carpenter JP, Holland GA, Baum RA, et al. Magnetic resonance venography for the detection of deep venous thrombosis: comparison with contrast venography and duplex Doppler ultrasonography. J Vasc Surg 1993;18(5):734–41.

[31] Prandoni P, Lensing AW, Cogo A, et al. The long-term clinical course of acute deep venous thrombosis. Ann Intern Med 1996;125(1):1–7.

[32] Wakefield TW, Myers DD, Henke PK. Mechanisms of venous thrombosis and resolution. Arterioscler Thromb Vasc Biol 2008;28(3):387–91.

[33] Meissner MH, Manzo RA, Bergelin RO, et al. Deep venous insufficiency: the relationship between lysis and subsequent reflux. J Vasc Surg 1993;18(4):596–605 [discussion: 606–8].

[34] Douketis JD, Crowther MA, Foster GA, et al. Does the location of thrombosis determine the risk of disease recurrence in patients with proximal deep vein thrombosis? Am J Med 2001;110(7):515–9.

[35] Kahn SR, Shrier I, Julian JA, et al. Determinants and time course of the postthrombotic syndrome after acute deep venous thrombosis. Ann Intern Med 2008;149(10): 698–707.

[36] Tsuji A, Yamada N, Ota S, et al. Early results of rheolytic thrombectomy in patients with proximal deep vein thrombosis. Circ J 2011;75(7):1742–6.

[37] Baekgaard N, Broholm R, Just S, et al. Long-term results using catheter-directed thrombolysis in 103 lower limbs with acute iliofemoral venous thrombosis. Eur J Vasc Endovasc Surg 2010;39(1):112–7.

[38] Watson L, Broderick C, Armon MP. Thrombolysis for acute deep vein thrombosis. Cochrane Database Syst Rev 2014;(1):CD002783.

[39] Manninen H, Juutilainen A, Kaukanen E, et al. Catheter-directed thrombolysis of proximal lower extremity deep vein thrombosis: a prospective trial with venographic and clinical follow-up. Eur J Radiol 2012;81(6):1197–202.

[40] Haig Y, Enden T, Slagsvold CE, et al. Determinants of early and long-term efficacy of catheter-directed thrombolysis in proximal deep vein thrombosis. J Vasc Interv Radiol 2013;24(1):17–24 [quiz: 26].

[41] Sharifi M, Bay C, Mehdipour M, et al. Thrombus Obliteration by Rapid Percutaneous Endovenous Intervention in Deep Venous Occlusion (TORPEDO) trial: midterm results. J Endovasc Ther 2012;19(2):273–80.

[42] Enden T, Haig Y, Kløw NE, et al. Long-term outcome after additional catheter-directed thrombolysis versus standard treatment for acute iliofemoral deep vein thrombosis (the CaVenT study): a randomised controlled trial. Lancet 2012;379(9810):31–8.

[43] Juhan CM, Alimi YS, Barthelemy PJ, et al. Late results of iliofemoral venous thrombectomy. J Vasc Surg 1997;25(3):417–22.

[44] Raju S, Darcey R, Neglen P. Unexpected major role for venous stenting in deep reflux disease. J Vasc Surg 2010;51(2):401–8 [discussion: 408].

[45] Tung CS, Soliman PT, Wallace MJ, et al. Successful catheter-directed venous thrombolysis in phlegmasia cerulea dolens. Gynecol Oncol 2007;107(1):140–2.

[46] Robinson DL, Teitelbaum GP. Phlegmasia cerulea dolens: treatment by pulse-spray and infusion thrombolysis. AJR Am J Roentgenol 1993;160(6):1288–90.

[47] Righini M. Is it worth diagnosing and treating distal deep vein thrombosis? No. J Thromb Haemost 2007;5(Suppl 1):55–9.

[48] Schellong SM. Distal DVT: worth diagnosing? Yes. J Thromb Haemost 2007;5(Suppl 1): 51–4.

[49] Oger E. Incidence of venous thromboembolism: a community-based study in Western France. EPI-GETBP Study Group. Groupe d'Etude de la Thrombose de Bretagne Occidentale. Thromb Haemost 2000;83(5):657–60.

[50] Galanaud JP, Sevestre-Pietri MA, Bosson JL, et al. Comparative study on risk factors and early outcome of symptomatic distal versus proximal deep vein thrombosis: results from the OPTIMEV study. Thromb Haemost 2009;102(3):493–500.

[51] Kahn SR, Ginsberg JS. The post-thrombotic syndrome: current knowledge, controversies, and directions for future research. Blood Rev 2002;16(3):155–65.

[52] Luxembourg B, Schwonberg J, Hecking C, et al. Performance of five D-dimer assays for the exclusion of symptomatic distal leg vein thrombosis. Thromb Haemost 2012;107(2): 369–78.

[53] Palareti G, Cosmi B, Lessiani G, et al. Evolution of untreated calf deep-vein thrombosis in high risk symptomatic outpatients: the blind, prospective CALTHRO study. Thromb Haemost 2010;104(5):1063–70.

[54] Lagerstedt CI, Olsson CG, Fagher BO, et al. Need for long-term anticoagulant treatment in symptomatic calf-vein thrombosis. Lancet 1985;2(8454):515–8.

[55] Galanaud JP, Quenet S, Rivron-Guillot K, et al. Comparison of the clinical history of symptomatic isolated distal deep-vein thrombosis vs. proximal deep vein thrombosis in 11,086 patients. J Thromb Haemost 2009;7(12):2028–34.

[56] Cogo A, Lensing AW, Koopman MM, et al. Compression ultrasonography for diagnostic management of patients with clinically suspected deep vein thrombosis: prospective cohort study. BMJ 1998;316(7124):17–20.

[57] Birdwell BG, Raskob GE, Whitsett TL, et al. The clinical validity of normal compression ultrasonography in outpatients suspected of having deep venous thrombosis. Ann Intern Med 1998;128(1):1–7.

[58] Bernardi E, Prandoni P, Lensing AW, et al. D-dimer testing as an adjunct to ultrasonography in patients with clinically suspected deep vein thrombosis: prospective cohort study. The Multicentre Italian D-dimer Ultrasound Study Investigators Group. BMJ 1998;317(7165): 1037–40.

[59] Wells PS, Anderson DR, Bormanis J, et al. Value of assessment of pretest probability of deep-vein thrombosis in clinical management. Lancet 1997;350(9094):1795–8.

[60] Perrier A, Desmarais S, Miron MJ, et al. Non-invasive diagnosis of venous thromboembolism in outpatients. Lancet 1999;353(9148):190–5.

[61] Kraaijenhagen RA, Piovella F, Bernardi E, et al. Simplification of the diagnostic management of suspected deep vein thrombosis. Arch Intern Med 2002;162(8):907–11.

[62] Righini M, Galanaud JP, Guenneguez H, et al. Anticoagulant therapy for symptomatic calf deep vein thrombosis (CACTUS): a randomised, double-blind, placebo-controlled trial. Lancet Haematol 2016;3(12):e556–62.

[63] Meissner MH, Caps MT, Bergelin RO, et al. Early outcome after isolated calf vein thrombosis. J Vasc Surg 1997;26(5):749–56.

[64] McLafferty RB, Moneta GL, Passman MA, et al. Late clinical and hemodynamic sequelae of isolated calf vein thrombosis. J Vasc Surg 1998;27(1):50–6 [discussion: 56–7].

[65] Browse NL, Clemenson G. Sequelae of an 125I-fibrinogen detected thrombus. Br Med J 1974;2(5917):468–70.

[66] Prandoni P, Villalta S, Polistena P, et al. Symptomatic deep-vein thrombosis and the post-thrombotic syndrome. Haematologica 1995;80(2 Suppl):42–8.

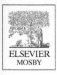

Advances in Surgery 52 (2018) 57–71

ADVANCES IN SURGERY

Proper Use of Cholecystostomy Tubes

Francesca M. Dimou, MD, MS[a], Taylor S. Riall, MD, PhD[b],*

[a]Department of Surgery, University of South Florida, 13220 USF Laurel Drive, 5th Floor, Tampa, FL 33612, USA; [b]Department of Surgery, University of Arizona, 1501 North Campbell Avenue, Room 4237, PO Box 245131, Tucson, AZ 85724-5131, USA

Keywords
• Gallstone disease • Gallbladder disease • Cholecystostomy
• Percutaneous cholecystostomy • Calculous cholecystitis • Acalculous cholecystitis

Key points

- The 2013 Tokyo Guidelines (TG13) provide consensus regarding cholecystostomy tube placement based on severity of cholecystitis but do not account for the severity of underlying illness/comorbidity. The 2018 Updated Tokyo Guidelines (TG18) management algorithms take comorbidity into account.
- Current practice in the United States does not follow TG13 in grade II and grade III disease, especially with regard to cholecystostomy tube placement, but are more aligned with the new TG18.
- After a cholecystostomy tube is placed, its subsequent management remains inconsistent and the literature reports various algorithms.
- Cholecystostomy tubes have short-term and long-term complications; once placed, patients should undergo interval cholecystectomy if their underlying medical condition can be optimized and cholecystectomy safely performed.

INTRODUCTION

Gallstone disease is one of the most common gastrointestinal diseases encountered by surgeons. As the incidence of gallstones increases with age, surgeons are increasingly faced with older patients with severe cholecystitis and associated physiologic decompensation due to both their gallbladder pathology and their underlying medical comorbidities.

Disclosure: The authors have nothing to disclose.

*Corresponding author. E-mail address: tsriall@surgery.arizona.edu

https://doi.org/10.1016/j.yasu.2018.03.011

The definitive treatment in patients presenting with acute cholecystitis is cholecystectomy, most often performed laparoscopically. The first ultrasound-guided cholecystostomy tube [1] was performed in 1979 and subsequently described in 1980 by Radder [2], who performed the procedure in a 54-year-old patient with gallbladder empyema. Cholecystostomy tube placement decompresses the gallbladder and allows for source control and is a viable option for patients who cannot tolerate a cholecystectomy. The primary indication for tube placement, as indicated in the US literature is the high-surgical risk patient often described as "debilitated" or "critically ill."

The establishment of the Tokyo Guidelines in 2007 (TG07) and subsequent revision in 2013 (TG13) were developed to provide consensus regarding the diagnosis and management of patients with severe gallstone disease [3,4]. The TG07 and TG13 guidelines primarily classify cholecystitis based on the severity of gallstone disease and do not account for a patient's medical comorbidities (Table 1). It is based on this classification that an algorithm for cholecystostomy tube placement has been derived. The guidelines specifically recommend the use of cholecystostomy tubes in patients with grade II cholecystitis with symptoms greater than 72 hours who fail antibiotic therapy or with grade III cholecystitis (Fig. 1). These guidelines were recently revised. The 2018 Tokyo Guidelines (TG18) recommend emergent gallbladder decompression with percutaneous cholecystostomy

Table 1
Tokyo Guidelines classification of acute cholecystitis based on disease severity

Grade	Definition
I (Mild)	• No findings of organ dysfunction and mild disease of the gallbladder • Cholecystectomy is deemed safe • Do not meet "moderate" or "severe" category

II (Moderate)	• Degree of inflammation is likely associated with operative difficulty if cholecystectomy is to be undertaken
	• Associated with any one of the following:
	  ○ Elevated WBC ($>18{,}000/mm^3$)
	  ○ Palpable tender mass in the right upper quadrant
	  ○ Symptoms >72 h
	  ○ Marked local inflammation (ie, gangrenous cholecystitis, pericholecystic abscess, hepatic abscess, biliary peritonitis, emphysematous cholecystitis)

III (Severe)	• Cholecystitis with associated organ dysfunction, which may include any one of the following:
	  ○ Circulatory failure (hypotension requiring treatment with dopamine >5 μg/kg per minute or any dose of norepinephrine)
	  ○ Neurologic disturbance (decreased level of consciousness)
	  ○ Respiratory failure ($PaO_2{:}FiO_2$ ratio <300)
	  ○ Renal failure (oliguria, creatinine >2.0 mg/dL)
	  ○ Hepatic failure (INR >1.5)
	  ○ Thrombocytopenia (platelet count $<100{,}000/mm^3$)

Abbreviations: INR, International Normalized Ratio; WBC, white blood cell count.

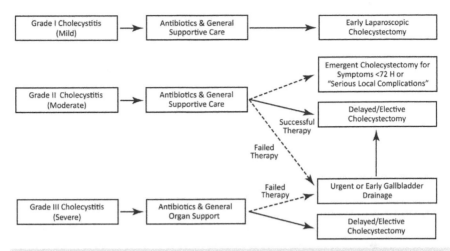

Fig. 1. TG13 algorithm for the management of acute calculous cholecystitis. Cholecystostomy tube placement is recommended in grade II and grade III disease when antibiotics and supportive care do not provide source control. Delayed elective cholecystectomy is recommended after tube placement. (*From* Mayumi T, Takada T, Kawarada Y, et al. Results of the Tokyo consensus meeting Tokyo guidelines. J Hepatobiliary Pancreat Surg 2007;14(1):121; with permission.)

tube in grade II and grade III cholecystitis when antibiotics and supportive care fails and comorbidity is such that laparoscopic cholecystectomy is high risk (Fig. 2).

There is an increasing body of literature supporting early cholecystectomy in patients presenting with complicated acute gallstone disease, with most studies recommending early cholecystectomy within 72 hours of symptoms [5,6]. Recent literature reports that cholecystectomy can safely be performed up to 10 days of symptom onset, and earlier surgery is associated with decreased morbidity and shorter hospital stays [7]. These studies are reflected in the TG18 management algorithms.

Although the use of cholecystostomy tubes in the United States has increased from 3.9% in 1996% to 9.7% in 2010 [8], a majority of patients with grade II disease are appropriately undergoing immediate cholecystectomy based on data regarding safety in this setting. In cases of grade III disease, cholecystostomy tubes are reserved for the sickest patients who cannot tolerate general anesthesia. Recent data reporting on Medicare beneficiaries with a diagnosis of gallstone disease between 1995 and 2011 found only 6.4% of patients with a diagnosis of grade III cholecystitis and only 5% of these patients actually underwent a cholecystostomy tube [8].

Despite the move toward early cholecystectomy in all patients presenting with acute calculous cholecystitis, there remains a subset of patients who present with a high anesthetic and surgical risk secondary to the severity of their gallstone disease, the complexity of their comorbid conditions, or a combination of both. It is in these cases that cholecystostomy tube placement is

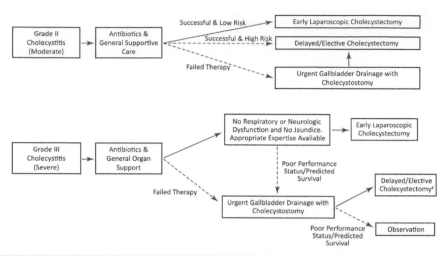

Fig. 2. TG18 algorithm for the management of patients with acute calculous cholecystitis. Cholecystostomy tube is now recommended in patients with grade II disease only if they fail antibiotics and supportive care and are not candidates for cholecystectomy based on poor performance status as measured by a CCI score greater than or equal to 6 or ASA class greater than or equal to 3. In grade III disease, cholecystostomy is recommended in patients who (1) fail antibiotics and supportive care, (2) have respiratory and/or neurologic dysfunction, and (3) do not rapidly resolve their cardiovascular and renal dysfunction. After cholecystostomy tube placement, cholecystectomy is recommended unless the CCI is greater than or equal to 4 and life expectancy is short, in which case patients can be observed. These management protocols assumed advanced centers who have ICU care, appropriate surgical expertise, and advanced endoscopy. (*Adapted from* Okamoto K, Suzuki K, Takada T, et al. Tokyo Guidelines 2018: flowchart for the management of acute cholecystitis. J Hepatobiliary Pancreat Sci 2018;25(1):66; with permission.)

indicated. There remains controversy, however, regarding indications, which may be addressed by the new TG18 guidelines.

INDICATIONS FOR CHOLECYSTOSTOMY TUBE PLACEMENT

It is important to understand that cholecystostomy tube placement is driven by 2 main components: gallbladder pathology and patient-related factors. Gallbladder pathology primarily refers to the presence or absence of stones (calculous or acalculous cholecystitis), the severity of the inflammatory process, and the duration of symptoms. The patient-related factors are less well defined, subjective, and primarily based on physician/surgeon judgment. These factors include underlying cardiac, respiratory, renal, and other systemic disease that increase surgical risk. Such comorbid conditions in the setting of acute gallbladder disease may lead to physiologic decompensation in the setting of manageable inflammation from the surgical standpoint. In the United States, cholecystostomy tube placement is generally performed in critically ill, debilitated, and/or high-surgical risk patients with calculous and acalculous disease.

Acute calculous cholecystitis

Acute gallbladder disease is most often related to gallstones. Complications from gallstones include acute calculous cholecystitis, choledocholithiasis, cholangitis, and gallstone pancreatitis [9–11]. The pathophysiology of acute cholecystitis is obstruction of the cystic duct by an impacted gallstone, leading to transmural edema, inflammation, and eventual necrosis. Cholecystostomy tube placement allows for gallbladder decompression in the setting of cystic duct obstruction without requiring a major anesthetic, because the procedure can be done under ultrasound guidance with minimal sedation. Decompression of the gallbladder reduces the inflammatory process, allowing the patient to recover from the infectious process and any underlying systemic decompensation related to decreased physiologic reserve or severity of cholecystitis; it also provides a bridge to definitive therapy with an interval cholecystectomy.

In the setting of acute calculous cholecystitis and need for cholecystostomy tube, studies conducted in the United States do not report severity of acute cholecystitis as the primary indication for tube placement (Table 2); rather, the indications for cholecystostomy tube placement are patient comorbidities, making the risk of anesthesia and surgery prohibitive. Some studies are nonspecific, simply recommending cholecystostomy tube in "poor surgical candidates" without clear definition. Other studies report specific patient-related factors as indications for cholecystostomy tube placement. In 2016, Boules and colleagues [12] did a retrospective review of 424 patients who underwent cholecystostomy tube placement. It was at the attending surgeon's discretion whether a patient was considered a high-risk surgical candidate; review of the data identified 5 risk factors for cholecystostomy tube placement: cardiac surgery within 2 months of symptom onset, pulmonary infection, end-stage liver disease with cirrhosis, new diagnosis of pulmonary embolism, use of systemic anticoagulation, and hemodynamic instability. Other retrospective reviews have reported indications, such as stage IV terminal cancer and coronary artery disease [13,14].

An earlier retrospective study identified patients who presented to an emergency department (ED) with severe cholecystitis or were inpatients for other conditions and developed severe cholecystitis and underwent cholecystostomy tube placement [15]. The investigators classified patients based on their own severity illness score: systemic inflammatory response syndrome (SIRS) classification in conjunction with radiographic findings (positive Murphy sign, air within the gallbladder wall, and gallbladder perforation). All patients in the study were deemed poor surgical candidates with more than 50% having either cardiovascular disease or underlying malignancy. The TG18 attempt to define this group at high risk for early operative intervention. In TG18, for grade II disease, cholecystostomy tube is recommended in patients who have a Charlson Comorbidity Index (CCI) score greater than or equal to 6 or American Society of Anesthesiologists (ASA) class greater than or equal to 3 and where antibiotics and supportive care have failed to control local inflammation. For grade III disease, cholecystostomy tube is recommended in patients who fail

Table 2
Studies reporting various indications for cholecystostomy tube placement

Author, year	Sample size	Study design	Reported indications
Bala et al [9], 2015	257	Retrospective	Physician discretion and either the presence of comorbid conditions and/or lack of clinical improvement with antibiotic therapy alone
Başaran et al [13], 2005	18	Retrospective	Medical comorbidity, including terminal cancer, uncontrolled hypertension and diabetes, CAD, HTN and CRI, ARF
Berber et al [33], 2000	15	Retrospective	High risk for general anesthesia secondary to comorbidities and/or chronic illness
Boules et al [12], 2016	380	Retrospective	Inflammation too severe during attempted laparoscopic cholecystectomy
			Cardiac surgery within 2 mo of symptom onset
			Pulmonary infection
			End-stage liver disease
			New diagnosis of PE
			Use of systemic anticoagulation
			Hemodynamic instability
Byrne et al [14], 2003	45	Retrospective	Medical comorbidities, including cardiovascular disease and malignancy
Cha et al [23], 2014	82	Retrospective	Patient comorbidities
Chang et al [22], 2014	60	Retrospective	Failure to respond to initial medical treatment in patients with high perioperative risk
			Impending rupture of a severely distended gallbladder that may cause clinical deterioration
			Suspected gallbladder necrosis or perforation in patients with severe comorbidities and no other treatments available
Hatzidakis [34], 2002	63	Prospective	Randomized to cholecystostomy tube group, but patients were referred to surgical team for possible tube placement
Hsieh [35], 2012	166	Retrospective	Septic shock/severe sepsis
			Gallbladder rupture
			Failed conservative treatment after 48 h
Horn et al [19], 2015	278	Retrospective	High burden of comorbidity
			Prolonged symptom duration reported as >5 d
Joseph et al [15], 2012	106	Retrospective	Poor surgical candidates

Study	N	Type	Indications
Khasawneh [36], 2015	245	Retrospective	Calculous cholecystitis Acalculous cholecystitis
Kim et al [11], 2017	144	Retrospective	Sepsis likely from a biliary source
Kortram [37], 2011	27	Retrospective	No specific indications except for decision for tube placement was a "multidisciplinary manner"
McKay et al [26], 2012	68	Retrospective	A component of 1 or more of the following: • Age • ASA • APACHE • Comorbidity Surgeon discretion
Nasim [38], 2011	62	Retrospective	ASA grade I/IV Significant sepsis resulting in hemodynamic instability Patients deemed moderate risk or high risk for general anesthesia
Nikfarjam [39], 2013	32	Prospective	Patients who were evaluated and deemed unable to tolerate general anesthesia Declined surgery
Pang et al [25], 2016	71	Retrospective	Severe sepsis/shock Gallbladder perforation Multiple comorbidities
Paran [40], 2006	54	Prospective	Poor surgical candidate secondary to comorbidities and/or symptoms >72 h
Saeed [41], 2010	41	Observational case series	Calculous cholecystitis Acalculous cholecystitis Gallbladder perforation and/or empyema
Spira [42], 2002	55	Retrospective	Biliary sepsis Septic shock Severe comorbidities
Wang [43], 2016	279	Retrospective	Patient preference Failure to respond to initial medical management Impending rupture of severely distended gallbladder Severe sepsis/septic shock
Wisemen [44], 2010	86	Retrospective	Comorbidities and age

Abbreviations: APACHE, assessment and chronic health evaluation; ARF, acute renal failure; CAD, coronary artery disease; CRI, chronic renal insufficiency; HTN, hypertension; PE, pulmonary embolism.

antibiotics and supportive care, who are jaundiced and have neurologic or respiratory dysfunction, and whose associated organ system failure is not rapidly reversible with therapy; cholecystostomy tube is also recommended in grade III disease where antibiotics and supportive care is effective and cardiovascular and renal organ system failure is reversed but patients have poor performance status (CCI score >4 and ASA class ≥3 [see Fig. 2]) [16].

Acalculous cholecystitis

Other studies have reported cholecystostomy tube placement in patients with acalculous cholecystitis (Table 3) [17–21]. Acalculous cholecystitis is not an obstructive process; this disease process primarily occurs in patients who are critically ill, including burn patients or chronic patients in the ICU who cannot tolerate surgical intervention. One of the larger retrospective studies on acalculous cholecystitis evaluated 704 patients who underwent percutaneous cholecystostomy and compared outcomes to those who underwent cholecystectomy [21]. Specifically, the study compared patients with a cholecystostomy tube to those who underwent a laparoscopic cholecystectomy converted to open cholecystectomy. In a multivariable logistic regression model, morbidity

Table 3
Studies primarily reporting outcomes in patients with acalculous cholecystitis who undergo percutaneous cholecystostomy placement

Author, year	Total acute acalculous cholecystitis (N)	Study design	Outcomes
Anderson et al [17], 2013	4329	Retrospective	Decreased mortality in patients undergoing cholecystectomy vs PC (HR 0.29, $P<.001$)
Chung et al [18], 2012	57	Retrospective	In-hospital mortality was 21% and 49% were managed nonoperatively; 31% underwent cholecystectomy; 7% had recurrent cholecystitis.
Horn et al [19], 2015	278	Retrospective	30-d mortality was 4.7%; 54.7% of patients were definitively treated with PC with a follow-up of 5 y; 23.5% of patients were readmitted for recurrent cholecystitis; 28% underwent an LC at some point in the study period.
Kirkegard et al [20], 2015	56	Observational	30-d mortality was 10.7%, with 80.4% definitively treated with PC; 9% underwent LC at some point in the study period.
Simorov et al [21], 2013	704	Retrospective	Compared with LC and OC, those who underwent PC had decreased LOS, morbidity, ICU stay, and cost. No difference in mortality.

Abbreviations: HR, hazard ratio; LC, laparoscopic cholecystectomy; LOS, length of stay; PC, percutaneous cholecystostomy; OC, open cholecystectomy.

was lower in the cholecystostomy tube group but mortality was similar. Based on these data, the investigators proposed cholecystostomy tube placement in those with acalculous cholecystitis as a permanent treatment or a bridge to cholecystectomy given the increased risk of converting to an open operation and its associated morbidity.

Mortality rates in those with acalculous cholecystitis and percutaneous cholecystostomy tubes remain high according to the data; 30-day and in-hospital mortality rates range from 9% to 21%. Even though these data propose cholecystostomy tubes as definitive treatment of those with acalculous cholecystitis who cannot tolerate cholecystectomy, one-third of patients eventually underwent definitive treatment with a cholecystectomy (see Table 3).

COMPLICATIONS OF TUBE PLACEMENT
Initial studies describing outcomes of cholecystostomy tube placement primarily report placement as "feasible" and "safe." Success rates of tube placement exceed 90% in most studies but primarily refer to immediate tube placement and no acute complications [10,22–24]. Yet, complications from tube placement can occur immediately after the procedure but often occur in the long-term, requiring multiple repeated interventions related to tube complications.

Complications
Immediate complications from cholecystostomy tube placement include biliary peritonitis, sepsis, and tube dislodgement. The incidence of cholecystostomy tube-related complications across observational studies is shown in Table 4. Studies reporting such complications are primarily small, single-institution retrospective reviews. In a study by Joseph and colleagues [15], 32% of critically ill patients who had a cholecystostomy tube placed did not improve or declined clinically after cholecystostomy tube placement. Another study, including 71 patients with acute calculus cholecystitis, reported a complication rate of 28% with reported severe complications, such as perforated viscus; 14% of these patients experienced tube dislodgement [25]. Another study done in Korea by Cha and colleagues reported outcomes of 82 patients who underwent cholecystostomy tube placement [23]. The reported technical success rate was 100% and clinical success reported as 98%; yet, 1 patient died secondary to cholecystitis-related sepsis. No other complications were reported in this cohort. Overall, complications specifically related to cholecystostomy tube placement ranged from 5% to 33% (see Table 4); again, complications were primarily related to bleeding, tube dislodgement, or catheter-associated pain.

Readmission and recurrence rates
Readmission rates are high in patients with cholecystostomy tubes placement secondary to dislodgement, dysfunction, or simply pain (see Table 4). Furthermore, there is associated greater cost with frequent hospital visits, radiologic

Table 4
Tube-related complications, readmission, and cholecystectomy rates associated with of chole-cystostomy tube placement

Author, year	Total (N)	Tube-related complications (%)	Readmission rates (%)	Recurrent cholecystitis (%)	Cholecystectomy (%)
Al-Jundi [45], 2012	30	9	NR	NR	36.7
Bala et al [9], 2015	257	31	15	NR	63.4
Başaran et al [13], 2005	18	5.6	NR	NR	42.8
Berber [34], 2000	15	13	NR	NR	80[a]
Boules et al [12], 2016	380	NR	3.7	NR	32.9
Byrne et al [14], 2003	45	2	NR	NR	37.8
Cha et al [23], 2014	82	NR	0	0	54.8
Chang et al [22], 2014	60	9.8	NR	11.7	5
Hatzidakis [34], 2002	63	5	NR	NR	25
Hsieh [35], 2012	166	16.3	NR	13.8	31.9
Horn et al [19], 2015	278	35.2	23.5	23.5	28.4
Jang [28], 2015	93	3.2	NR	19.3	33
Joseph et al [15], 2012	106	5	NR	NR	27
Khasawneh [36], 2015	245	NR	NR	NR	83
Kim et al [11], 2017	144	21.4	NR	9.7	27.9
Kortram [37], 2011	27	3.7	NR	19.7	16
McKay et al [26], 2012	68	14.7	41	41	30
Nasim [38], 2011	62	1.6	NR	9.7	37
Nikfariam [39], 2013	32	19	NR	NR	28
Pang et al [25], 2016	71	28	NR	NR	45
Paran [40], 2006	54	33	19[b]	NR	51.8
Saeed [41], 2010	41	25	NR	NR	22
Spira [42], 2002	55	16	19.2	19.2	56.4
Wang [43], 2016	279	NR	NR	9.2	33
Wisemen [44], 2010	86	21	NR	NR	54.6

Abbreviation: NR, not reported.
[a]Unknown denominator.
[b]Percent of patients who had PC and never underwent surgery because deemed unfit.

interventions, and overall increased hospital days. Studies demonstrate that recurrence of cholecystitis ranges from 9% to 41% (see Table 4) and readmissions rates are as high as 41% [19,26]. Causes for readmission rates in these patients are not clearly reported but likely secondary to tube dislodgement, pain, and/or recurrence of their disease.

Long-term survival
In a study of long-term outcomes in Medicare beneficiaries with grade III cholecystitis, 30-day, 90-day, and 2-year survival rates were significantly lower in patients who underwent cholecystostomy tube placement compared with propensity matched controls. Specifically, 2-year survival rates were 35% versus 41% in those with a tube compared with those without a tube, respectively [8].

TUBE MANAGEMENT

Cholecystostomy tube removal

Literature is limited and varied when reporting management of cholecystostomy tubes after placement. The are no published guidelines regarding tube management; however, the Tokyo Guidelines clearly recommend delayed cholecystectomy after tube placement, regardless of initial grade of the cholecystitis. Studies reporting postprocedure tube management are inconsistent. For example, Cha and colleagues [23] reported a proposed algorithm of patients who underwent cholecystostomy tube placement. Patients were evaluated for biliary tract patency via cholangiogram once their symptoms and clinical status improved during the index hospitalization. If patency was demonstrated via contrast emptying into the duodenum, the catheter was clamped; patients who tolerated clamping trials and had clinical improvement had their tube removed prior to discharge. If the cystic duct was not patent, patients had their tube kept to external drainage and discharged with the tube in place. Patients with recurrent cholecystitis, worsening laboratory values, or worsening symptoms with clamping trials had their catheter placed back to drainage for 7 days and were reassessed. The median length of time that the tube remained in place was not reported nor was the time to cholecystectomy.

> Zarour and colleagues [27] reviewed outcomes of 119 patients who underwent cholecystostomy tube placement for acute cholecystitis. They reported that all patients who underwent tube placement were discharged with the tube in place and underwent follow-up cholangiogram 2 weeks to 3 weeks later; if a patient was deemed an appropriate surgical candidate, the tube was clamped, left in place, and the patient subsequently underwent cholecystectomy. In patients who were not deemed fit but had biliary tract patency, the tube was removed. Overall, patients in the study had varying times in which the tube remained in place and were dependent on resolution of symptoms or whether they underwent a cholecystectomy

Other studies have reported the duration of drainage with a cholecystostomy tube but have not proposed an algorithm. Times ranged up to 70 days if patients did not undergo definitive treatment with a cholecystectomy compared with only 10 days in those who eventually underwent cholecystectomy [28]. These data demonstrate the variability in physician practices when managing patients who undergo cholecystostomy tube placement. Most studies recommend drainage for 3 weeks to 6 weeks because this allows a tract to develop [29]; however, patients with uncontrolled diabetes, persistent infection, or malnutrition and those on steroids may hinder the healing process and tube drainage is recommended for a longer period of time [30,31].

Ultimately, tube removal is dependent on resolution of a patient's symptoms and reported pain resolution. This is done through evaluation of laboratory values, abdominal examination, and patient report of resolved abdominal pain. If the patient's clinical status improves, the patient should have the biliary tree evaluated prior to tube removal. Specifically, there must be patency of the patient's cystic duct or the likelihood of recurrent episodes of cholecystitis is extremely high. The timeline in which a cholangiogram is done in these patients varies anywhere from 1 week to 6 weeks. It is reasonable to consider cholangiogram once a patient's clinical status improves. If cholangiogram demonstrates a patent cystic duct, the next step is clamping of the cholecystostomy tube, with removal in the absence of recurring symptoms. As discussed later, however, every attempt to optimize patient comorbidities and provide definitive treatment with cholecystectomy should be made [32].

The criterion of cystic duct patency does not necessarily apply to those with acalculous cholecystitis because the pathophysiology is different, but patients should at least undergo clamping trials prior to removal to reduce the risk of patients having recurrent symptoms after tube removal and requiring an additional procedure.

Definitive treatment

The only definitive treatment of patients with acute cholecystitis is cholecystectomy. In patients who undergo cholecystostomy tube placement, the Tokyo Guidelines recommend delayed interval cholecystectomy after tube placement (see Fig. 2), except for patients with initial grade III disease and poor performance status and predicted survival. These recommendations apply to those with calculous cholecystitis, but other reports on patients with acalculous cholecystitis agree that cholecystectomy may not be necessary [21].

Despite the Tokyo Guidelines and recommendation for cholecystectomy, the data vary widely, with cholecystectomy rates ranging from 15% to 80% after cholecystostomy tube placement (see Table 4). In this setting, cholecystectomy is primarily done in the elective setting after a patient's clinical status has improved. Cholecystectomy may also be required if cholecystostomy tube placement fails to control local inflammation and systemic sepsis. Data published in Medicare beneficiaries undergoing cholecystostomy tube placement for grade III cholecystitis demonstrate that only one-third of these patients undergo definitive treatment with a delayed cholecystectomy [8]. The recurrence of acute cholecystitis in those who do not undergo definitive therapy ranges from 11% to 41% (see Table 4); therefore, definitive therapy should be sought after if a patient's clinical status allows.

PROPOSED ALGORITHM FOR CHOLECYSTOSTOMY TUBE PLACEMENT AND MANAGEMENT

The proper use of cholecystostomy tubes includes temporary treatment of patients with cholecystitis, calculous, or acalculous who cannot tolerate surgery according to the TG18 guidelines. The severity of cholecystitis or the duration of symptoms are not absolute contraindications for cholecystectomy and do not mandate cholecystostomy tube placement. Potential reasons for a patient's inability to tolerate surgery include severe systemic disease including cardiovascular disease, underlying malignancy, and any condition that precludes general anesthesia.

Cholecystostomy tubes do not serve as definitive therapy for patients with cholecystitis and complications, including disease recurrence, remain high in these patients. Once placed, a follow-up evaluation of a patient's clinical status and interrogation of the cholecystostomy tube should be undertaken prior to removal. If possible, once the acute episode has resolved, the patient's underlying medical conditions should be optimized and cholecystectomy performed.

The TG18 algorithm for management of patients with acute cholecystitis is shown in Fig. 2. Initial evaluation should include assessment of patients' clinical status and severity of their gallbladder disease. If patients are hemodynamically stable and able to tolerate a general anesthetic, cholecystectomy should be performed as soon as possible during the index admission regardless of the Tokyo grade. Cholecystostomy tubes should be reserved for patients who do not rapidly respond to antibiotics and supportive care and are not candidates for cholecystectomy due to underlying comorbidity and physiologic decompensation due to acute illness. In cases of grade III disease, if a patient improves with antibiotics and organ support, re-evaluation should be undertaken during the index hospitalization for possible cholecystectomy at a center that has appropriate surgical expertise, anesthesia support, and ICU support. If not performed on the index admission, then delayed or elective cholecystectomy should be done on patients who have a life expectancy of greater than a year because recurrence rates are high. Incorporating models that predict patient survival into the treatment algorithms for patients with grade II and grade III cholecystitis may help guide decision making. Regardless, as with all interventions, there are risks and benefits; therefore, physicians must consider the risks and benefits of this intervention and its long-term consequences.

References

[1] Elyaderani M, Gabriele OF. Percutaneous cholecystostomy and cholangiography in patients with obstructive jaundice. Radiology 1979;130(3):601–2.

[2] Radder RW. Ultrasonically guided percutaneous catheter drainage for gallbladder empyema. Diagn Imaging 1980;49(6):330–3.

[3] Takada T, Strasberg SM, Solomkin JS, et al. TG13: updated Tokyo guidelines for the management of acute cholangitis and cholecystitis. J hepato-biliary-pancreatic Sci 2013;20(1):1–7.

[4] Mayumi T, Takada T, Kawarada Y, et al. Results of the Tokyo consensus meeting Tokyo guidelines. J hepato-biliary-pancreatic Surg 2007;14(1):114–21.

[5] Cao AM, Eslick GD, Cox MR. Early laparoscopic cholecystectomy is superior to delayed acute cholecystectomy: a meta-analysis of case-control studies. Surg Endosc 2016;30(3): 1172–82.

[6] Gurusamy K, Samraj K, Gluud C, et al. Meta-analysis of randomized controlled trials on the safety and effectiveness of early versus delayed laparoscopic cholecystectomy for acute cholecystitis. Br J Surg 2010;97(2):141–50.

[7] Ansaloni L, Pisano M, Coccolini F, et al. 2016 WSES guidelines on acute calculous cholecystitis. World J Emerg Surg 2016;11(1):25.

[8] Dimou FM, Adhikari D, Mehta HB, et al. Outcomes in older patients with grade iii cholecystitis and cholecystostomy tube placement: a propensity score analysis. J Am Coll Surg 2017;224(4):502–11.e1.

[9] Bala M, Mizrahi I, Mazeh H, et al. Percutaneous cholecystostomy is safe and effective option for acute calculous cholecystitis in select group of high-risk patients. Eur J Trauma Emerg Surg 2015;42(6):1–6.

[10] Alvino DML, Fong ZV, McCarthy CJ, et al. Long-term outcomes following percutaneous cholecystostomy tube placement for treatment of acute calculous cholecystitis. J Gastrointest Surg 2017;21(5):761–9.

[11] Kim D, Iqbal SI, Ahari HK, et al. Expanding role of percutaneous cholecystostomy and interventional radiology for the management of acute cholecystitis: an analysis of 144 patients. Diagn Interv Imaging 2017; https://doi.org/10.1016/j.diii.2017.04.006.

[12] Boules M, Haskins IN, Farias-Kovac M, et al. What is the fate of the cholecystostomy tube following percutaneous cholecystostomy? Surg Endosc 2016;31(4):1707–12.

[13] Başaran O, Yavuzer N, Selçuk H, et al. Ultrasound-guided percutaneous cholecystostomy for acute cholecystitis in critically ill patients: one center's experience. Turk J Gastroenterol 2005;16(3):134–7.

[14] Byrne MF, Suhocki P, Mitchell RM, et al. Percutaneous cholecystostomy in patients with acute cholecystitis: experience of 45 patients at a US referral center. J Am Coll Surg 2003;197(2): 206–11.

[15] Joseph T, Unver K, Hwang GL, et al. Percutaneous cholecystostomy for acute cholecystitis: ten-year experience. J Vasc Interv Radiol 2012;23(1):83–8.e1.

[16] Okamoto K, Suzuki K, Takada T, et al. Tokyo guidelines 2018: flowchart for the management of acute cholecystitis. J Hepatobiliary Pancreat Sci 2018; https://doi.org/10.1002/jhbp.516.

[17] Anderson JE, Chang DC, Talamini MA. A nationwide examination of outcomes of percutaneous cholecystostomy compared with cholecystectomy for acute cholecystitis, 1998-2010. Surg Endosc 2013;27(9):3406–11.

[18] Chung YH, Choi ER, Kim KM, et al. Can percutaneous cholecystostomy be a definitive management for acute acalculous cholecystitis? J Clin Gastroenterol 2012;46(3):216–9.

[19] Horn T, Christensen SD, Kirkegård J, et al. Percutaneous cholecystostomy is an effective treatment option for acute calculous cholecystitis: a 10-year experience. HPB (Oxford) 2015;17(4):326–31.

[20] Kirkegard J, Horn T, Christensen SD, et al. Percutaneous cholecystostomy is an effective definitive treatment option for acute acalculous cholecystitis. Scand J Surg 2015;104(4): 238–43.

[21] Simorov A, Ranade A, Parcells J, et al. Emergent cholecystostomy is superior to open cholecystectomy in extremely ill patients with acalculous cholecystitis: a large multicenter outcome study. Am J Surg 2013;206(6):935–40 [discussion: 940–1].

[22] Chang YR, Ahn Y-J, Jang J-Y, et al. Percutaneous cholecystostomy for acute cholecystitis in patients with high comorbidity and re-evaluation of treatment efficacy. Surgery 2014;155(4):615–22.

[23] Cha BH, Song HH, Kim YN, et al. Percutaneous cholecystostomy is appropriate as definitive treatment for acute cholecystitis in critically ill patients: a single center, cross-sectional study. Korean J Gastroenterol 2014;63(1):32–8.

[24] van Overhagen H, Meyers H, Tilanus HW, et al. Percutaneous cholecystectomy for patients with acute cholecystitis and an increased surgical risk. Cardiovasc Intervent Radiol 1996;19(2):72–6.

[25] Pang KW, Tan CHN, Loh S, et al. Outcomes of percutaneous cholecystostomy for acute cholecystitis. World J Surg 2016;40(11):2735–44.

[26] McKay A, Abulfaraj M, Lipschitz J. Short- and long-term outcomes following percutaneous cholecystostomy for acute cholecystitis in high-risk patients. Surg Endosc 2012;26(5): 1343–51.

[27] Zarour S, Imam A, Kouniavsky G, et al. Percutaneous cholecystostomy in the management of high-risk patients presenting with acute cholecystitis: Timing and outcome at a single institution. Am J Surg 2017; https://doi.org/10.1016/j.amjsurg.2017.01.030.

[28] Jang WS, Lim JU, Joo KR, et al. Outcome of conservative percutaneous cholecystostomy in high-risk patients with acute cholecystitis and risk factors leading to surgery. Surg Endosc 2015;29(8):2359–64.

[29] McGillicuddy EA, Schuster KM, Barre K, et al. Non-operative management of acute cholecystitis in the elderly. Br J Surg 2012;99(9):1254–61.

[30] Picus D, Burns MA, Hicks ME, et al. Percutaneous management of persistently immature cholecystostomy tracts. Journal of vascular and interventional radiology. JVIR 1993;4(1): 97–101 [discussion: 101–2].

[31] Corbett CR, Fyfe NC, Nicholls RJ, et al. Bile peritonitis after removal of T-tubes from the common bile duct. Br J Surg 1986;73(8):641–3.

[32] Little MW, Briggs JH, Tapping CR, et al. Percutaneous cholecystostomy: the radiologist's role in treating acute cholecystitis. Clin Radiol 2013;68(7):654–60.

[33] Berber E, Engle KL, String A, et al. Selective use of tube cholecystostomy with interval laparoscopic cholecystectomy in acute cholecystitis. Archives of Surgery 2000;135(3):341–6.

[34] Hatzidakis AA, Prassopoulos P, Petinarakis I, et al. Acute cholecystitis in high-risk patients: percutaneous cholecystostomy vs conservative treatment. European Radiology 2002;12(7): 1778–84.

[35] Hsieh YC, Chen CK, Su CW, et al. Outcome after percutaneous cholecystostomy for acute cholecystitis: a single-center experience. J Gastrointest Surg 2012;16(10):1860–8.

[36] Khasawneh MA, Shamp A, Heller S, et al. Successful laparoscopic cholecystectomy after percutaneous cholecystostomy tube placement. The Journal of Trauma and Acute Care Surgery 2015;78(1):100–4.

[37] Kortram K, de Vries Reilingh TS, Wiezer MJ, et al. Percutaneous drainage for acute calculous cholecystitis. Surg Endosc 2011;25(11):3642–6.

[38] Nasim S, Khan S, Alvi R, et al. Emerging indications for percutaneous cholecystostomy for the management of acute cholecystitis—a retrospective review. Int J Surg 2011;9(6):456–9.

[39] Nikfarjam M, Shen L, Fink MA, et al. Percutaneous cholecystostomy for treatment of acute cholecystitis in the era of early laparoscopic cholecystectomy. Surgical Laparoscopy, Endoscopy & Percutaneous Techniques 2013;23(5):474–80.

[40] Paran H, Zissin R, Rosenberg E, et al. Prospective evaluation of patients with acute cholecystitis treated with percutaneous cholecystostomy and interval laparoscopic cholecystectomy. Int J Surg 2006;4(2):101–5.

[41] Saeed SA, Masroor I. Percutaneous cholecystostomy (PC) in the management of acute cholecystitis in high risk patients. J Coll Physicians Surg Pak 2010;20(9):612–5.

[42] Spira RM, Nissan A, Zamir O, et al. Percutaneous transhepatic cholecystostomy and delayed laparoscopic cholecystectomy in critically ill patients with acute calculus cholecystitis. Am J Surg 2002;183(1):62–6.

[43] Wang C-H, Wu C-Y, Yang JC-T, et al. Long-term outcomes of patients with acute cholecystitis after successful percutaneous cholecystostomy treatment and the risk factors for recurrence: a decade experience at a single center. PLoS ONE 2016;11(1):e0148017.

[44] Wiseman JT, Sharuk MN, Singla A, et al. Surgical management of acute cholecystitis at a tertiary care center in the modern era. Archives of Surgery 2010;145(5):439–44.

[45] Al-Jundi W, Cannon T, Antakia R, et al. Percutaneous cholecystostomy as an alternative to cholecystectomy in high risk patients with biliary sepsis: a district general hospital experience. Annals of the Royal College of Surgeons of England 2012;94(2):99–101.

Advances in Surgery 52 (2018) 73–87

ADVANCES IN SURGERY

Is Maintenance of Certification Working in Surgery?

Spence M. Taylor, MD

Greenville Health System, 300 East McBee Street, Greenville, SC 29601, USA

Keywords

- Surgical maintenance of certification • MOC controversy • Physician burnout

Key points

- Medical knowledge is increasing at an exponential pace; a process of continuous learning for physicians is essential.
- Time-honored, continuous learning requirements to maintain American Board of Surgery (ABS) certification (recertification examination required since 1976) are criticized as burdensome, expensive, and irrelevant to practice.
- Controversy is fueled by unprecedented rates of physician burnout, where the administrative burden of practice (including Maintenance of Certification [MOC]) is a major contributor.
- The ABS is taking steps to make MOC less onerous, more user friendly, and more applicable—to include replacing the 10-year recertification examination.

INTRODUCTION

For most health professionals, American Board of Medical Specialties (ABMS) board certification signifies the pinnacle of a long educational process and the ultimate goal of medical training. Surgery is no exception. The ABMS consists of 24 member boards certifying physicians in 39 specialties and 86 subspecialties—resulting in more than 880,000 physician diplomates, 27% of whom are surgical subspecialists. For years, beginning in the 1930s, board certification represented a brand of excellence, a milestone to be achieved at the beginning of practice and a distinction earned forever. With the explosion of new medical knowledge in the latter half of the twentieth century, however, several member boards questioned the premise that completion of an examination process at

---

Disclosures: None.

E-mail address: staylor@ghs.org

https://doi.org/10.1016/j.yasu.2018.04.002

the end of training could assure lifelong competency in a given medical specialty. Verification of ongoing competency became a reality in the 1970s when member boards began introducing the idea of recertification for senior diplomates. Recertification in the form of a written summative examination was adopted and proactively enacted by various specialties including surgery. Over time, all member boards adopted some process to prove maintenance of certification (MOC) for diplomates and by 2005 MOC became an ABMS expectation.

The purpose of this article is to address the question, "Is MOC working in surgery?" Before this question is debated, it may be important to consider the value of board certification in general. Although board certification, as discussed later, has increasingly become a minimum standard for various credentialing bodies and processes, the ABMS ostensibly considers certification and MOC a voluntary process, chosen by a physician or surgeon as a means to document expertise in a medical specialty by meeting the profession-driven standards and requirements. Or, as stated on the ABMS Web site, "…(board certification is a) highly-visible indicator that physicians know today's standards of practice." Originally, hospitals, patients, payors, and other institutions, such as the medical-legal system, considered board certification a distinction beyond that of basic medical licensure (not a minimum standard), especially for specialty care–a peer-controlled standard of excellence. Therefore, the question posed by this article is an interesting and of considerable debate.

At the outset, to ask if board certification "is working" infers that the process is actually designed to accomplish some meaningful purpose or task. Currently, the ABMS and its member boards are struggling with this–how can (or even should) attainment of a measurable standard of medical knowledge and professionalism, which the boards ostensibly accomplish, equate to some outcome? And what outcome should be accomplished and measured? Currently, most member boards, including the American Board of Surgery (ABS), target lifelong learning and assessment as the task to be accomplished. If the outcome desired, however, is improved patient care, then data to support board certification in these terms are only minimally supportive. There have been a few published systematic reviews of the literature and clinical outcome correlation studies that have suggested board certification and MOC result in better clinical outcomes, but none of these has been in surgical practices [1–3]. Additionally, there have been several trade journals suggesting that board certification correlated with higher surgeon reimbursement and personal income–hardly an altruistic call for wide-scale endorsement. As such, endorsement of board certification and MOC are mostly intuitive; it makes sense that surgeons who stay current with the latest medical and professional trends will be better doctors. Despite this, there is no consensus as to the value of MOC. This article provides an overview regarding the need for monitored lifelong learning as well as a historical perspective on licensure, credentialing, and board certification. Next, it reviews the current controversies related to MOC, the association of MOC and physician well-being, and, finally, it the actions taken by the ABS to address the controversies, the measures taken to improve the MOC process, and plans to validate its value.

UNDERSTANDING MAINTENANCE OF CERTIFICATION: ITS NEED AND ITS HISTORY

There are more than 30,000 surgical diplomates with an active primary certificate in general and/or vascular surgery. Each graduated medical school, attained the professional standards to become licensed by the state, completed training in a residency approved by the Accreditation Council for Graduate Medical Education, achieved institutional credentials to practice surgery, passed a written board-qualifying examination, and successfully completed an oral certifying examination. Becoming a diplomate of the ABS represents successful completion of one of the most rigorous academic and professional processes. From the beginning, board certification was considered a privilege reserved for the most competent, not a minimum standard for all surgeons to achieve. Certificates are issued and revoked at the discretion of the ABS, with the goal of maintaining a standard of quality and accountability to the public. As surgical training became more refined, the treatment and outcomes more available, and medical information more accessible, expectations of the public have become more sophisticated. Contemplate the following: in 1950 it took 50 years to double medical knowledge; in 1980, it took 7 years; in 2010, it took 3.5 years; and the 2020 projection is that it will take 73 days. Approximately 7300 new clinical articles with pertinent information are published monthly, requiring an estimated 627.5 hours per month (of a total 730.5 hours in a month) to stay current [4,5]. Although the general public may not be aware of the extraordinary rate of which medical knowledge turns over, they are aware that this is in an age of information where new ideas and thoughts flow constantly. It is then probably unreasonable to assume that the general public will accept the premise that a doctor can be certified as competent at the completion of training and then not need to demonstrate maintenance of competency until retirement.

Gallup data from 2003 showed that 98% of those polled believed that their doctor should be board certified and 79% believed their doctor should undergo periodic recertification [6]. That same audience might be troubled to learn that physicians are frequently reticent to adopt new treatments, their funds of knowledge often lagging up to 17 years behind evidence-based therapies [7,8]. Furthermore, a 2006 systematic review of the literature published in the *Journal of the American Medical Association* (*JAMA*) found a poor or inverse correlation between physicians' self-assessment of their current medical practice compared with external observations of their competency. Most troubling, the lowest correlation between self-assessment and external validation occurred among physicians least skilled and most confident in their own abilities [9]. From these data, it is difficult to deny a need for processes that encourage or require lifelong learning and document adoption of current best practices for health professionals. As well, externally validated mechanisms to assure that these practices are successfully adopted are essential. Without both, there is no assurance that current medical care is acceptably practiced. Lastly, intuition dictates that patients, many of who are subject to periodic external validation of their own vocational competencies, would be appalled to learn that their surgeons were not subject to similar, or more stringent, periodic validation. After all, if plumbers are required to document continuing education to maintain licensure—and they are—why should not doctors? As such, questions regarding verification of competence are less one of "if" and more of "how" and "what."

Traditionally, there have been 3 mechanisms to assess professional competency for medical practitioners: state licensure, staff credentialing, and specialty board certification. Within this construct, assurance of the basic level of professionalism and medical competence rests with state licensure and local credentialing. Credentialing, the oldest form of competency assessment, dates back to the Middle Ages and licensure in America to post–Civil War nineteenth century. Although these important institutions continue today, it was in 1933 with the development of the Advisory Board for Medical Specialties—the precursor to the ABMS—that specialty physician competency was assessed. Initially meant to be considered a step above basic licensure and credentialing, board certification was a voluntary system—an indicator of excellence and exceptional professional achievement until the 1980s–1990s, when consumer activists and managed care insurance panels began to recognize board certification as a desirable and differentiating distinction for providers. As a consequence, the reimbursement implications of not being board certified created enormous financial pressure on physicians to become certified. In 1972, the American Board of Family Medicine, followed by the ABS in 1976, began limiting the duration of certification—requiring a written examination every 7 years to 10 years to maintain certification. As such, the early vestiges of MOC were beginning to materialize [10]. Other specialties followed suit and by 2005 the ABMS formally introduced its requirements of MOC for all specialty boards: Part I, Professionalism and Professional Standing; Part II, Lifelong Learning and Self-Assessment; Part III, Assessment of Knowledge, Judgment, and Skills; and Part IV, Improvement in Medical Practice. Over the next decade the ABMS component boards, including the ABS, were allowed to independently develop standards, acceptable practices, and implementation timelines for each element, with oversite by the ABMS. Unlike other specialties, the ABS, on its own volition, developed and implemented many of the requirements long before the 2005 ABMS directive (Part I in 1937, Part II in 2000, Part III in 1976, and Part IV in 2005). The ABS officially began enrolling diplomates into the 3-year MOC administrative cycle in 2005 [11].

At face value, the ABMS MOC process seems logical and manageable, addressing the information explosion that challenges its diplomates by motivating practice-based learning and self-assessment of practice habits. It protects the public, whom the diplomates serve, and it meant self-directed learning by its diplomates. Despite its merits, few could have predicted the intensity and breadth of the backlash that has occurred, crescendoing in nature, against both the MOC process and the ABMS member boards. In retrospect, there were 2 critical miscalculations: the timing of implementation of MOC and the executors of the process—physicians during a time of looming unprecedented burnout. Currently, MOC has escalated to become one of the most controversial ABMS initiatives ever. Given such, a review of the controversy is warranted.

MAINTENANCE OF CERTIFICATION: THE CONTROVERSY

Over the past decade, changes in American health care have arguably affected the practicing physician more than any other time in history. Financial pressures, narrow insurance networks, hospital employment, challenging productivity expectations, loss of autonomy, the electronic health record (EHR), burdensome and often inexplicable regulatory requirements, increased patient volumes, complexity of aging baby boomers, and physician workforce shortages have all increased the work load beyond what could ever have been anticipated [12]. In recent years, a relatively new hazard in the work place has been discovered, *occupational burnout syndrome*—a condition first described in the mid-1970s disproportionately affecting those whose work involves interaction with people (teachers, health workers, soldiers, and so forth) [13]. Burnout is characterized by a symptom complex that includes emotional exhaustion, depersonalization (cynicism), and decreased effectiveness (inefficiency). According to survey data, burnout is widespread and increasing, affecting as many as 54% of practicing physicians in 2015 compared with 45% in 2011 [14,15]. It involves all specialties, including surgery. In a recent editorial published in *JAMA*, investigators described burnout as a consequence of excessive workload, increased clerical burden, loss of control of work environment, practice inefficiency, problems with work-life balance, and a feeling of loss of purpose [12]. The true impact of burnout on the overall condition of US health care is not completely understood, but experts believe its effect to be both impactful and significant. High rates of burnout can be considered both a marker of dysfunction in the health care system as well as a contributing factor to dysfunction—not to mention a driver of provider attrition [16]. In other studies, the top 3 causes for burnout, in order, include the increasingly bureaucratic nature of practice, computerization of practice, and excessive work hours (no doubt related to bureaucracy and computers) [17].

Particularly incriminating is the EHR. Unlike other industries where computerization has significantly improved operational efficiency, the EHR has done just the opposite in health care. Although magnificent in capturing data and documenting treatment, EHR data input, for some reason, has been relegated to health professionals (labeled as best practice by the computer vendors), thus assigning to the most sophisticated, expensive and critically short workforce resource (doctors and nurses) the most menial task of clerical documentation. The consequences of such practices in many cases have created massive access bottlenecks and patient dissatisfaction, not to mention professional burnout. In a recently published time-motion study where 57 physicians were observed for more than 430 work hours, approximately 50% of the physician time was spent doing nonclinical clerical work (eg, EHR related tasks) compared with 33% spent doing direct patient care (with 37% of this time associated with a doctor in front of an open computer at a patient's side). For every hour spent performing clinical work, 2 hours were spent performing clerical work [18]. Some have suggested that the EHR may ultimately prove the most significant occupational health hazard (burnout) in medicine since the radiograph developed in the early twentieth century.

It is within this environment that the ABMS introduced MOC. Like the EHR, it was a new process administratively assigned to the physician, significantly adding to the nonclinical burden and no doubt contributing to burnout. Also like the EHR, the value of MOC has been significantly questioned and difficult to prove. Although many physicians, including surgeons, accept the theoretic rationale for MOC and are familiar with data showing the benefits of initial certification, most have concerns about the relevance and effectiveness of current MOC programs [2,19–22]. MOC has sparked major controversy in the medical community, as evidenced by editorials, letters, petitions, opinion polls, and even efforts to create an alternative certification board [20,23–33]. In a recent survey of more than 800 physicians, more than 80% agreed that MOC is a burden; the vast majority consider MOC activities, such as self-assessment continuing medical education (CME) and examination preparation, of little value for practice improvement or patient care. Dissatisfaction was pervasive across all practice settings and all specialties, including surgery [34].

That the current MOC controversy could potentially collapse the ABMS is evident by the unresolved conflict between the American Board of Internal Medicine (ABIM) and its diplomates. Widely reported in the lay press, this conflict represents a perfect storm where a specialty of diplomates, already experiencing significant clinical burnout, were informed in January 2014 that their requirements to maintain certification were going to substantially broaden. Although bemoaning the additional administrative burden posed by the new requirements, the diplomates' objection took a different angle: alleging that the new MOC requirements were financially motivated, with the ABIM reaping millions of dollars in new profits on the backs of its diplomates. A sequence of events—a near revolt followed, including the formation of a competing certifying board not requiring MOC, the National Board of Physicians and Surgeons (NBPAS); several embarrassing news articles, including in *Newsweek* magazine; a call from the American Medical Association to scrap MOC; a public apology by the ABIM temporarily suspending MOC; and multistate legislative efforts to eliminate MOC.

Regarding the legislative efforts to eliminate MOC, past ABS director Dr J. Patrick Walker gave an in-depth report to the Board of Governors and Board of Regents of ABS in October 2017 at its Clinical Congress in San Diego, California. Dr Walker chronicled the events leading up to the passage of Texas Bill 1148, a bill designed to restrict the use of MOC as a credentialing tool. The bill, driven by physician members of the Texas Medical Association in an emotionally intense debate, fell short of its primary goal to completely outlaw MOC, leaving the use of MOC for credentialing up to the hospitals. Dr Walker stressed that the effort to restrict the use of MOC for credentialing is an organized multistate effort. At this time, 5 states (Texas, Maine, Maryland, Tennessee, and Georgia) have passed some form of legislation eliminating or restricting the use of MOC as the sole criteria for credentialing physicians by hospitals and/or insurance panels. In his report, Dr Walker conveyed that 15 other states (Oregon, California, Oklahoma, Missouri, Arkansas, Mississippi, Florida, South Carolina, Ohio, Michigan, New Jersey, Rhode Island, Massachusetts, Alaska, and New York) have debated or are actively considering or have anti-MOC legislation in progress (Fig. 1). These efforts underscore the intensity of the debate and question whether MOC can survive in its current form. As well, some investigators believe the debate even jeopardizes the future of the ABMS itself. In the meantime, the NBPAS continues its fight to gain legitimacy with credentialing bodies and diplomate opposition continues to escalate. At present, the controversy seems far from resolved.

MAINTENANCE OF CERTIFICATION FOR SURGERY: A CALL TO ACTION

Institutionally, the ABS has followed the debate over MOC with interest. As an early adopter of the recertification process, the ABS has supported the efforts of the ABMS to make certification more than a 1-time assessment. Since 1976,

LEGISLATION PASSED
Georgia, Maine, Maryland, Tennessee, Texas

LEGISLATION PENDING
California, Massachusetts, Michigan, Ohio, New Jersey

LEGISLATION STALLED
New York, Rhode Island

LEGISLATION DEAD/WITHDRAWN
Alaska, Arkansas, Florida, Mississippi, Missouri,

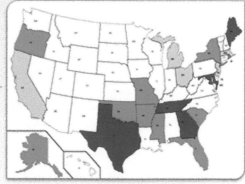

Fig. 1. States with anti-MOC legislation.

approximately 1500 diplomates dutifully register each fall to take a written examination, known as the ABS MOC examination. The 200-question multiple-choice examination tests broad-based surgical knowledge in a variety of subspecialty areas as well as principles common to all of areas of surgery. Diplomates through the years have fared well, with historical pass rates of approximately 95%. Until recently, complaints to the ABS have been few. Most practicing surgeons have grown up in the current certification paradigm where initial certification with a written and oral examination is followed by a recertification examination every 10 years. As the controversy around MOC intensified, mostly within other medical specialties, the ABS directors were uncertain about the opinions and degree of dissatisfaction among current surgery diplomates. Although the ABS has maintained its position that it needs to be responsive to the concerns of its diplomates, its primary accountability is to the general public, the patients whom surgeons serve and treat. To that end, the ABS has had difficulty accepting the premise of alternative boards that all forms of MOC should be abandoned. For reasons discussed previously, the ABS supports lifelong learning and assessment of diplomates as an essential cornerstone of the surgical profession. The board, however, has also officially maintained a position of openness to change, exploring new, different, and more effective ways to assess its diplomates.

To better understand the opinions of its diplomates, the ABS conducted a targeted cross-sectional survey of 1500 surgery diplomates during the summer of 2016. The top priorities for improving MOC identified by the diplomates included modification of the self-assessment CME requirements, improved practice relevance of the MOC examination, and cost reduction of the process. The majority (76%) of respondents favored continuation of the 10-year examination process but also favored a modular approach geared to the specific practice of the diplomate. Although the Likert scale portion of the survey seemed to support current practices, the comments, which were voluminous in nature, unmasked a consistent and concerning theme of dissatisfaction with the current MOC process. Much of the dissatisfaction mirrored the anti-MOC rhetoric expressed within other specialties and was consistent with independent feedback received by many directors. As a consequence, the ABS directors, after a year-long review, voted in June 2017 to replace MOC with a new lifelong learning and continuous certification process—one to be developed that eventually eliminates or makes optional the 10-year recertification examination, reduces CME requirements, and explores new summative evaluation methods for its diplomates. As well, during its deliberations the directors believed that the term, MOC, and taxonomy had become a liability and should be avoided in the future.

Also at the June meeting, the board appointed a sprint team of directors and staff to devise a new continuous learning process to be considered and approved before its 2018 winter retreat.

As part of the board directive, a comprehensive survey was constructed and sent to all diplomates in the late summer 2017. The results of that survey included responses from approximately 10,000 diplomates (33%) and are shown in Figs. 2–5. Similar to the 2016 survey, more than 80% of diplomate responders preferred a process tailored to both core surgical principles and practice-specific content. When specifically queried, however, approximately 60% of diplomates preferred a more frequent, lower-stakes, open book assessment process than the current 10-year summative assessment model. Only 13% favored the 10-year examination interval, whereas most diplomates preferred a shorter interval (every 2 years) as long as the assessment was low stakes in nature.

To the sprint team, the survey findings provided a clear case for exploration of alternatives to the 10-year summative examination process (MOC Part III). Accordingly, the sprint team studied other approaches currently used by other ABMS member boards. The options ranged from high-stakes examinations at

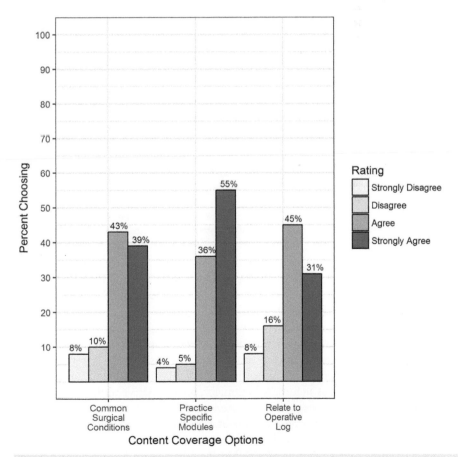

Fig. 2. Response from an ABS poll, 2017: content coverage for a new MOC examination. (*Courtesy of* American Board of Surgery, Philadelphia, PA.)

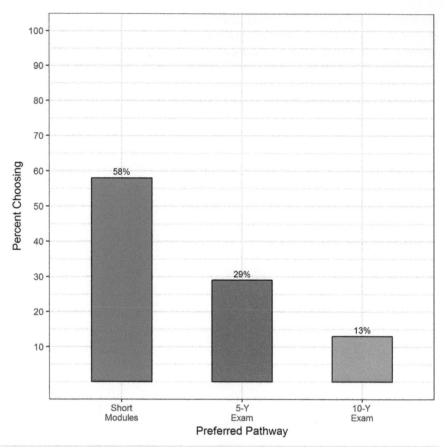

Fig. 3. Response from an ABS poll, 2017: preferred pathway for a new MOC examination. (*Courtesy of* American Board of Surgery, Philadelphia, PA.)

shorter intervals, similar to the current ABS MOC Part III process, to daily low-stakes on-line question formats (MOC Anesthesiology or MOCA Minute). After careful consideration, the sprint team settled for a middle-of-the-road approach similar to processes adopted by other surgical boards. In the fall of 2017, the sprint team proposed and the directors approved a new MOC process for general surgery. Features of the new process include attestation as to the maintenance of professional bearing (MOC Part I) and documentation of CME (MOC Part II) as before. Additionally, an alternative to the 10-year summative examination process was proposed as a pilot: a 40-question, open book examination to be taken every 2 years at home with immediate feedback and an opportunity to retake if a failing grade is assigned. The goal for the new process is to combine elements of MOC Part II with those of MOC Part III. Thus, the questions will focus on the most current practice guidelines and will feature short, in-depth critiques after each question, making the process equally as

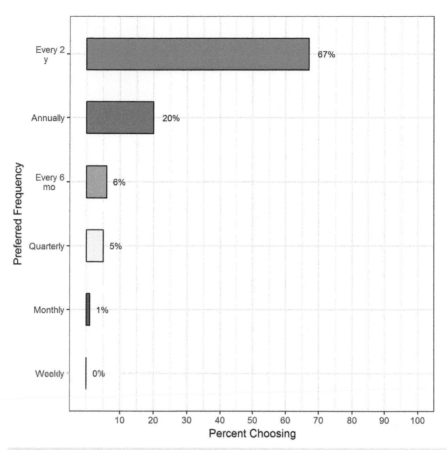

Fig. 4. Response from an ABS poll, 2017: testing intervals for the MOC process. (*Courtesy of American Board of Surgery, Philadelphia, PA.*)

formative as it is summative. If diplomates choose to participate in the every 2-year process, they will be exempt from the 10-year summative examination. In addition, participation in the every 2-year process will obviate the current requirement for self-assessment CME. The ABS pilot was approved by the ABMS Committee on Continuous Certification in November 2017 and is expected to be considered by the full ABMS Board with immediate implementation in the winter of 2018 if approved. If the pilot is successful, it is anticipated that the new process will eventually entirely replace the 10-year summative MOC Part III examination.

IS MAINTENANCE OF CERTIFICATION WORKING IN SURGERY? A SUMMARY

In summary, when assessing whether MOC in surgery is working or not, there are 2 primary considerations. First is acknowledgment that there exists a

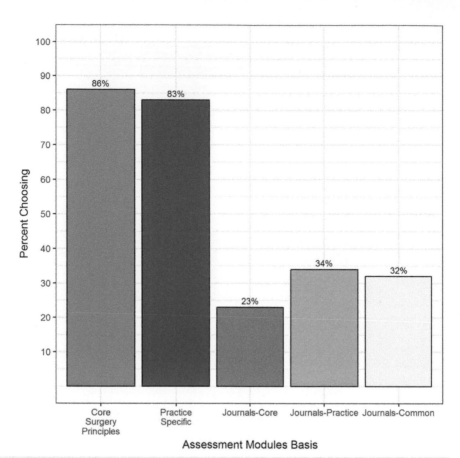

Fig. 5. Response from an ABS poll, 2017: assessment module basis for a new MOC examination. (*Courtesy of* American Board of Surgery, Philadelphia, PA.)

general need for ongoing continuous learning and assessment for surgeons. It is the opinion of the author that the public deserves and expects their surgeons to be enrolled in processes that assure the latest treatment options and techniques are adopted into practice, especially given the amount and rapidity of information turnover today. Therefore, critics, such as the NBPAS, who espouse the suspension of all formal MOC activities, should be viewed with skepticism and caution. That said, it is conceded that defending an onerous and burdensome process with little proved value is equally nonsensical. Thus, the ABMS member boards, including the ABS, need to continuously monitor processes for effectiveness, especially given the extraordinary nonclinical administrative burden shouldered by its diplomates today. MOC must be embraced as value-added and essential, not burdensome and bureaucratic. To meet this goal, the ABS—in addition to the changes in its MOC program—is currently undertaking a comprehensive strategic plan and governance redesign. From this, an ABS office of education capable of assessing the ongoing effectiveness of its certification/assessment practices is being discussed. Therefore, future changes in assessment practices such the new 2-year MOC pilot will not be based on supposition but on analysis of ongoing organizational and implementation science data.

Next, when asking whether or not MOC is working, there needs to be an understanding as to what is meant by the term, *working*. This is a complex issue that starts with an understanding of surgical competency. Most surgical diplomates believe that the ABMS appropriately characterized the attributes of physician competency when it created its definition of MOC in 2005: maintenance of personal professionalism, documentation of practiced-based continuous learning, and objective periodic assessment of knowledge and clinical outcomes. Although the ABMS, through its 4-part MOC process, ostensibly claims to monitor all these competencies, the member boards, including the ABS, do not possess the ability to effectively do so. If "working" means that the ABS alone comprehensively monitors all of these competencies, then the answer to whether MOC is working is most likely "no." When contemplating the question, however, it the interdependence among the ABMS specialty boards, the state medical licensing agencies, and the various institutional credentialing panels must be considered. Collectively, these bodies work in tandem and do a reasonable job accomplishing the objective. For instance, although the ABS monitors professional standing, it is the state boards that are best suited to monitor new and ongoing breaches of professionalism. The ABS credentials committee is usually made aware of such breaches only after diplomates lose their state medical licenses (a requirement of board certification). Action taken on the board certificate in question by the ABS almost always mimics that of the state on a diplomate's medical license. Likewise, although the ABS endorses processes where diplomates monitor their surgical outcomes, it is the credentialing bodies of hospitals that are held accountable by governmental agencies, accrediting bodies, and payors for individual patient safety and practitioner outcomes. Clearly, the ABS must rely on these processes to address questions of clinical competency based on patient outcomes for its diplomates. And lastly, although state boards and hospitals monitor lifelong learning and assessment, they have become more and more reliant on the specialty boards for enforcement of standards around each. Therefore, it can be concluded that if the objective of MOC is to maintain and document surgeon competency as defined by the ABMS, the process is indeed "working"—and working well—through the interdependent efforts of the state medical boards, the medical specialty certifying boards, and the hospital credentials committees.

If, however, "working" is defined as diplomate satisfaction with the process, then clearly there are opportunities for improvement. Although the recent actions taken by the ABS to change MOC seem to be steps in the right direction, time will tell if they will completely address all the issues. In the meantime, there is little doubt that the MOC process is contributing to the overall administrative burden and the current occupational health hazard of clinician burnout, the effects of which are no doubt major impediments to patient access, professional revenue generation, patient satisfaction, teaching, and research. Any improvements in health care that impose more administrative burden on clinicians will likely be unsuccessful. Most physicians believe there is a crisis that must be addressed: a need for immediate deployment of administrative support for providers—clinician support specialists who are capable of relieving administrative burden. Surely the financial investment for such individuals will offset their cost. A priority must be moving physicians from behind the EHR to back in front of their patients; to re-engineer work flows that center on the patient and not the health record; to make the focus access to care and not mundane documentation; to develop interprofessional practice teams where clinicians provide care using their most advanced terminal degree, accepting that it does not require an MD, DO, or BSN to type information into a computer; and above all to eliminate unnecessary, nonclinical, burdensome tasks from clinicians—which include MOC. Only then will continuous certification be accepted and assume its appropriate role, the administrative duty only physicians can do—embraced as desirable and not rebuked as onerous.

References

[1] Sharp L, Bashook P, Lipsky M, et al. Specialty board certification and clinical outcomes: the missing link - American board of medical specialties. Acad Med 2002;77(6):534–42.

[2] Lipner RS, Hess BJ, Phillips RL Jr. Specialty board certification in the United States: issues and evidence. J Contin Educ Health Prof 2013;33(Suppl 1):S7–35.

[3] Nichols D. Maintenance of certification and the challenge of professionalism. Pediatrics 2017;139(5):e20164371.

[4] Densen P. Challenges and opportunities facing medical education. Trans Am Clin Climatol Assoc 2011;122:48–58.

[5] Alper BS, Hand JA, Elliot SG, et al. How much effort is needed to keep up with the literature relevant for primary care? J Med Libr Assoc 2004;92(4):429–37.

[6] Brennan TA, Horwitz RI, Duffy FD, et al. The role of physician specialty board certification status in the quality movement. JAMA 2004;292:1038–43.

[7] Morris ZS, Wooding S, Jonathan Grant J. The answer is 17 years, what is the question: understanding time lags in translational research. J R Soc Med 2011;104(12):510–20.

[8] Fuchs VR, Milstein A. The $640 billion question—why does cost-effective care diffuse so slowly? N Engl J Med 2011;364:1985–7.

[9] Davis D, Mazmanian P, Fordis M, et al. Accuracy of physician self-assessment compared with observed measures of competence: a systematic review. JAMA 2006;269(9):1094–102.

[10] Cassel CK, Holmboe ES. Professionalism and accountability: the role of specialty board certification. Trans Am Clin Climatol Assoc 2008;119:295–304.

[11] Malangoni MA, Shiffer CD. The American board of surgery maintenance of certification program: the first 10 years. Bull Am Coll Surg 2015;100(7):15–9.

[12] Shanafelt TD, Dyrbye LN, West CP. Viewpoint: addressing physician burnout: the way forward. JAMA 2017;317(9):901–2. Available at: http://jamanetwork.com/pdfaccess.ashx?url=/data/journals/jama/0/. Accessed February 14, 2017.

[13] Maslach C, Jackson S, Leiter M. Maslach burnout inventory manual. 3rd edition. Palo Alto (CA): Consulting Psychologists Press; 1996.

[14] Shanafelt TD, Boone S, Tan L, et al. Burnout and satisfaction with work-life balance among US physicians relative to the general US population. Arch Intern Med 2012;172(18):1377–85.

[15] Shanafelt TD, Hasan O, Dyrbye LN, et al. Changes in burnout and satisfaction with work-life balance in physicians and the general US working population between 2011 and 2014. Mayo Clin Proc 2015;90(12):1600–13.

[16] Wallace JE, Lemaire JB, Ghali WA. Physician wellness: a missing quality indicator. Lancet 2009;374(9702):1714–21.

[17] Shanafelt TD, Noseworthy JH. Executive leadership and physician well-being: nine organizational strategies to promote engagement and reduce burnout. Mayo Clin Proc 2017;92(1):129–46.

[18] Sinsky C, Colligan L, Li L, et al. Allocation of physician time in ambulatory practice: a time and motion study in 4 specialties. Ann Intern Med 2016;165(11):753–60.

[19] Hawkins RE, Lipner RS, Ham HP, et al. American Board of medical specialties maintenance of certification: theory and evidence regarding the current framework. J Contin Educ Health Prof 2013;33(suppl 1):S7–19.

[20] Drazen JM, Weinstein DF. Considering recertification. N Engl J Med 2010;362(10): 946–7.

[21] Lipner RS, Bylsma WH, Arnold GK, et al. Who is maintaining certification in internal medicine and why? A national survey 10 years after initial certification. Ann Intern Med 2006;144(1):29–36.

[22] Culley DJ, Sun H, Harman AE, et al. Perceived value of Board certification and the Maintenance of Certification in Anesthesiology Program (MOCA_). J Clin Anesth 2013;25(1): 12–9.

[23] Iglehart JK, Baron RB. Ensuring physicians' competence: is maintenance of certification the answer? N Engl J Med 2012;367(26):2543–9 [Erratum appears in N Engl J Med 2013;368(8):781].

[24] Cook DA, Holmboe ES, Sorensen KJ, et al. Getting maintenance of certification to work: a grounded theory study of physicians' perceptions. JAMA Intern Med 2015;175(1):35–42.

[25] Levinson W, King TE Jr, Goldman L, et al. Clinical decisions. American Board of Internal Medicine maintenance of certification program. N Engl J Med 2010;362(10):948–52.

[26] Weiss KB, Bryant LE Jr, Morgan LB, et al. The ABIM and recertification. N Engl J Med 2010;362(25):2428–9 [author reply: 2429–30].

[27] Steele R. Maintenance of certification. Clin Pediatr (Phila) 2011;50(7):584–6.

[28] Strasburger VC. Ain't misbehavin': is it possible to criticize maintenance of certification (MOC)? Clin Pediatr (Phila) 2011;50(7):587–90.

[29] Teirstein PS. Boarded to deathdwhy maintenance of certification is bad for doctors and patients. N Engl J Med 2015;372(2):106–8.

[30] Kritek PA, Drazen JM. Clinical decisions: American Board of Internal Medicine maintenance of certification programdpolling results. N Engl J Med 2010;362(15):e54.

[31] Physicians for Certification Change. Petitions and pledge of non-compliance. Available at: http://nomoc.org/. Accessed March 18, 2016.

[32] Baron R. ABIM announces immediate changes to MOC program. Available at: http://www.abim.org/news/abim-announces-immediatechanges-to-moc-program.aspx. Accessed February 25, 2015.

[33] National Board of Physicians and Surgeons website. Available at: https://nbpas.org/. Accessed March 18, 2016.

[34] Cook DA, Blachman MJ, West CP, et al. Physician attitudes about maintenance of certification: a cross-specialty national survey. Mayo Clin Proc 2016;91(10):1336–45.

Advances in Surgery 52 (2018) 89–100

ADVANCES IN SURGERY

ELSEVIER
MOSBY

How Should Gallbladder Cancer Be Managed?

Teviah E. Sachs, MD, MPH[a],*, Oluseyi Akintorin, MD[b], Jennifer Tseng, MD, MPH[a]

[a]Department of Surgery, Boston University School of Medicine, 88 East Newton Street, Collamore – C500, Boston, MA 02118, USA; [b]Department of Surgery, Harvard University School of Medicine, Beth Israel Deaconess Medical Center, Lowry Medical Office Building, 110 Francis Street, Suite 9B, Boston, MA 02215, USA

Keywords
- Gallbladder cancer • Cholecystectomy • Liver resection
- Risk factors for gallbladder cancer • Recurrent gallbladder cancer

Key points
- Gallbladder cancer is highly malignant and rarely curable when symptomatic.
- Surgical resection is appropriate in early-stage disease.
- A multidisciplinary approach is appropriate for later-stage disease.
- When diagnosed, patients should be referred to a high-volume center.
- When appropriate, patients should be offered to enroll in clinical trials.

INTRODUCTION
Background
- Gallbladder cancer is a highly malignant and rarely curable disease that affects approximately 5000 new patients in the United States each year [1,2]. Due to the rarity of the disease, it is difficult to determine the overall survival rate, which varies between 5% and 12% [1,3,4]. For incidental gallbladder cancer, most commonly found on laparoscopic resection for biliary colic or symptomatic cholelithiasis, cure is possible and survival rates are far better [5]. A higher incidence of gallbladder cancer is seen in certain populations,

---

Disclosure Statement: The authors have nothing to disclose.

*Corresponding author. Department of Surgical Oncology, Boston Medical Center, 820 Harrison Avenue, FGH Building - Suite 5007, Boston, MA 02118. E-mail address: teviah.sachs@bmc.org

https://doi.org/10.1016/j.yasu.2018.04.003

including Native Americans in both North America and South America, especially Chile, Bolivia, and New Mexico [6].

Anatomy

- The gallbladder sits underneath the liver in the right upper quadrant of the abdomen (Fig. 1A)
- The gallbladder has 4 distinct anatomic zones: fundus, body/infundibulum, neck, and cystic duct (see Fig. 1B)
- The layers of the gallbladder wall, which are important in T stage, include the epithelium, the lamina propria, the muscularis, the perimuscular connective tissue, and the serosa (see Fig. 1C)
- A majority of cancers arise in the fundus (60%), followed by the body and infundibulum (30%) and the neck and cystic duct (10%)

Risk factors

- Cholelithiasis and chronic cholecystitis are the most common risk factors for gallbladder cancer [7]. It is believed that the chronic irritation and resultant inflammation leads to gallbladder cancer in a dysplasia to carcinoma sequence [8]. Gallstones are the leading cause of inflammation and irritation of the gallbladder epithelium. Therefore, risk factors for gallbladder cancer mimic those of gallstone disease, including female gender, obesity, and age, among others.
- Larger gallstones (>2–3 cm) have higher association with gallbladder cancer [9] (Fig. 2).

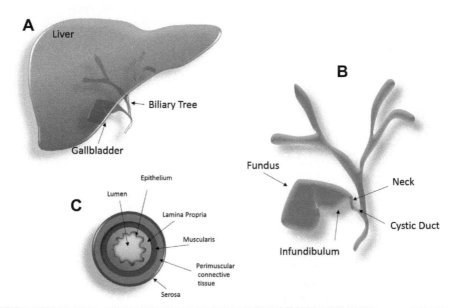

Fig. 1. Depiction of (A) location of the gallbladder beneath the liver, (B) the anatomy of the gallbladder as it relates to the biliary tree, and (C) cross-section of the gallbladder revealing the layers of the gallbladder wall.

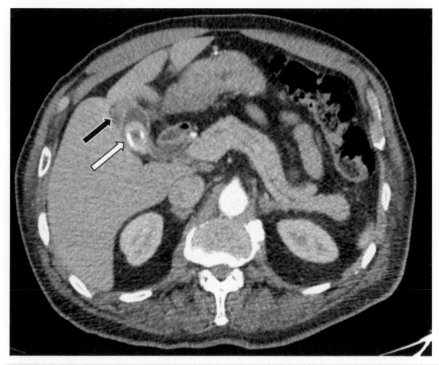

Fig. 2. Patient with an asymptomatic, large calcified gallstone in the gallbladder (*white arrow*), with an associated soft tissue mass in the fundus (*black arrow*), which is concerning for malignancy.

- Chronic bacterial infection (most commonly *Helicobacter* and *Salmonella* species) is also associated with increased risk of gallbladder cancer [10].
- Aflatoxin, more commonly associated with hepatocellular cancer, is also believed a risk factor for gallbladder cancer [11].
- Chronic inflammation can lead to calcium deposition within the wall of the gallbladder, also referred to as porcelain gallbladder (Fig. 3), which is often associated with gallbladder cancer [12].
- Anomalous pancreatobiliary duct junction is a congenital condition in which the pancreatic duct and biliary duct join more proximally in their course than is normal. This is hallmarked by an elongated common channel in imaging. This malformation is associated with an increase in all biliary tract cancers, including gallbladder cancer, although the relative risk is uncertain [13].
- Polyps, most commonly adenomatous polyps, are believed a precursor to gallbladder cancer and an adenoma to carcinoma sequence similar to that of colonic polyps has been suggested [14]. Adenomas greater than 1 cm in size, or those that are growing over time or have suspicious features, are of particular risk and warrant cholecystectomy.

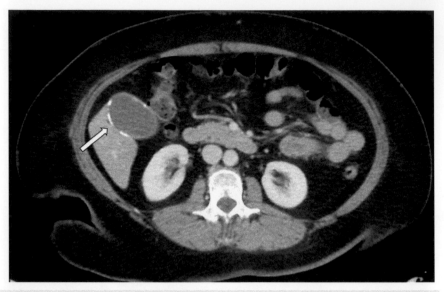

Fig. 3. Axial CT image revealing calcifications (*arrow*) in the gallbladder wall, progressive over time and concerning for malignancy.

Presentation

- Due to the distensability of the gallbladder, cancers are rarely identified early, unless discovered incidentally on imaging or for symptoms.
- Those who do have symptoms generally have symptoms similar to that of cholelithiasis, cholecystitis, or biliary colic.
- More advanced tumors may present with unintentional weight loss, right upper quadrant fullness, jaundice, or—in cases of adjacent duodenal involvement—duodenal obstruction.
- Gallbladder cancers identified incidentally on cholecystectomy account for less than 1% of cholecystectomy specimens [15,16].
- If very early stage (stage Ia or less), then cholecystectomy alone is considered curative.
- If discovered intraoperatively, open resection or termination of the operation and referral to a high-volume center is appropriate to minimize the risk of inadequate resection or peritoneal or port-site seeding.
- Later-stage cancers that are usually identified due to symptoms should be appropriately staged prior to resection.

Staging

- Gallbladder cancer is staged based on the TNM staging system [17,18].
- T stage is based on depth of invasion of the layers of the gallbladder (see Fig. 1C), whereas N stage is based on lymph node involvement and M stage represents metastatic disease.
  - Prior American Joint Committee on Cancer (AJCC) (seventh edition) staging reflected a bias toward location of involved lymph nodes (Table 1).

Table 1
T,N,M Staging of gallbladder cancer, adapted from the AJCC 7th edition

Stage Grouping		T Stage		N Stage		M Stage
Not stageable	X 0	Cant be assessed No evidence of primary tumor	X	Cant be assessed	X	Cant be assessed
0	is	Carcinoma in situ				
I	1a	Tumor invades lamina propria				
	1b	Tumor invades muscular layer	0	No regional Lymphnodes involved		
II	2	Tumor invades into perimuscular tissue but not through serosa				
IIIA	3	Tumor invades through serosa, either into liver parechnyma or other adjacent organs	1	Metastatic disease involving nodes along the cystic duct, common bile duct, hepatic artery or portal vein	0	No distant metastatic disease
IIIB						
IVA^a	4	Tumor invades main portal vein, hepatic artery or invades two or more adjacent organs				
IVB^b			2	Metastatic disease involving nodes along the aorta, vena cava, superior mesenteric artery or celiac artery	1	Distant metastatic disease

^aStage IVA disease T4N0 or T4N1.
^bStage IVB disease is any T stage, with either N2 or M1 disease present
  From Compton CC, Byrd DR, Garcia-Aguilar J, et al. Gallbladder. In: Compton CC, editor. AJCC Cancer Staging Atlas. 2nd edition. New York: Springer; 2012. p. 259–68; with permission.

- Recent AJCC (eighth edition) staging concentrates more on number of nodes) involved and distinguishes T2 disease based on location of invasion (T2a: visceral side of gallbladder, T2b: hepatic side of gallbladder) (Table 2).

Work-up
- Preoperatively suspected cancer
  - Patients who present with symptoms and are identified as having a concern for gallbladder cancer should undergo imaging to evaluate for extent of disease. This may include right upper quadrant ultrasound, CT, or MRI. PET, although not routinely used and not recommended in the preoperative assessment of gallbladder cancer, may be of use in select cases of suspected metastatic disease when the results would alter management [19].
  - Laboratory testing, including complete blood cell count, comprehensive metabolic panel including liver function tests, and coagulation factors, are appropriate. Tumor markers common for biliary malignancy, such as cancer

Table 2
T,N,M Staging of gallbladder cancer, adapted from the AJCC 8th edition

Stage Grouping		T Stage	N Stage	M Stage
Not stageable	X	Cant be assessed	X Cant be assessed	X Cant be assessed
	0	No evidence of primary tumor		
0	is	Carcinoma in situ		
I	1a	Tumor invades lamina propria		
	1b	Tumor invades muscular layer		
II	2a	Tumor invades into perimuscular tissue on the visceral peritoneal side, but not through serosa	0 No regional lymph nodes involved	0 No distant metastatic disease
	2b	Tumor invades into perimuscular tissue on the hepatic side, but not through serosa		
IIIA	3	Tumor invades through serosa either into liver parchnyma or		
IIIB			1 Metastatic disease involving 1-3 lymph nodes	
IVA[a]	4	Tumor invades main portal vein, hepatic artery or invades two or more adjacent organs	2 Metastatic disease involving >4 lymph nodes	1 Distant metastatic disease
IVB[b]				

[a]Stage IVA disease T4N0 or T4N1.
[b]Stage IVB disease is any T stage, with either N2 or M1 disease present.
From Zhu AX, Pawlik TM, Kooby DA, et al. Gallbladder. In: Amin MB, editor. AJCC Cancer Staging Manual. 8th edition. Chicago; AJCC; 2017. p. 303; with permission.

antigen (CA) 19-9 can be helpful in both diagnosis and prognosis. Sensitivity and specificity of CA 19-9 are 72% and 96% respectively [20]. Other tumor markers, such as carcinoembryonic antigen (CEA) (12% and 97%) and CA 242 (64% and 99%), are less sensitive but more specific.
- ○ Endoscopic ultrasound can be useful for assessing depth of invasion [21] and for fine-needle aspiration of the lesion in question, should biopsy be warranted [22].
- Perioperatively suspected or postoperatively diagnosed
  - ○ In patients who are diagnosed incidentally, after resection, appropriate laboratory testing and staging should be performed prior to attempt at further resection, when warranted.
  - ○ In cases of gallbladder cancer suspected intraoperatively, conversion to an open operation is appropriate, to minimize risk of peritoneal seeding. If

advanced disease is suspected, peritoneal washings, biopsy of metastatic lesions, and abandonment of cholecystectomy are appropriate. If a surgeon does not feel comfortable with the disease, then cessation of the operation and referral to a higher volume center are recommended.
- Consideration for referral
  - Long-term survival in patient with disease stage Ib or higher is low and for advanced disease is extremely poor [5,23], but surgical resection is still possible for patients whose disease is not distantly metastatic. Referral to an experienced surgeon or center is recommended for these cases, because a multidisciplinary approach is favored.

Operative considerations
- Early-stage disease
  - For cancers that are diagnosed incidentally on pathologic evaluation of cholecystectomy, those that are T1a (Fig. 4) or in situ disease and those where the cystic duct margin is negative do not require further surgical intervention [24]. It is important, however, to appropriately work-up the patient to rule out distant disease and properly stage the patient.
- Locally advanced disease
  - For patients whose disease is nonmetastatic and does not invade beyond the serosa (T stage 1b, 2, or 3), guidelines from the National Comprehensive Cancer Network recommend surgical resection with en bloc liver resection (extended cholecystectomy) [25]. This should include portal lymphadenectomy and, depending on the extent of the disease, possible common bile duct resection to obtain negative margins.
  - These patients should receive appropriate adjuvant therapy as well, which is associated with improved survival. Data from the National Cancer Database have shown that appropriate extended cholecystectomy performed with adjuvant therapy improves median survival by more than 50% compared with extended cholecystectomy alone [24].
  - Adjuvant therapy is most commonly gemcitabine based or fluoropyrimidine (5-fluorouracil or capecitabine) based in combination with a platinum agent (cisplatin or oxaliplatin) [23].

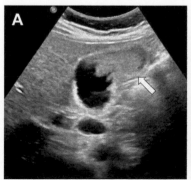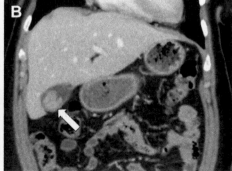

Fig. 4. Asymptomatic lesion (*white arrow*) identified incidentally in the gallbladder fundus as seen on (A) ultrasound and (B) CT of the abdomen. This lesion was resected and was a T1a lesion. No further treatment was required.

- For R1 or R2 resections, radiation is appropriate to control disease. In the adjuvant setting with R0 resections, the data are less clear, but radiation in addition to chemotherapy can be considered in a multidisciplinary setting with significant results [26].
- Port-site resection
  - Port-site recurrence (Fig. 5) after initial cholecystectomy generally portends peritoneal spread of gallbladder cancer. Resection of port site at the time of definitive resection is not mandatory and likely does not improve survival [27,28].
  - If recurrence occurs at the port site after definitive resection, radiation and chemotherapy may provide both symptomatic relief and clinical response, although this should be considered palliative.
- Metastatic or locally unresectable disease
  - Median survival for patients with metastatic or locally unresectable disease is less than 6 months [23], so treatment, if any, should focus on the patient's wishes.
  - If available, and warranted, palliative care consultation should be considered, with a goal of managing patient symptoms.
  - Outside of palliative intentions, surgical intervention should be avoided.
  - If jaundice is present, biliary drainage via endoscopic or percutaneous routes is appropriate.

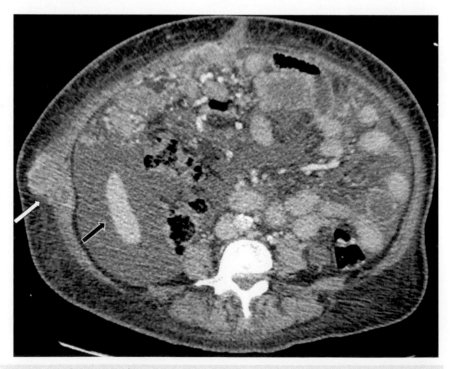

Fig. 5. Axial CT image showing a patient with port-site recurrence of her gallbladder cancer (*white arrow*) as well as diffuse malignant ascites around the liver (*black arrow*).

○ Chemotherapy, radiation, or both are appropriate and demonstrate improved survival and palliation of symptoms, although patients with poor performance status may not tolerate these treatment modalities [29–31].
○ Clinical trials, if available, are also appropriate in select cases.

Postoperative treatment and follow-up
- Adjuvant therapy
  ○ Patients with disease that is T2 or greater, who have undergone definitive resection, seem to benefit most from adjuvant therapy [23–26].
  ○ National Comprehensive Cancer Network guidelines state that adjuvant therapy with chemotherapy (gemcitabine-based or fluoropyrimidine-based regimen) with or without radiation be considered [25].
- Recurrence/failure of therapy
  ○ Second-line therapy often uses whichever first-line therapy was not used initially (gemcitabine-based or fluoropyrimidine-based therapy) but progression-free survival and overall survival are poor [32].
  ○ Patients who recur early with local or distant recurrence should be managed similar to those with metastatic disease. Multidisciplinary discussion, screening for trial eligibility, and involvement of palliative care should be offered to the patient.
  ○ Late recurrence is even less well understood, and management in these patients can be approached in a personalized fashion.
- Follow-up
  ○ Similar to many other aspects of care for patients with gallbladder cancer, consensus on follow-up of these patients is lacking in the absence of randomized trials.
  ○ Most centers agree that close follow-up is necessary, with 3-month to 6-month intervals for at least 5 years, and for long-term survivors, yearly follow-up may be recommended.
  ○ In addition to clinical examination, laboratory studies that include liver function tests and tumor markers (CA 19-9, CA 242, and CEA) can be followed if elevated preoperatively. In addition, surveillance imaging is recommended to include the regional and distant spread of disease (CT of the abdomen, pelvis, and chest) [33].

Survival
- With the exception of T1a or carcinoma in situ, gallbladder cancer survival is poor. Data from the National Cancer Database and the American College of Surgeons reveal that even early-stage cancers have limited 5-year survival [5] (Table 3).
- Extended cholecystectomy with adjuvant therapy in appropriately selected patients offers the best long-term survival [24].

Future directions
- Current therapies have not led to a dramatic change in the overall survival of patients with gallbladder cancer.
- Current trials are examining the role of second line therapy in previously treated patients with locally advanced or metastatic biliary tract cancers [34].
- Most trials examine symptom control, or recurrent disease, rather than adjuvant or targeted therapy.

Table 3
Survival of patients with gallbladder cancer based on stage at presentation

Stage	Five-year survival (%)
0/in situ	80
I	50
II	28
IIIA	8
IIIB	7
IVA	4
IVB	2

From Cancer.org. Survival statistics for gallbladder cancer by stage. American Cancer Society. Available at: https://www.cancer.org/cancer/gallbladder-cancer/detection-diagnosis-staging/survival-rates.html. Accessed December 3, 2017; with permission.

- The role of targeted molecular therapy for gallbladder cancer, as for all biliary tract malignancies, is still in its infancy.
- Glucose oncometabolism, abnormal DNA methylation, and noncoding RNAs may offer some promise as foci for future targeted therapies [35–37].
- The HER2 and (erbB2) and K-ras signaling pathways also offer potential for future treatments [38,39].

SUMMARY

Gallbladder cancer is a terrible disease and survival in all but the earliest-stage cancers is poor. Although significant advances have been made in the diagnosis, operative resection, and adjuvant therapy for these cancers, little impact has been made on overall survival. Patients should be assessed in a multidisciplinary fashion, and patient selection is critical for best outcomes. When applicable, clinical trials should be offered to patients to advance the understanding of this disease. For patients with advanced or recurrent disease, clinical trials or best supportive care is appropriate. Future targeted therapies likely offer the best hope for improving survival in these patients.

References

[1] Carriaga MT, Henson DE. Liver, gallbladder, extrahepatic bile ducts, and pancreas. Cancer 1995;75(1 Suppl):171–90.
[2] Pandey M. Risk factors for gallbladder cancer: a reappraisal. Eur J Cancer Prev 2003;12(1):15–24.
[3] Cubertafond P, Gainant A, Cuchiaro G. Surgical treatment of 724 carcinomas of the gallbladder. Results of the French surgical association survey. Ann Surg 1994;219:275–80.
[4] Smith GC, Parks RW, Madhavan KK, et al. A 10-year experience in the management of gallbladder cancer. HPB (Oxford) 2003;5(3):159–66.
[5] Survival Statistics for Gallbladder Cancer by Stage. Available at: https://www.cancer.org/cancer/gallbladder-cancer/detection-diagnosis-staging/survival-rates.html. Accessed November 17, 2017.
[6] Shaffer EA. Gallbladder cancer, the basics. Gastroenterol Hepatol 2008;4(10):737–41.
[7] Misra S, Chaturvedi A, Misra NC, et al. Carcinoma of the gallbladder. Lancet Oncol 2003;4(3):167–76.

[8] Lewis JT, Talwalkar JA, Rosen CB, et al. Prevalence and risk factors for gallbladder neoplasia in patients with primary sclerosing cholangitis: evidence for a metaplasia-dysplasia-carcinoma sequence. Am J Surg Pathol 2007;31(6):907–13.

[9] Diehl AK. Gallstone size and the risk of gallbladder cancer. JAMA 1983;250(17):2323–6.

[10] Kumar S. Infection as a risk factor for gallbladder cancer. J Surg Oncol 2006;93(8):633–9.

[11] Koshiol J, Gao YT, Dean M, et al. Association of aflatoxin and gallbladder cancer. Gastroenterology 2017;153(2):488–94.

[12] Stephen AE, Berger DL. Carcinoma in the porcelain gallbladder: a relationship revisited. Surgery 2001;129(6):699–703.

[13] Kang CM, Kim KS, Choi JS, et al. Gallbladder carcinoma associated with anomalous pancreaticobiliary duct junction. Can J Gastroenterol 2007;21(6):383–7.

[14] Trivedi V, Gumaste VV, Liu S, et al. Gallbladder cancer adenoma-carcinoma or dysplasia-carcinoma sequence? Gastroenterol Hepatol 2008;4(10):735–7.

[15] Dorobisz T, Dorobisz K, Chabowski M, et al. Incidental gallbladder cancer after cholecystectomy: 1990 to 2014. Onco Targets Ther 2016;9:4913–6.

[16] Choi SB, Han HJ, Kim CY, et al. Incidental gallbladder cancer diagnosed following laparoscopic cholecystectomy. World J Surg 2009;33(12):2657–63.

[17] Compton CC, Byrd DR, Garcia-Aguilar J, et al. Gallbladder. In: Compton CC, editor. AJCC cancer staging atlas. 2nd edition. New York: Springer; 2012. p. 259–68.

[18] Zhu AX, Pawlik TM, Kooby DA, et al. Gallbladder. In: Amin MB, editor. AJCC cancer staging manual. 8th edition. Chicago (IL): AJCC; 2017. p. 303.

[19] Butte J, Redondo F, Waugh E, et al. The role of PET-CT in patients with incidental gallbladder cancer. HPB (Oxford) 2009;11(7):585–91.

[20] Wang YF, Feng FL, Zhao XH, et al. Combined detection tumor markers for diagnosis and prognosis of gallbladder cancer. World J Gastroenterol 2014;20(14):4085–92.

[21] Sadamoto Y, Kubo H, Harada N, et al. Preoperative diagnosis and staging of gallbladder carcinoma by EUS. Gastrointest Endosc 2003;58(4):536–41.

[22] Costache M, Iordache S, Karstensen J, et al. Endoscopic ultrasound-guided fine needle aspiration: from the past to the future. Endosc Ultrasound 2013;2(2):77–85.

[23] Duffy A, Capanu M, Abou-Alfa GK, et al. Gallbladder cancer (GBC): 10-year experience at Memorial Sloan-Kettering Cancer Centre (MSKCC). J Surg Oncol 2008;98(7):485–9.

[24] Kasumova GG, Tabatabaie O, Najarian RM, et al. Surgical management of gallbladder cancer simple versus extended cholecystectomy and the role of adjuvant therapy. Ann Surg 2017;266:625–31.

[25] National Comprehensive Cancer Network. NCCN clinical practice guidelines in oncology: hepatobiliary cancers. Version 4.2017. Available at: www.nccn.org. Accessed November 17, 2017.

[26] Wang SJ, Lemieux A, Kalpathy-Cramer J, et al. Nomogram for predicting the benefit of adjuvant chemoradiotherapy for resected gallbladder cancer. J Clin Oncol 2011;29(35):4627.

[27] Maker AV, Butte JM, Oxenberg J, et al. Is port site resection necessary in the surgical management of gallbladder cancer? Ann Surg Oncol 2012;19(2):409–17.

[28] Fuks D, Regimbeau JM, Pessaux P, et al. Is port-site resection necessary in the surgical management of gallbladder cancer? J Visc Surg 2013;150(4):277–84.

[29] Houry S, Barrier A, Huguier M. Irradiation therapy for gallbladder carcinoma: recent advances. J Hepatobiliary Pancreat Surg 2001;8(6):518–24.

[30] Houry S, Haccart V, Huguier M, et al. Gallbladder cancer: role of radiation therapy. Hepatogastroenterology 1999;46(27):1578–84.

[31] Ishii H, Furuse J, Yonemoto N, et al. Chemotherapy in the treatment of advanced gallbladder cancer. Oncology 2004;66(2):138–42.

[32] Lamarca A, Hubner RA, David Ryder W, et al. Second-line chemotherapy in advanced biliary cancer: a systematic review. Ann Oncol 2014;25:2328–38.

[33] Valle JW, Borbath I, Khan S, et al. On behalf of the ESMO Guidelines Committee Biliary cancer: ESMO clinical practice guidelines for diagnosis, treatment and follow-up. Ann Oncol 2016;27(Suppl 5):v28–37.
[34] Valle J. The Christie NHS Foundation Trust. Active Symptom Control Alone or With mFOL-FOX Chemotherapy for Locally Advanced/Metastatic Biliary Tract Cancers (ABC06). NCT01926236. Available at: https://clinicaltrials.gov. Accessed November 17, 2017.
[35] Khandelwal A, Malhotra A, Jain M, et al. The emerging role of long non-coding RNA in gallbladder cancer pathogenesis. Biochimie 2017;132:152–60.
[36] Tekcham DS, Tiwari PK. Non-coding RNAs as emerging molecular targets of gallbladder cancer. Gene 2016;588(1):79–85.
[37] Oyasiji T, Zhang J, Kuvshinoff B, et al. Molecular targets in biliary carcinogenesis and implications for therapy. Oncologist 2015;20(7):742–51.
[38] O'Dell MR, Huang JL, Whitney-Miller CL, et al. Hezel AF Kras(G12D) and p53 mutation cause primary intrahepatic cholangiocarcinoma. Cancer Res 2012;72(6):1557–67.
[39] Kiguchi K, Carbajal S, Chan K, et al. Constitutive expression of ErbB-2 in gallbladder epithelium results in development of adenocarcinoma. Cancer Res 2001;61(19):6971–6.

Advances in Surgery 52 (2018) 101–111

ADVANCES IN SURGERY

How to Predict 30-Day Readmission

Tyler S. Wahl, MD, MSPH[a], Mary T. Hawn, MD, MPH[b],*

[a]Department of Surgery, University of Alabama at Birmingham, 1722 7th Avenue South, Kracke Building 217, Birmingham, AL 35249, USA; [b]Surgery, Stanford University, Alway Building M121, 300 Pasteur Drive, MC 5115, Stanford, CA 94305, USA

Keywords

• Readmission • Predict • Surgical outcomes

Key points

• Factors influencing surgical readmissions are multifactorial and can generally be summarized into biologic, social, surgical, and health care factors.

• Surgical readmissions are complex with patient risk profiles largely unique to the surgical procedure performed.

• Surgical readmissions are challenging to predict despite using granular perioperative patient-centered data known to providers at the time of discharge.

INTRODUCTION

Health care utilization through hospital readmission following hospital discharge within 30 days is publically reported and associated with both clinical and economic implications. According to a 2009 study using Medicare claims data, one-fifth of all hospitalized patients were rehospitalized within 30 days of discharge [1]. Of readmitted patients, 67.1% and 51.5% of medical and surgical patients, respectively, were readmitted or died within the first year of an index hospital discharge, costing an estimated $17 billion per year. Specifically, one in 7 patients are readmitted within 30 days following major surgery using similar Medicare claims data [2]. It is no surprise that the Affordable Care Act [3] implemented the Hospital Readmission Reduction Program in 2012 to incentivize hospitals with higher than expected 30-day readmission rates to adopt strategies to reduce costly readmissions and improve quality of care. The Centers for Medicare and Medicaid Services (CMS) targeted its first surgical procedure

Disclosure: The authors have nothing to disclose.

*Corresponding author. E-mail address: mhawn@stanford.edu

https://doi.org/10.1016/j.yasu.2018.03.015
0065-3411/18/Published by Elsevier Inc.

with total hip and knee arthroplasty in 2015 and coronary artery bypass grafting in 2017 with plans for other surgical procedures likely to follow in the future. Clinical leaders have urged investigators to respond with a call-to-action for feasible and cost-effective strategies to reduce readmissions [4,5]. It has been long debated whether surgical readmissions are predictable and thereby preventable with intervention. A brief review of previously described predictors, reasons for readmission, and interventions to prevent readmissions are described elsewhere [6]. The purpose of this article is to update discussion on the ensuing challenges in predicting surgical readmission.

PREDICTORS OF READMISSION

Understanding the events that drive surgical readmission remains a constant challenge for policymakers and clinical leaders. Investigators have identified various multifactorial associations with readmission that are used in regression analyses to predict 30-day readmission. Thorough reviews describing unique patient risk profiles for readmission by procedure case-mix have been described [7–9]. Patient readmission risk profiles generally reflect biologic factors such as patient biology and comorbid conditions, social determinants of health, surgical factors including education or acuity of disease and perioperative management, and healthcare system factors involving multidisciplinary care components contributing to readmission. [6,10]

Biologic and social factors

Patient disease and comorbidity are known to place patients at increased risk of surgical readmission [11]. Readmission risk scores using granular data have been developed accounting for patient comorbidity [12,13]. Frail patients and those with dependent functional status are also more likely to experience readmission after surgery [14–17]. The modified frailty index (mFI) is a validated deficit-accumulation frailty tool using 11 preoperative characteristics including comorbidities and functional status tracked by the American College of Surgeons National Surgical Quality Improvement Project (ACS-NSQIP) [18]. Although the mFI has been associated with morbidity and mortality following major surgery across various specialties, its association with readmissions and how the individual components contribute to readmission following surgery were unclear until investigators used a large national retrospective cohort of 118 Veterans Affairs medical centers comprising 236,957 surgeries from 2007 to 2014 [15]. An mFI was calculated based on preoperative patient comorbidities and functional status for veteran patients undergoing general, orthopedic, and vascular surgery having a postoperative length of stay of at least 2 days. The mFI, when measured as a continuous proportional variable, was associated with 30-day readmission with an 11% increase in odds of readmission for each incremental increase in the index. When analyzed using individual components, impaired functional status with dependent status or having any residual deficit from a prior stroke contributed most to the predictive ability of the mFI for readmission. Although there are many measures and definitions of frailty, both retrospective and prospective, frailty present at the time of surgery is likely associated with readmission. Prospective studies are needed to understand preoperative measures of frailty and their relationship to readmission risk in real time.

Patients with diminished estimated glomerular filtration rates without a reported history of chronic kidney disease (CKD) experience poor surgical outcomes, including surgical readmission [19]. Biggs and colleagues [20] investigated 62,332 patients undergoing elective abdominal aortic aneurysm repair with 5678 having CKD and 688 having end-stage renal disease (ESRD). Patients with advanced age, female sex, blood loss anemia, chronic pulmonary disease, diabetes with complications, open approach, CKD, and ESRD were significantly associated with 30-day readmission with ESRD patients having the highest risk. Proteinuria, also known as microalbuminuria, is a marker for renal dysfunction associated with long-term CKD among patients with proteinuria who experience acute kidney injury (AKI) [21]. The authors' group investigated the association of preoperative proteinuria with postoperative predischarge AKI and readmission among patients with and without known renal dysfunction at the time of surgery. Preoperative proteinuria data were obtained from 153,767 surgeries with heterogeneous case-mix using Veteran Health Administration (VHA) and Veterans Affairs Surgical Quality Improvement Project (VASQIP) data from 119 Veterans Affairs facilities between 2007 and 2014. Overall, 11.2% of surgeries resulted in AKI with a dose-dependent increase in AKI with increasing proteinuria levels. Patients with proteinuria tended to have diabetes mellitus, black ethnicity, CKD, dependent functional status, and more comorbidity. Interestingly, patients with normal preoperative renal function having proteinuria experienced a dose-dependent association with postoperative AKI. After adjusting for perioperative variables, preoperative proteinuria was independently associated with predischarge AKI and 30-day unplanned readmission in a dose-dependent fashion in patients with or without preoperative renal dysfunction.

Although readmission rates vary by procedure mix, the indication for surgery may further explain readmission variance within similar specialties and procedures. Readmission rates varied by indication for lower extremity arterial bypass with higher readmission risk among critical limb ischemia with rest pain or tissue loss compared with claudication or other indications [22,23]. Further studies are needed to understand indications among other surgical procedures, and providers should consider indications for surgery during preoperative patient education and risk assessment.

Patient factors account for 95% of the variation in readmission following hepatobiliary surgery at 300 hospitals with hospital and provider factors showing little impact on readmission [24]. Gonzalez and colleagues [23] studied 479,047 Medicare vascular surgery patients undergoing lower extremity revascularization and found that readmissions were attributed to hospital patient-mix rather than hospital quality. Merkow and colleagues [16] investigated a more heterogeneous patient population and case-mix from a national sample of 498,875 operations performed in 2012 at 346 ACS-NSQIP hospitals. Patient-level factors alone explained most of the risk for readmissions compared with models using only inpatient complications, discharge destination, or hospital characteristics. Gani and colleagues [25] found that 82.8% of the variability in 30-day readmissions is attributed to patient-level factors, 14.5% attributed to surgical specialty, and 2.8% to individual surgeons among 22,559 patients from 2009 to 2013 among various specialties. Furthermore, Morris and colleagues [17] looked at 237,441 VASQIP procedures among noncardiac general, orthopedic, and vascular surgery from 2007 to 2014. Preoperative patient-level factors contributed most to a predictive model for readmission with modest predictive improvement using operative and postoperative information before discharge. Prior health care utilizations with an inpatient admission or emergency department visit within 6 months of an index operation are also associated with surgical readmission.

Patient demographics and social determinants impacting readmission highlight disparities in surgery. Race is a known independent predictor associated with poor outcomes, including readmission. Black patients experience higher mortality, complication, and readmission rates compared with patients of different races [25,26]. Patients at minority-serving hospitals are more likely to be readmitted following major surgery than patients at non-minority-serving hospitals [27]. Studies have shown Asian, black, and Hispanic patients experience higher readmission rates compared with whites following surgery despite adjusting for patient, procedure, and hospital factors [17,25,26,28,29]. Low socioeconomic status and disadvantaged social determinants of health, financial stress, substance abuse, limited education, mental health, poor social support, homelessness, poor self-efficacy, medication nonadherence, or lack of self-management skills contribute to readmission [11,30–33].

Surgery/health care factors

Whether complications occur, high patient-reported pain scores greater than 8 (lowest 0 to highest 10) at time of discharge were highly associated with readmission among Veterans Affairs patients undergoing major surgery and warrants further investigation [17]. Hernandez-Boussard and colleagues [34] investigated the association of inpatient pain control and postoperative readmission using 211,231 unique surgeries from 121 Veteran Affairs medical centers between 2007 and 2012. Patient-reported pain score assessments (lowest 0 to highest 10) were summarized daily from vital sign assessments from the time of surgery until discharge and identified 6 significant pain trajectories to time of discharge. Trajectories ranged from low (0–2), mild (2–4), to low, mild, moderate (4–6), to low, moderate, and high (>6). They found a significant dose-dependent effect with increasing inpatient postoperative pain scores/trajectories with hospital utilization through pain-related emergency care or readmission. Patients with the highest pain score trajectory (>6) until time of discharge were roughly 4 times more like to experience a pain-related readmission compared with patients with the lowest postoperative pain trajectory.

Perioperative glycemic control is a predictor of not only postoperative complications but also surgical readmission according to a 2017 Jones and colleagues [35] study of 23,094 surgeries at 117 Veteran Affairs facilities. Patients with peak postoperative blood glucose levels greater than 250 mg/dL within 48 hours of surgery were significantly associated with 30-day readmission. Elevated preoperative hemoglobin A1c was not significantly associated with readmission likely because of increased vigilance among diabetic patients. The frequency of surveillance for hyperglycemia was higher with lower thresholds to use insulin among patients with preoperative hemoglobin A1c >6.5%. A small single-institutional study showed that among patients without a diagnosis of diabetes before medical admission, 59% undergo glucose monitoring with only 54% of those patients treated with insulin for hyperglycemia [36].

It is well known that postoperative complications place patients at increased risk for prolonged length of stay, morbidity, readmission, and mortality. Similar to various studies using single-institution datasets, Kassin and colleagues [37] studied ACS-NSQIP outcomes among 1442 general surgery patients from 2009 to 2012. They showed that having any postoperative complication, independent of patient- or procedure-specific factors, increased risk of readmission by a factor of 4. Gani and colleagues [25] used administrative claims data from 2009 to 2013 of 22,559 patients undergoing major surgery and found patient comorbidity, race, having a postoperative complication, and extended length of stay predicted readmission. A systematic review of 35 studies involving vascular, general, bariatric, and colorectal surgery found reliable predictors of readmission involving postoperative complications, medication-related issues, comorbidity, and postoperative length of stay [38]. Among Veterans Affairs patients undergoing 59,273 colorectal, arthroplasty, vascular, and gynecology procedures from 2005 to 2009, more than a quarter of assessed VASQIP complications occurred after discharge and ultimately resulted in readmission [39].

Regarding provider care and disposition location at time of discharge, multicomorbid patients with or without predischarge complications often require additional resources during their recovery and are at risk for readmission [16]. Greenblatt and colleagues [40] in 2010 showed that vascular patients were 2.5 times more likely to experience a readmission when discharged to a skilled nursing facility. Among general surgery, orthopedic, and vascular Veteran Affairs patients, patients admitted from skilled nursing facilities or transferred from another hospital preoperatively were more likely to be readmitted in addition to those who were discharged to locations other than home [17]. Rather than poor clinical care delivered at ancillary care facilities, disposition to locations other than original admission source may reflect a sicker population with a reduced capacity to regain homeostasis following surgery. On the other hand, social support and available resources remain a topic of interest because homeless patients discharged to skilled nursing facilities or locations other than home are less likely to be readmitted, a finding contradictory to non–homeless patients.

Hong and colleagues [41] investigated surgery readmissions following major gastrointestinal cancer operations among 110,857 patients in California from

355 hospitals in 2004 to 2011, 44 of which were vulnerable hospitals (safety-net or high Medicaid payer systems). Vulnerable hospital systems and teaching status were significantly associated with 30-day readmission; however, the number of beds and procedure volume were not significantly associated with increased readmission. Vulnerable hospitals by definition care for minority or more comorbid populations that likely result in poor outcomes [27,41]. Goodney and colleagues [42] showed that hospital volume was not significantly associated with readmission among 2.5 million cardiovascular and cancer surgeries within Medicare.

Among bariatric surgeries, hospital teaching status and provider procedural volume are associated with readmissions. A low-volume bariatric surgeon (<25 cases/y) had 15 times higher risk of readmission than medium-volume bariatric surgeons (26–150 cases/y) [43]. Furthermore, low hospital volume, specifically facilities that perform less than 300 bariatric cases/y, was significantly associated with increased 30-day [44] and 1-year [45] readmission. High volume facilities having improved outcomes with lower readmission rates may reflect structural processes of care and available resources. These bariatric outcomes led to a CMS policy for bariatric surgery to be performed at only centers of excellence (COE). Dimick and colleagues [46] showed that there were no significant differences in rates of complications before and after CMS policy implementation, meaning non-COE facilities performed bariatric surgery with similar outcomes. Although readmissions were not included in analysis, hospital and surgeon volume likely did not explain outcomes and point to patient case-mix. In order to understand whether surgical readmissions represent global hospital effects or a sum of team and patient-level effects, Hollis and colleagues [47] investigated 100,086 Veteran Affairs patients undergoing general, orthopedic, and vascular surgery at 84 facilities from 2007 to 2014. Hospitals varied by the number of specialties above or below a national median readmission rate, yet this variation was not attributed to hospital volume, region, operative complexity, or procedure mix. Upon adjustment for patient factors, little variation in readmission could be explained by facility or specialty-specific factors. Patient and procedure case-mix factors contributed most as opposed to broader team/facility level effects.

READMISSION REASONS

Understanding how postdischarge events impact readmission has led to investigators to focus on why patients are readmitted, rather than whether they were readmitted. Early single-institutional reports of reasons for readmission are largely influenced by patient risk profiles and procedure case-mix influence [7–9]. Generally, reasons for readmissions range from wound complications, including infection and seroma, gastrointestinal disturbances, nutrition, postoperative pain, exacerbations of known medical conditions, or procedure related with or without exacerbation of comorbidities.

It was not until large-national cohorts that more generalizable reasons for readmission were understood that support single institutional findings and may prove worthy targets for intervention. Merkow and colleagues [16] highlight reasons for readmission nationally among bariatric, colectomy, ventral hernia repair, hysterectomy, total hip/knee arthroplasty, and lower extremity vascular bypass. Surgical site infection (19.5%) and gastrointestinal derangements with ileus obstruction (10.3%) were among the most common reasons for 30-day readmission followed by complications with less than 5% event rates (bleeding, pulmonary, venous thromboembolism, dehydration/poor nutrition, sepsis, stroke, or pain). Readmission rates were uniform in distribution over the postoperative period without a particular peak postdischarge day or readmission reason. Morris and colleagues [17] support surgical site infection and wound complications as the most frequent reasons for surgical readmission among general, orthopedic, and vascular procedures. Most wound complications occurred within the first week of discharge and increase during the second week among vascular patients. As mentioned above, surgical patients with increasing patient-reported pain score trajectories before discharge were more likely to use health care through emergency care visits or readmissions for pain related reasons [34].

As stated previously, postoperative events add to prediction models' ability to predict surgical readmissions, however, are not available at the time of discharge. Predischarge perioperative factors are all that are available to providers during disposition planning. Postdischarge data are useful, however, to guide discharge planning for commonly experienced problems patients encounter postdischarge that make them more likely to be readmitted. Predicting readmissions for more common reasons for readmission are feasible through continued characterization of associated patient and procedural factors. The ability to predict who will and who will not return remains a challenge needing continued improvement.

QUALITY IMPROVEMENT

The Hospital Readmission Reduction Program considers rehospitalizations a reflection of suboptimal care that when improved to the standard of care would mitigate readmission rates, again highlighting the challenge of classifying unplanned readmissions as predictable or avoidable. Readmissions may not always reflect poor quality of care delivered predischarge because only 42% of all unplanned medical and surgical readmissions within the VHA were identified as clinically related in a 2014 study of 2,069,804 VHA hospital discharges [48]. Of surgery-related readmissions, 71% were clinically related. Overall, most of all unplanned readmissions were likely unrelated to index hospitalization. Although surgical readmissions may be more clinically relevant, efforts to characterize clinically unrelated unplanned readmissions remain an area of continued investigation. Readmissions may reflect quality care to facilitate proactive intervention for brewing complications rather than monitoring potentially deadly complications in the outpatient setting [16,49]. Disparities in care may continue to grow under the current readmission policy because potentially unidentified or unmodifiable patient factors lead to readmissions and penalize hospitals with sicker more disadvantaged patients [27,49].

Readmissions are challenging to predict and therefore difficult to prevent calling into question whether this metric is an adequate indicator of surgical quality. Surgical readmissions related to surgical quality are difficult to identify given that surgical readmissions are not always indicative of complications that occurred during the index hospitalization [16,48]. Until a new nationally reported marker for surgical quality is proposed, the current readmission definition requires revision. Because reasons for readmission continue active characterization, quality tracking improvement programs, including ACS-NSQIP and VASQIP, do not account for reasons for readmission [39]. Almost half of readmissions are not captured with a complication currently assessed by national quality improvement programs such as VASQIP. Furthermore, definitions of readmission should capture 30-day all-cause readmission and be standardized to ensure universal interpretation and reporting [8].

CHALLENGES OF PREDICTION

Despite involving multifactorial and granular data in sophisticated regression models, current prediction models fail to confidently predict surgical readmission. Kansagara and colleagues [11] reviewed 30 studies with readmission prediction models yielding fairly poor discriminatory abilities with c-statistics ranging within 0.50-0.60 and few above 0.70. Previously described large national cohorts of hundreds of thousands of patients undergoing heterogeneous surgeries using elaborate prediction models yielded Royston (R^2) values of 10.3% [17] and 27% [16]. What is most notable about these studies is that even with the size of the cohort and complexity of information available to predict readmissions at the time of discharge, researchers were unable to attain an adequate model predicting readmission. Granular prediction models in these large studies explained less than one-third of readmissions and reflect continued unmeasured confounding bias within the limitations of large retrospective databases. Morris and colleagues improved pre-discharge readmission prediction models from a c-statistic of 0.71 at the time of discharge to a c-statistic of 0.76 or R^2 of 19.6% from 10.3% after including post-discharge complications in post-hoc analyses [17]. Because postdischarge surgical complications are associated with readmission [39], the ability to predict readmissions is improved once postdischarge information is included; however, this is not pragmatic because postdischarge information is not known at the time of discharge. Understanding how postdischarge factors contribute to readmission allows for projected clinical courses, resource utilization, and intervention; however, this remains a continued area of investigation. Overall, readmissions are challenging to predict despite using granular perioperative patient-centered data known to providers at the time of discharge.

In summary, although readmissions are strongly associated with surgical complications, the contribution of underlying patient comorbidity, social determinants, and health care delivery systems challenges all to contribute to whether a patient is more likely to be readmitted following a surgical procedure. Because readmission is a nonspecific outcome as compared with more specific complications such as surgical site infection, it is much more difficult to predict, and as such, less likely to be improved with a single intervention.

References

[1] Jencks SF, Williams MV, Coleman EA. Rehospitalizations among patients in the Medicare fee-for-service program. N Engl J Med 2009;360(14):1418–28.

[2] Tsai TC, Joynt KE, Orav EJ, et al. Variation in surgical-readmission rates and quality of hospital care. N Engl J Med 2013;369(12):1134–42.

[3] Patient Protection and Affordable Care Act of 2010. Vol Pub. L. No 111–148, 124 Stat. 119, amended by Health Care and Education Reconciliation Act of 2010, Pub. L. No. 111-152, 124 Stat. 1029 (codified as amended in scattered sections of 42 U.S.C.)2010.

[4] Postel M, Frank PN, Barry T, et al. The cost of preventing readmissions: why surgeons should lead the effort. Am Surg 2014;80(10):1003–6.

[5] Horwitz LI, Partovian C, Lin Z, et al. Development and use of an administrative claims measure for profiling hospital-wide performance on 30-day unplanned readmission. Ann Intern Med 2014;161(10 Suppl):S66–75.

[6] Wahl TS, Hawn MT. How do we prevent readmissions after major surgery? Adv Surg 2017;51(1):89–100.

[7] Lee TJ, Martin RC 2nd. Readmission rates after abdominal surgery: can they be decreased to a minimum? Adv Surg 2012;46:155–70.

[8] Lucas DJ, Pawlik TM. Readmission after surgery. Adv Surg 2014;48:185–99.

[9] Brown EG, Bold RJ. Hospital readmissions: are they preventable? Adv Surg 2015;49: 15–29.

[10] Lucas DJ, Haider A, Haut E, et al. Assessing readmission after general, vascular, and thoracic surgery using ACS-NSQIP. Ann Surg 2013;258(3):430–9.

[11] Kansagara D, Englander H, Salanitro A, et al. Risk prediction models for hospital readmission: a systematic review. JAMA 2011;306(15):1688–98.

[12] Piper GL, Kaplan LJ, Maung AA, et al. Using the Rothman index to predict early unplanned surgical intensive care unit readmissions. J Trauma Acute Care Surg 2014;77(1):78–82.

[13] Bradley EH, Yakusheva O, Horwitz LI, et al. Identifying patients at increased risk for unplanned readmission. Med Care 2013;51(9):761–6.

[14] Robinson TN, Walston JD, Brummel NE, et al. Frailty for surgeons: review of a National Institute on Aging conference on frailty for specialists. J Am Coll Surg 2015;221(6):1083–92.

[15] Wahl TS, Graham LA, Hawn MT, et al. Association of the modified frailty index with 30-day surgical readmission. JAMA Surg 2017;152(8):749–57.

[16] Merkow RP, Ju MH, Chung JW, et al. Underlying reasons associated with hospital readmission following surgery in the United States. JAMA 2015;313(5):483–95.

[17] Morris MS, Graham LA, Richman JS, et al. Postoperative 30-day readmission: time to focus on what happens outside the hospital. Ann Surg 2016;264(4):621–31.

[18] Velanovich V, Antoine H, Swartz A, et al. Accumulating deficits model of frailty and postoperative mortality and morbidity: its application to a national database. J Surg Res 2013;183(1):104–10.

[19] Blitz JD, Shoham MH, Fang Y, et al. Preoperative renal insufficiency: underreporting and association with readmission and major postoperative morbidity in an academic medical center. Anesth Analg 2016;123(6):1500–15.

[20] Biggs JH, Kim RJ, Dombrovkiy VY, et al. Association of renal disease and readmission after abdominal aortic aneurysm repair in the Medicare population. J Am Coll Surg 2017;225(4S1):S223–4.

[21] James MT, Pannu N, Hemmelgarn BR, et al. Derivation and external validation of prediction models for advanced chronic kidney disease following acute kidney injury. JAMA 2017;318(18):1787–97.

[22] Jones CE, Richman JS, Chu DI, et al. Readmission rates after lower extremity bypass vary significantly by surgical indication. J Vasc Surg 2016;64(2):458–64.

[23] Gonzalez AA, Cruz CG, Dev S, et al. Indication for lower extremity revascularization and hospital profiling of readmissions. Ann Vasc Surg 2016;35:130–7.

[24] Hyder O, Dodson RM, Nathan H, et al. Influence of patient, physician, and hospital factors on 30-day readmission following pancreatoduodenectomy in the United States. JAMA Surg 2013;148(12):1095–102.

[25] Gani F, Lucas DJ, Kim Y, et al. Understanding variation in 30-day surgical readmission in the era of accountable care: effect of the patient, surgeon, and surgical subspecialties. JAMA Surg 2015;150(11):1042–9.

[26] Tsai TC, Orav EJ, Joynt KE. Disparities in surgical 30-day readmission rates for Medicare beneficiaries by race and site of care. Ann Surg 2014;259(6):1086–90.

[27] Shih T, Ryan AM, Gonzalez AA, et al. Medicare's hospital readmissions reduction program in surgery may disproportionately affect minority-serving hospitals. Ann Surg 2015;261(6): 1027–31.

[28] Girotti ME, Shih T, Revels S, et al. Racial disparities in readmissions and site of care for major surgery. J Am Coll Surg 2014;218(3):423–30.

[29] Gunnells DJ Jr, Morris MS, DeRussy A, et al. Racial disparities in readmissions for patients with inflammatory bowel disease (IBD) after colorectal surgery. J Gastrointest Surg 2016;20(5):985–93.

[30] Arbaje AI, Wolff JL, Yu Q, et al. Postdischarge environmental and socioeconomic factors and the likelihood of early hospital readmission among community-dwelling Medicare beneficiaries. Gerontologist 2008;48(4):495–504.

[31] McIntyre LK, Arbabi S, Robinson EF, et al. Analysis of risk factors for patient readmission 30 days following discharge from general surgery. JAMA Surg 2016;151(9):855–61.

[32] Jiang HJ, Boutwell AE, Maxwell J, et al. Understanding patient, provider, and system factors related to Medicaid readmissions. Jt Comm J Qual Patient Saf 2016;42(3):115–21.

[33] Martin RC, Brown R, Puffer L, et al. Readmission rates after abdominal surgery: the role of surgeon, primary caregiver, home health, and subacute rehab. Ann Surg 2011;254(4): 591–7.

[34] Hernandez-Boussard T, Graham LA, Desai K, et al. The fifth vital sign: postoperative pain predicts 30-day readmissions and subsequent emergency department visits. Ann Surg 2017;266(3):516–24.

[35] Jones CE, Graham LA, Morris MS, et al. Association between preoperative hemoglobin A1c levels, postoperative hyperglycemia, and readmissions following gastrointestinal surgery. JAMA Surg 2017;152(11):1031–8.

[36] Levetan CS, Passaro M, Jablonski K, et al. Unrecognized diabetes among hospitalized patients. Diabetes Care 1998;21(2):246–9.

[37] Kassin MT, Owen RM, Perez SD, et al. Risk factors for 30-day hospital readmission among general surgery patients. J Am Coll Surg 2012;215(3):322–30.

[38] Wiseman JT, Guzman AM, Fernandes-Taylor S, et al. General and vascular surgery readmissions: a systematic review. J Am Coll Surg 2014;219(3):552–69.e2.

[39] Morris MS, Deierhoi RJ, Richman JS, et al. The relationship between timing of surgical complications and hospital readmission. JAMA Surg 2014;149(4):348–54.

[40] Greenblatt DY, Weber SM, O'Connor ES, et al. Readmission after colectomy for cancer predicts one-year mortality. Ann Surg 2010;251(4):659–69.

[41] Hong Y, Zheng C, Hechenbleikner E, et al. Vulnerable hospitals and cancer surgery readmissions: insights into the unintended consequences of the patient protection and affordable care act. J Am Coll Surg 2016;223(1):142–51.

[42] Goodney PP, Stukel TA, Lucas FL, et al. Hospital volume, length of stay, and readmission rates in high-risk surgery. Ann Surg 2003;238(2):161–7.

[43] Weller WE, Rosati C, Hannan EL. Relationship between surgeon and hospital volume and readmission after bariatric operation. J Am Coll Surg 2007;204(3):383–91.

[44] Nguyen NT, Paya M, Stevens CM, et al. The relationship between hospital volume and outcome in bariatric surgery at academic medical centers. Ann Surg 2004;240(4): 586–93 [discussion: 593–4].
[45] Zingmond DS, McGory ML, Ko CY. Hospitalization before and after gastric bypass surgery. JAMA 2005;294(15):1918–24.
[46] Dimick JB, Nicholas LH, Ryan AM, et al. Bariatric surgery complications before vs after implementation of a national policy restricting coverage to centers of excellence. JAMA 2013;309(8):792–9.
[47] Hollis RH, Graham LA, Richman JS, et al. Hospital readmissions after surgery: how important are hospital and specialty factors? J Am Coll Surg 2017;224(4):515–23.
[48] Rosen AK, Chen Q, Shin MH, et al. Medical and surgical readmissions in the Veterans Health Administration: what proportion are related to the index hospitalization? Med Care 2014;52(3):243–9.
[49] Hawn MT. Unintended consequences of the hospital readmission reduction program. Ann Surg 2015;261(6):1032–3.

Advances in Surgery 52 (2018) 113–126

ADVANCES IN SURGERY

Nipple-Sparing Mastectomy

Barbara L. Smith, MD, PhD*,
Suzanne B. Coopey, MD

Division of Surgical Oncology, Massachusetts General Hospital, 55 Fruit Street, Boston, MA 02114, USA

Keywords

• Nipple-sparing mastectomy • Breast cancer • Risk reduction

Key points

• Today's nipple-sparing mastectomy (NSM), also called total skin-sparing mastectomy, preserves the entire skin envelope of the breast and includes standard, complete excision of breast tissue.

• Results to date have found NSM oncologically safe for risk reduction and cancer treatment.

• The central reason for preservation of the nipple is to improve the cosmetic outcome over what could be achieved with skin-sparing mastectomy and nipple reconstruction.

• Experience to date has found favorable patient satisfaction measures after NSM for cancer treatment or risk reduction.

BACKGROUND

Preservation of the nipple during mastectomy provides a superior cosmetic result compared with nipple excision and reconstruction. Today's nipple-sparing mastectomy (NSM), also called total skin-sparing mastectomy, preserves the entire skin envelope of the breast and includes standard, complete excision of breast tissue and removal of axillary nodes. Experience to date has found favorable patient satisfaction measures after NSM for cancer treatment or risk reduction. Howard and colleagues [1] found that patient satisfaction with breast appearance and overall psychosocial well-being were actually higher after NSM with reconstruction than at the preoperative, baseline

Disclosure: The authors have nothing to disclose.

*Corresponding author. Massachusetts General Hospital Center for Breast Cancer, Yawkey 9A, 55 Fruit Street, Boston, MA 02114. E-mail address: blsmith1@mgh.harvard.edu

https://doi.org/10.1016/j.yasu.2018.03.008

assessment. When Metcalfe and coworkers [2] compared outcomes among NSM and skin-sparing mastectomy patients 4 years after surgery, NSM patients had higher satisfaction with their reconstructed breasts and higher sexual well-being scores compared with skin-sparing mastectomy patients.

NSM was initially explored when immediate breast reconstruction became possible but was largely abandoned in the 1980s because of concerns about the oncologic safety of preserving the nipple [3].

More recently, with an increasing number of women choosing bilateral mastectomies for breast cancer risk reduction and treatment, there has been renewed interest in nipple-sparing options. The safety of skin-sparing mastectomy techniques that remove only the nipple and areola have been established [4]. There are also a few reports of areola-sparing mastectomy techniques that remove the nipple but preserve the pigmented areola skin [5]. Skin-sparing approaches, although technically challenging, have become standard of care for most surgeons who regularly perform breast surgery. Development of oncologically safe NSM approaches has been the next technical challenge.

NIPPLE ANATOMY
Early approaches to NSM were based on the premise that preservation of the blood supply to the nipple required leaving at least 0.5 to 1 cm of breast tissue beneath the nipple and areola [6]. This "subcutaneous mastectomy" technique reliably preserved nipple perfusion but was ultimately deemed oncologically unsafe. Anecdotal reports of local recurrence and development of new cancers in breast tissue retained beneath the nipple areola complex (NAC) [3,7] led to abandonment of this approach.

To help guide development of an oncologically safe NSM procedure our group performed a detailed study of nipple microanatomy. This work identified several previously unrecognized features of nipple anatomy relevant to nipple-sparing surgery [8,9]. Awareness of these features has allowed development of techniques for thorough resection of ducts beneath and within the nipple while preserving nipple perfusion [10,11], described in subsequent sections.

Duct bundle anatomy
The mean number of nipple ducts is 23 with a mean duct bundle diameter of 5 to 5.5 mm centered within the nipple papilla. This diameter is fairly uniform and independent of external nipple diameter [8].

Vessel anatomy
Nipple skin perfusion is predominantly from the skin. Only one-third of vessels to the nipple travel within the duct bundle, whereas two-thirds travel in nipple skin preserved during NSM [9]. Perfusion of the areola is almost exclusively through skin vessels.

Skin flap anatomy
There are no Cooper ligaments under the nipple and areola. The subcutaneous fat layer present under breast skin does not extend under the nipple and areola

and there are no subcutaneous vessels immediately under nipple and areola skin.

Nipple sensation

As in skin-sparing mastectomies, development of skin flaps during NSM results in numbness of central breast skin. Patients should be informed that the nipple will be numb with loss of light touch sensation in central breast skin. Deeper pressure sensation is preserved via other chest wall structures. With longer follow-up, return of some limited skin sensation is being noted, but only in a minority of NSM patients.

CURRENT ISSUES IN NIPPLE-SPARING MASTECTOMY

Modern NSM approaches require consideration of oncologic safety, surgical technique, and cosmetic outcome as they apply to the individual patient. As for any new technique, it is important for each surgeon to monitor their own results and modify routines to optimize outcomes.

ONCOLOGIC SAFETY

In patients with breast cancer, the primary goal of any mastectomy surgery is removal of all areas of malignancy with clear margins. An important secondary goal is removal of all normal breast tissue that could give risk to a new cancer in the future. For unaffected high-risk patients undergoing mastectomy for risk reduction, thorough removal of breast tissue is the primary goal. Results to date have found NSM oncologically safe for risk reduction and cancer treatment.

Prophylactic nipple-sparing mastectomy

Several groups have now published oncologic outcomes after NSMs performed for risk reduction. Hartmann and colleagues [7] reported results in a cohort of 639 women undergoing prophylactic mastectomy at the Mayo Clinic from 1960 to 1993 for a family history of breast cancer or for high-risk atypia. Approximately 90% of mastectomies in this series were nipple sparing. Prophylactic mastectomy reduced the risk of breast cancer by 90% to 95% at 14 years median follow-up compared with matched control subjects undergoing surveillance alone. Details of surgical technique were not reported, but no tumors developed in any retained NAC. Of note, 26 patients in the series were subsequently identified as having a BRCA1 or BRCA2 gene mutation. None of these BRCA mutation carriers had developed breast cancer at 13 years median follow-up, although six to eight breast cancers would have been expected based on estimates of risk of malignancy with surveillance alone [12].

To date, outcomes of more than 1200 NSM performed in BRCA mutation carriers have been reported with no recurrences in the NAC to date. Jakub and colleagues [13] identified 551 prophylactic NSM performed at nine institutions among 203 patients undergoing bilateral prophylactic mastectomies and 145 undergoing contralateral prophylactic mastectomy. Their series included 201 BRCA1 and 144 BRCA2 mutation carriers. At 56 months mean follow-up no tumors had developed in any retained NAC. Yao and colleagues [14] reported results of 397 NSM in 201 BRCA mutation carriers performed at two institutions, including 125 BRCA1 and 76 BRCA2 mutation carriers. Among these, 51 patients had a known breast cancer at the time of mastectomy. At 33 months median follow-up there were no new or recurrent cancers in any retained NAC. Peled and colleagues [15] reported no NAC recurrences at 51 months among 106 NSM in BRCA mutation carriers, including 27 patients with cancer. Manning and colleagues [16] found no NAC recurrences at 28 months among 177 NSM in BRCA mutation carriers, including 26 patients with cancer.

Therapeutic nipple-sparing mastectomy

NSMs have become increasingly common in patients with breast cancer. Rates of tumor recurrence in the retained NAC are less than 1% in all recent series, with no recurrences at all in most series (Table 1), although follow-up remains short.

Two Italian series provide the largest experience to date of NSM for breast cancer treatment. Lohsiriwat and colleagues [17] reported results of 861 NSM performed for breast cancer. Their surgical technique retained at least 5 mm of glandular tissue beneath the NAC, allowed positive nipple margins, and included a single 11-Gy fraction of intraoperative radiation to the NAC in some patients. At 50 months median follow-up the rate of tumor recurrence in the NAC was 0.8%, with some recurrences presenting as Paget disease of the nipple. Orzalesi and colleagues [18] reviewed a national multi-institutional Italian NSM registry that included 1006 patients. Among 755 cases included in the locoregional recurrence analysis, five (0.7%) had developed a recurrence in the NAC at 36 months mean follow-up. Details of surgical technique and nipple margin assessment were not reported.

Rates of NAC recurrence are extremely low in series where surgical technique involved an attempt to remove all subareolar and nipple duct tissue and obtain clear nipple/areola margins. There has been only a single report of tumor recurrence in the retained NAC to date among series from institutions

Table 1
Rates of locoregional and NAC recurrence after nipple-sparing mastectomy

Series	# Breasts	Follow-up (mo)	Locoregional recurrence (%)	# NAC recurrence
Lohsiriwat et al, [17] 2012	861	50	4.2	7
Orzalesi et al, [18] 2016	755	36	2.9	5
Peled et al, [19] 2012	412	28	2	0
Coopey et al, [20] 2016	312	42	2.9	0
Krajewski et al, [21] 2015	226	24	1.7	0
Benediktsson and Perbeck, [22] 2008	216	156	20.8	0
Filho et al, [23] 2011	157	10	0	0
Boneti et al, [24] 2011	152	25	4.6	0
Jensen et al, [25] 2011	127	60	0	0
Gerber et al, [26] 2009	60	101	11.7	1

that strive to remove all breast tissue under the NAC, although median follow-up is short in many series (see Table 1).

Disease-free and overall survival after NSM seems equivalent to survival after mastectomy without reconstruction. De la Cruz and colleagues [27] performed a review and meta-analysis of 20 NSM series published in 2006 to 2014 that included patients treated from 1985 to 2012, separating studies based on length of follow-up. Disease-free survival was 93% in series with less than 3 years follow-up, 92% in series with 3 to 5 years follow-up, and 76% in series with greater than 5 years follow-up, noting that patients in the oldest series received their care in the 1980 and 1990. Recent matched cohort studies found no difference in local recurrence or survival between patients who underwent NSM compared with those undergoing mastectomy without reconstruction. Adam and colleagues [28] matched 67 NSM-reconstruction patients with 203 mastectomies without reconstruction patients and found no difference in estimated 5-year disease-free survival (94.1% and 82.5%, respectively; $P = .068$) or overall survival (96.2% and 91.3%, respectively; $P = .166$). Park and colleagues [29] compared 114 patients who underwent NSM or skin-sparing mastectomy with reconstruction to matched patients undergoing mastectomy without reconstruction. There was no significant difference in recurrence rates between the two groups, with 96.4% and 96.1% 5-year locoregional recurrence-free survival, respectively ($P = .552$) [29].

Management of a positive nipple margin

In patients with no clinical or radiographic evidence of nipple involvement by tumor, rates of microscopic tumor involvement on final pathology range from 2.5% to 10% in therapeutic mastectomies [23,24,30–34] and 0% to 3% [23,32,34] in prophylactic mastectomies. At present, nipple removal is recommended for patients with tumor at their final nipple margin, with the option of retaining the areola [32]. Most nipples excised for positive margins have no residual tumor detected on histopathology analysis [32,34]. There has been some discussion of selective use of radiation and/or systemic therapy or even observation alone for a positive nipple margin, although this remains investigational [34]. Among patients with positive nipple margins treated with excision, there have been no recurrences to date around the site of the excised nipple [32,34].

SURGICAL TECHNIQUE

Current NSM techniques require thorough excision of breast tissue and nipple/subareolar ducts while preserving blood supply to the nipple and skin flaps, often through a small or peripherally located incision. Important technical elements include appropriate selection of the skin incision, careful dissection in the Cooper ligament plane, thorough removal and histopathology evaluation of nipple and subareolar duct tissue, and assessment of skin flaps for retained breast tissue.

Incision selection

NSM is performed through a variety of incisions. Selection among incision options is based on skin perfusion and cosmetic factors. Our group favors the inferolateral approach for its cosmetic advantages and lower risk of nipple skin necrosis compared with circumareolar incisions [35], but several approaches can work well. Old biopsy and lumpectomy incisions can generally be ignored.

Inferolateral inframammary fold

Inferolateral inframammary fold incisions provide good access to the axilla and avoid injury to vessels in the medial portion of the inframammary fold [35]. With any inframammary fold approach, separating the breast from the pectoralis major and serratus anterior muscles early in the dissection allows the breast specimen to be mobilized downward through the incision and facilitates access to the superior and superior-medial skin flaps.

Inframammary fold

Inframammary fold incisions have the cosmetic advantage of being hidden in the upright position, but may make exposure of the upper portion of the breast flaps more difficult and usually require a separate incision for axillary node removal. Inframammary fold incisions that extend medially beyond the 6:00-o'clock position may also compromise perfusion to lower inner quadrant skin flap areas.

Vertical radial

NSM may be performed through a vertical radial incision extending from the 6:00-o'clock position of the areola border to the inframammary fold. Some plastic surgeons find that a vertical radial incision that includes excision of a curved ellipse of skin allows upward positioning of the nipple for ptosis correction. In women with prior Wise pattern reduction mammaplasty scars, the vertical portion of the scar usually provides sufficient exposure, with the option of extending the incision 90° around the lateral aspect of the old circumareolar incision.

Circumareolar with lateral extension

Surgeons who routinely perform skin-sparing mastectomies through a circumareolar incision may find that performing NSM through a periareolar incision with a lateral extension provides a more familiar view than an inframammary fold approach. However, the periareolar approach creates a visible scar in the center of the breast. In addition, retraction on areola skin can result in increased rates of skin necrosis [36], change in areola contour, and deviation of the NAC laterally [37]. Although a few centers favor periareolar incisions, many prefer inframammary incisions or vertical radial incisions.

Preexisting scars

NSM may be performed through preexisting incisions, including the inferior or vertical portion of Wise pattern reduction scars. However, inferolateral or inframammary fold incisions are often preferable even in patients with old biopsy and lumpectomy scars and risk of flap ischemia remains low [36].

Creation of flaps

Skin flaps are developed in the Cooper ligament plane as for all mastectomy surgery. Exposure and development of tension during NSM is with standard use of skin hooks and facelift retractors to hold the skin taut while the surgeon provides countertraction on the breast specimen. In many areas, it may be easier to protect the skin flaps if the surgeon retracts the skin flap while the assistant provides tension on the breast specimen with a facelift retractor or clamp (Fig. 1). For peripheral incisions, separating the breast from the pectoralis major as an early step in the dissection allows the breast specimen to be pulled out of the incision, allowing better exposure of the superior and medial flap areas.

Taking the nipple margin

Standard mastectomy skin flaps are raised in the Cooper ligament plane to the edge of the areola. The subcutaneous fat layer disappears under the areola and the dissection plane becomes the deep side of the areola dermis. Dissection stops underneath the nipple, leaving the fibrous tissue of the nipple duct bundle intact. Using blunt dissection, a curved clamp is then passed around the intact duct bundle and a second clamp is then used to grasp the bundle. With the convex side of the clamp toward the skin, the clamp is moved as close to the skin as possible without catching skin in the clamp (Fig. 2). The clamp is then rotated 90° toward the surgeon and the bundle sharply divided above

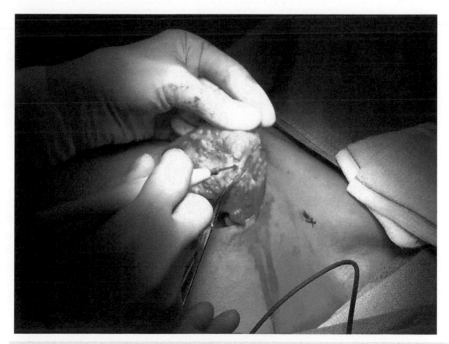

Fig. 1. Skin retraction by surgeon with retraction of breast specimen by assistant.

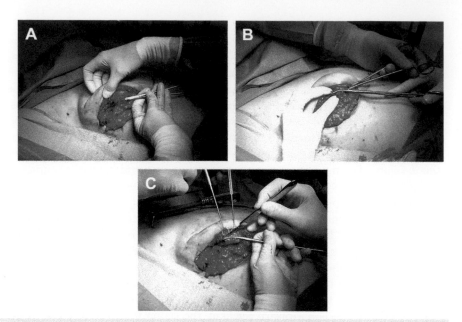

Fig. 2. (*A*) Blunt and sharp dissection allows clamp to be passed around nipple duct bundle. (*B*) Nipple duct bundle grasped in clamp. (*C*) Nipple duct bundle sharply divided from areola skin. The clamp is sharply divided from the underlying breast to obtain the nipple/subareolar margin.

and below the clamp. This maneuver removes most of the duct tissue from within the nipple, exposing the underside of the nipple and areola dermis while leaving the skin vessels intact. Excised nipple/subareolar margin tissue is sent for histologic analysis.

Other techniques for nipple margin assessment separate the nipple and areola skin completely from the underlying breast parenchyma using sharp dissection. A nipple margin specimen is then taken from the underside of the nipple and areola, removing breast and ductal tissue that remains for histologic assessment.

Final assessment of flaps

Most NSM are performed through peripheral or small central incisions that make exposure and flap development difficult. It is important to recognize that retraction on breast tissue while developing NSM skin flaps can expose the anterior surface of a superficial tumor. This makes the anterior margin appear positive to the pathologist and may result in a recommendation for postmastectomy radiation. To avoid creating this false impression that the margin is positive, the surgeon can clarify margin status by taking a thin shaved margin of tissue from the underside of the mastectomy flap directly over any areas of superficial primary tumor. If this specimen designated "additional margin anterior to mass" is free of tumor, the anterior margin should be considered negative and no additional intervention is required.

Reconstruction options

Any reconstruction approach may be used after NSM. Implant-based reconstructions are often chosen, especially after bilateral NSM. Preservation of the entire skin envelope with NSM enables single-stage implant reconstruction in many women with small to moderate size breasts, shortening the overall reconstruction process compared with tissue expander reconstruction and subsequent expander to implant exchange. For patients undergoing free flap reconstructions, the incision used for NSM must provide access for the microscope if needed.

SURGICAL COMPLICATIONS

NSM procedures are at risk for the same perioperative complications that occur with skin-sparing mastectomies and reconstruction. Skin flap necrosis and expander/implant loss are the most serious surgical complications after NSM. Rates of these major complications may be higher early in a surgeon's experience with NSM but decrease with experience [11,38].

Piper and colleagues [39] reviewed 16 NSM series and found that the average rate of partial or full-thickness skin flap necrosis was 9.5% and the rate of expander/implant loss was 3.9%. Colwell and colleagues [36] reviewed complications in nearly 500 NSM plus implant or expander reconstructions at Massachusetts General Hospital and found a 1.9% rate of implant loss. Increasing body mass index, smoking, periareolar incisions, and preoperative radiation were significant predictors of NSM complications.

COSMETIC CONSIDERATIONS

The central reason for preservation of the nipple is to improve the cosmetic outcome over what could be achieved with skin-sparing mastectomy and nipple reconstruction. Retained nipples are usually insensate, making their function purely cosmetic. More patients are excluded from nipple preservation based on cosmetic factors than for oncologic factors, although work continues on strategies to improve NSM options for women with significant ptosis or very large breasts.

Nipple position and ptosis correction

Expectation of a poor nipple position on the final reconstruction is a contraindication to nipple sparing. It was initially believed that NSM was only feasible in patients with small to moderate size breasts and minimal ptosis. However, it has become clear that NSM can provide an excellent cosmetic result in ptotic breasts. With single-stage submuscular implant reconstruction, the nipple routinely falls into a higher position, providing significant ptosis correction (Fig. 3). With tissue expander reconstruction, the expander can initially be underinflated, allowing contraction of the skin envelope, with or without tacking the NAC into a higher position, with subsequent expansion creating a better final nipple position. The expander can also be placed in a slightly lower position on the chest wall to preferentially expand the lower breast skin and effectively raise nipple position.

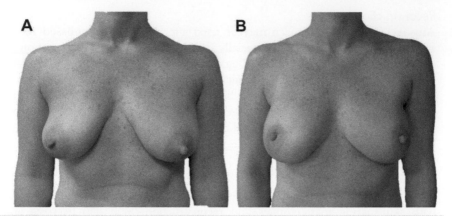

Fig. 3. (A) Preoperative ptosis. (B) Ptosis correction with bilateral nipple-sparing mastectomies with single-stage implant reconstruction.

Breast size

Nipple preservation remains challenging in patients with very large breasts and in women who desire significant reduction in breast size. There are no simple approaches that remove significant amounts of skin, raise nipple position, and maintain nipple perfusion. For patients where time is not an issue, such as prophylactic mastectomy patients, standard reduction mammaplasty is performed first to adjust size, with NSM performed through the vertical portion of the reduction scars 2 to 3 months later [40]. This 2- to 3-month delay is usually not feasible for patients with cancer, and nipple and skin resection with delayed nipple reconstruction may be the best option. Others have suggested NSM with autologous flap reconstruction followed by delayed mastopexy of the reconstructed breast for management of ptosis [41].

PATIENT SELECTION ISSUES

At present, most patients who require mastectomy are eligible for nipple sparing [38]. Direct involvement of the nipple by tumor on physical examination or imaging is an absolute contraindication to nipple sparing. Some authors also consider pathologic nipple discharge an absolute contraindication. In addition, the expectation of a poor location of the retained nipple excludes some patients from nipple sparing.

Tumor factors

Prior NSM guidelines excluded patients with tumors within 2 cm of the nipple from NSM. Increasing data on the safety of nipple-sparing approaches has led to revision of these guidelines. At present, patients with no direct tumor involvement of the nipple and/or areola on imaging or physical examination are eligible if a microscopically clear margin is obtained. Brachtel and colleagues [42] noted higher rates of unexpected nipple involvement by tumor in mastectomies with extensive high-grade ductal carcinoma in situ (DCIS) and for invasive lobular cancer, with lowest rates for invasive ductal cancer that contained minimal DCIS. However, if clear margins are obtained, any tumor histology can be considered for NSM.

Patients with higher stage breast cancers remain eligible for NSM. Peled and colleagues [43] reported a low risk of local recurrence among 139 patients with stage 2B or stage 3 breast cancer who underwent NSM, with only 5% developing isolated local recurrences at 41 months follow-up. No recurrence involved the retained NAC.

Patient factors

Tang and colleagues [44] analyzed patient factors associated with complications in 982 NSM performed at a single institution. Risk factors for complications included radiation, smoking, age older than 55 years, breast volume greater than 800 mL and a periareolar incision. Complication rates increased among patients with multiple risk factors. There was no association of reconstruction type or use of chemotherapy with risk of complications. Increasing body mass index is a risk for increased complications in some series [36] but not others [44]. It was concluded that complications could be minimized with appropriate patient selection and careful surgical technique [11,44].

Radiation and nipple-sparing mastectomy

Although prior radiation and postmastectomy radiation increase the risk of complications with any reconstruction, patients with prior radiation and those who need postmastectomy radiation remain eligible for NSM, and most do well. Tang and colleagues [44] at our institution compared 816 NSM with no radiation with 69 NSM in previously irradiated breasts. Prior radiation increased the rate of total nipple necrosis from 0.9% to 4.3% and increased the rate of implant failure from 2% to 3%. When postmastectomy radiation was required, the rate of total nipple necrosis increased from 0.9% to 4.1% and the rate of implant loss increased from 2% to 8.2% compared with no radiation.

PERIOPERATIVE AND FOLLOW-UP CARE

As in patients undergoing skin-sparing mastectomies with reconstruction, prevention of perioperative infections is important. Strategies to reduce infections include preoperative antibacterial skin cleansing by patients, meticulous surgical technique, and perioperative antibiotics. Postoperatively, it is important to strike a balance between limiting patient activity to reduce seroma formation and flap irritation while maintaining shoulder range of motion.

Some patients develop a scab or eschar on their nipple and/or areola because of partial nipple necrosis. It is important to avoid premature debridement of these partially ischemic nipples because most heal with time, with a good cosmetic outcome.

No routine breast imaging is needed for screening after NSM. For patients who underwent NSM for breast cancer, physical examinations are performed every 4 to 6 months as part of their regular oncologic follow-up. For patients undergoing NSM for DCIS or for risk reduction, annual physical examinations are standard. All NSM patients are instructed to report any new skin or subcutaneous nodules found on self-examination.

SUMMARY

- Nipple sparing provides a superior cosmetic result for patients who require mastectomy for breast cancer treatment or for risk reduction, with high levels of patient satisfaction.
- Rates of new or recurrent tumor in the retained nipple and areola are extremely low when a clear nipple/areola margin is obtained
- Meticulous surgical technique is essential to preserve the blood supply to the nipple and skin flaps, while also ensuring thorough excision of breast and nipple duct tissue.
- In appropriately selected patients the risk of complications after NSM is acceptably low.
- Most patients who require mastectomy are now eligible for nipple sparing.

References

[1] Howard MA, Sisco M, Yao K, et al. Patient satisfaction with nipple-sparing mastectomy: a prospective study of patient reported outcomes using the BREAST-Q. J Surg Oncol 2016;114:416–22.

[2] Metcalfe KA, Cil TD, Semple JL, et al. Long-term psychosocial functioning in women with bilateral prophylactic mastectomy: does preservation of the nipple-areolar complex make a difference? Ann Surg Oncol 2015;22:3324–30.

[3] Kasprzak L, Mesurolle B, Tremblay F, et al. Invasive breast cancer following bilateral subcutaneous mastectomy in a BRCA2 mutation carrier: a case report and review of the literature. World J Surg Oncol 2005;3:52.

[4] Yi M, Kronowitz SJ, Meric-Bernstam F, et al. Local, regional, and systemic recurrence rates in patients undergoing skin-sparing mastectomy compared with conventional mastectomy. Cancer 2011;117:916–24.

[5] Harness JK, Vetter TS, Salibian AH. Areola and nipple–areola sparing mastectomy for breast cancer treatment and risk reduction: report of an initial experience in a community hospital setting. Ann Surg Oncol 2011;18:917–22.

[6] Rice CO, Strickler JH. Adeno-mammectomy for benign breast lesions. Surg Gynecol Obstet 1951;93(6):759–62.

[7] Hartmann LC, Schaid DJ, Woods JE, et al. Efficacy of bilateral prophylactic mastectomy in women with a family history of breast cancer. N Engl J Med 1999;340:77–84.

[8] Rusby JE, Brachtel EF, Michaelson JS, et al. Breast duct anatomy in the human nipple: three dimensional patterns and clinical implications. Breast Cancer Res Treat 2007;106:171–9.

[9] Rusby JE, Brachtel EF, Taghian AG, et al. Microscopic anatomy within the nipple: implications for nipple sparing mastectomy. Am J Surg 2007;194:433–7.

[10] Rusby JE, Kirstein LJ, Brachtel EF, et al. Nipple-sparing mastectomy: lessons from ex vivo procedures. Breast J 2008;14:464–70.

[11] Wang F, Peled AW, Garwood E, et al. Total skin-sparing mastectomy and immediate breast reconstruction: an evolution of technique and assessment of outcomes. Ann Surg Oncol 2014;21:3223–30.

[12] Hartmann LC, Sellers TA, Schaid DJ, et al. Efficacy of bilateral prophylactic mastectomy in BRCA1 and BRCA2 gene mutation carriers. J Natl Cancer Inst 2001;93:1633–7.

[13] Jakub J, Peled A, Gray R, et al. Multi-institutional study of the oncologic safety of prophylactic nipple-sparing mastectomy in a BRCA population [Abstract]. Proceedings from

the 17th Annual Meeting of the American Society of Breast Surgeons. Dallas, Texas, April 13–17, 2016.

[14] Yao K, Liederbach E, Tang R, et al. Nipple-sparing mastectomy in brca1/2 mutation carriers: an interim analysis and review of the literature. Ann Surg Oncol 2015;22:370–6.

[15] Peled AW, Irwin CS, Hwang ES, et al. Total skin-sparing mastectomy in BRCA mutation carriers. Ann Surg Oncol 2014;21:37–41.

[16] Manning AT, Wood C, Eaton A, et al. Nipple-sparing mastectomy in patients with BRCA1/2 mutations and variants of uncertain significance. Br J Surg 2015;102(11):1354–9.

[17] Lohsiriwat V, Martella S, Rietjens M. Paget's disease as a local recurrence after nipple-sparing mastectomy: clinical presentation, treatment, outcome, and risk factor analysis. Ann Surg Oncol 2012;19:1850–5.

[18] Orzalesi L, Casella D, Santi C, et al. Nipple sparing mastectomy: surgical and oncological outcomes from a national multicentric registry with 913 patients (1006 cases) over a six year period. The Breast 2016;25:75–81.

[19] Peled AW, Foster RD, Stover AC, et al. Outcomes after total skin-sparing mastectomy and immediate reconstruction in 657 breasts. Ann Surg Oncol 2012;19:3402–9.

[20] Smith BL, Tang R, Rai U, et al. Oncologic safety of nipple-sparing mastectomy in women with breast cancer. J Am College Surg 2017;225:361–5.

[21] Krajewski AC, Boughey JC, Degnim AC, et al. Expanded indications and improved outcomes for nipple-sparing mastectomy over time. Ann Surg Oncol 2015;22:3317–23.

[22] Benediktsson KP, Perbeck L. Survival in breast cancer after nipple sparing subcutaneous mastectomy and immediate reconstruction with implants: a prospective trial with 13 years median follow-up in 216 patients. Eur J Surg Oncol 2008;34:143–8.

[23] Filho PA, Capko D, Barry JM, et al. Nipple-sparing mastectomy for breast cancer and risk-reducing surgery: the Memorial Sloan-Kettering Cancer Center experience. Ann Surg Oncol 2011;18:3117–22.

[24] Donell C, Yuen J, Santiago C, et al. Oncologic safety of nipple skin-sparing or total skin-sparing mastectomies with immediate reconstruction. J Am Coll Surg 2011;212:686–95.

[25] Jensen JA, Orringer JS, Giuliano AE. Nipple-sparing mastectomy in 99 patients with a mean follow-up of 5 years. Ann Surg Oncol 2011;18:1665–70.

[26] Gerber B, Krause A, Dieterich M, et al. The oncological safety of skin sparing mastectomy with conservation of the nipple-areola complex and autologous reconstruction: an extended follow-up study. Ann Surg 2009;249:461–8.

[27] De La Cruz L, Moody AM, Tappy EE, et al. Overall survival, disease-free survival, local recurrence, and nipple–areolar recurrence in the setting of nipple-sparing mastectomy: a meta-analysis and systematic review. Ann Surg Oncol 2015;22:3241–9.

[28] Adam H, Bygdeson M, De Boniface J. The oncological safety of nipple-sparing mastectomy: a Swedish matched cohort study. Eur J Surg Oncol 2014;40:1209–15.

[29] Park SH, Han W, Yoo TK, et al. Oncologic safety of immediate breast reconstruction for invasive breast cancer patients: a matched case control study. J Breast Cancer 2016;19:68–75.

[30] Crowe JP, Patrick RJ, Yetman RJ, et al. Nipple-sparing mastectomy update: one hundred forty-nine procedures and clinical outcomes. Arch Surg 2008;143(11):1106–10.

[31] Petit JY, Veronisi U, Orecchia R, et al. Nipple sparing mastectomy with nipple areola intraoperative radiotherapy: one thousand and one cases of a five years experience at the European Institute of Oncology of Milan (EIO). Breast Cancer Res Treat 2009;117:333–8.

[32] Tang R, Coopey SB, Merrill AL, et al. Positive nipple margins in nipple-sparing mastectomies: rates, management, and oncologic safety. J Am Coll Surg 2016;222:1149–55.

[33] Camp MS, Coopey SB, Tang R, et al. Management of positive sub-areolar/nipple duct margins in nipple-sparing mastectomies. Breast J 2014;20:402–7.

[34] Amara D, Peled AW, Wang F, et al. Tumor involvement of the nipple in total skin-sparing mastectomy: strategies for management. Ann Surg Oncol 2015;22:3803–8.

[35] Colwell AS, Gadd M, Smith BL, et al. An inferolateral approach to nipple-sparing mastectomy. Ann Plast Surg 2010;65:140–3.

[36] Colwell AS, Tessler O, Lin AM, et al. Breast reconstruction following nipple-sparing mastectomy: predictors of complications, reconstruction outcomes, and 5-year trends. Plast Reconstr Surg 2014;133:496–506.

[37] Djohan R, Gage E, Gatherwright J, et al. Patient satisfaction following nipple-sparing mastectomy and immediate breast reconstruction: an 8-year outcome study. Plast Reconstr Surg 2010;125:818–29.

[38] Coopey SB, Tang R, Lei L, et al. Increasing eligibility for nipple-sparing mastectomy. Ann Surg Oncol 2013;20:3218–22.

[39] Piper M, Peled AW, Foster RD, et al. Total skin-sparing mastectomy: a systematic review of oncologic outcomes and postoperative complications. Ann Plast Surg 2013;70:435–7.

[40] Spear SL, Rottman SJ, Seiboth LA, et al. Breast reconstruction using a staged nipple-sparing mastectomy following mastopexy or reduction. Plast Reconstr Surg 2012;129:572–81.

[41] DellaCroce FJ, Blum CA, Sullivan SK, et al. Nipple-sparing mastectomy and ptosis: perforator flap breast reconstruction allows full secondary mastopexy with complete nipple areolar repositioning. Plast Reconstr Surg 2015;136(1):1e–9e.

[42] Brachtel EF, Rusby JE, Michaelson JS, et al. Occult nipple involvement in breast cancer: clinicopathologic findings in 316 consecutive mastectomy specimens. J Clin Oncol 2009;27:4948–54.

[43] Peled AW, Wang F, Foster FD, et al. Expanding the indications for total skin-sparing mastectomy: is it safe for patients with locally advanced disease? Ann Surg Oncol 2016;23:87–91.

[44] Tang R, Coopey SB, Colwell AS, et al. Nipple-sparing mastectomy in irradiated breasts: selecting patients to minimize complications. Ann Surg Oncol 2015;22:3331–7.

Advances in Surgery 52 (2018) 127–135

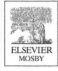

ADVANCES IN SURGERY

Should the Management of a Ruptured Abdominal Aortic Aneurysm Be Regionalized?

Courtney J. Warner, MD[a], Steven C. Stain, MD[b],
R. Clement Darling III, MD[c],*

[a]Albany Medical College, The Vascular Group, The Institute for Vascular Health and Disease, 391 Myrtle Avenue, Suite 5, Albany, NY 12208, USA; [b]Department of Surgery, Albany Medical Center Hospital, Albany Medical College, 50 New Scotland Avenue (MC194), Albany, NY 12208, USA; [c]Division of Vascular Surgery, Albany Medical College, Albany Medical Center Hospital, The Vascular Group, 391 Myrtle Avenue, Suite 5, Albany, NY 12208, USA

Keywords
• Ruptured aortic aneurysm • Aortic aneurysm • Regionalization • EVAR

Key points

- Regionalization of high-risk vascular emergencies is critically important to optimize patient outcomes.
- Transferring patients to rAAA repair center did not impact the low mortality of rEVAR at the tertiary care center.
- National consideration of the development of standards and possible accreditation of centers capable of caring for rAAA.

INTRODUCTION

Over the last two decades, there has been a paradigm shift in the treatment of ruptured abdominal aortic aneurysms (rAAA). Without surgical repair, a ruptured aneurysm is a universally fatal event. For many years mortality for rAAA has remained unchanged, with mortality reported between 35% and 70%. Endovascular aneurysm repair (EVAR) for rAAA has expanded, with multiple recent reports documenting lower short-term morbidity and mortality in patients treated with EVAR instead of open repair [1–4]. Although EVAR

Disclosure: The authors have nothing to disclose.

*Corresponding author. E-mail address: darlingc@albanyvascular.com

https://doi.org/10.1016/j.yasu.2018.03.010

has become generally accepted as a first-line therapy in the setting of rAAA, safe and efficient EVAR requires not only surgical expertise, but also advanced infrastructure including immediate availability of an operating room (OR) and experienced staff with fluoroscopy training. Historically, patients have been treated at the hospital of initial presentation, either by a trained vascular surgeon or a general surgeon in a rural setting, most often by the open technique. An emerging model of care delivery is the transfer of patients with rAAA to a tertiary medical center with the necessary expertise. Several centers have published experiences developing a multidisciplinary protocol to expedite EVAR for ruptured aneurysms [3,5,6]. Some practices have undertaken a strategy of regionalizing and consolidating rAAA care, based on the realization that it is more efficient to transfer the patients to an academic medical center with advanced imaging and immediate availability of an OR with endovascular capability.

BACKGROUND

In the late 20th century, trauma care delivery was modernized with advances in triage and regionalization to provide patients with appropriate high-level care in the fastest time possible. The mortality for traumatic gunshot wounds in New York State at the highest volume center is around 11%. In 1968, The American Trauma Society led a fight for nationwide quality trauma care. Its foundational goals were to prevent injury and trauma, and when trauma occurs, to ensure the injured victim is to be cared for by "the right people in the right place at the right time." In the mid-1980s the American Trauma Society worked with Congress to develop a new program to support trauma centers and systems resulting in the passage of the 1990 Trauma Systems Development Act. This has been successful and likely contributes to the low mortality for gunshot wounds in New York State.

Historically, advances in regionalization for high-level trauma have not been duplicated in emergent vascular surgery. High-quality data have shown that hospital volume is an important factor in achieving good outcomes for aneurysm repair. With the advent of EVAR for elective and ruptured aneurysms, many studies have shown that the mortality for rAAA treated with EVAR is less than open repair but requires significant resources to have the equipment, trained staff, and hospital infrastructure to reduce mortality to the 20% range.

- In 2007, Holt and colleagues [7] published in an extensive meta-analysis of more than 421,000 elective aneurysm repairs and 45,796 rAAA repairs demonstrating that higher volumes correlate with lower mortality.
- Veith and Ohki [8] were the first to perform EVAR for rAAA. In their collective world experience published in 2008, they performed 1000 cases with mortality of 22%.
- Ullery and colleagues [9] evaluated the effect of an endovascular-first protocol for the treatment of rAAA and found this to be associated with reductions in perioperative morbidity and mortality, a higher likelihood of discharge to home, and even improved long-term survival at 1 year.

It seems illogical that systems for ruptured aneurysm treatment do not more closely follow the regionalization paradigms popular in trauma surgery. Aortic pathology, whether caused by a ruptured aneurysm or a bullet, is eventually fatal unless treated by an adequately trained vascular surgeon or trauma surgeon in the case of trauma. One reason that rAAA mortality has been unchanged in the last 40 years may be that many regions do not have a system to deal with this highly lethal problem.

DISCUSSION

Does regionalization of ruptured abdominal aortic aneurysms really work? The Upstate New York example

As we branched out to provide vascular surgery coverage for numerous hospitals over 100 square miles in upstate New York, we started to regionalize vascular emergencies for efficiency and to streamline delivery of emergent vascular care. To examine the outcomes for regionalization of care for rAAA, we recently performed a retrospective study of all rAAA patients treated by The Vascular Group, which is a group of 20 board-certified vascular surgeons in eastern upstate New York.

Some key methodology points

- The management of rAAA in eastern upstate New York is by a single group of vascular surgeons over a 12-hospital geographic area.
- This study included all patients presenting to these hospitals with rAAA over a 13-year time period. The 12 hospitals included one academic medical center and 11 community hospitals.
  - The tertiary care center is Albany Medical Center Hospital, a 725-bed facility and Level 1 Trauma Center with 24-hour OR availability.
  - The community hospitals ranged from 173 to 487 beds.
- The Vascular Group were the only surgeons with vascular surgery privileges at the 12 hospitals, performed all operations, and directed the decision for transfer to the tertiary center.

During the study period, a protocol for the care of patients presenting with rAAA was developed by a multidisciplinary team consisting of surgeons, emergency physicians, anesthesiologists, nurses, and radiology technicians. For all patients presenting with suspected rupture, the vascular surgery on-call team is alerted. Patients with systolic blood pressure greater than 80 mm Hg on multiple reads are sent for emergent computed tomography angiogram. All patients are then transferred to an OR with endovascular capability and support staffing.

Medical records were reviewed from each hospital to gather demographic data and transfer-related data, including lowest systolic blood pressure during transfer, need for advanced cardiovascular life support (ACLS) protocol during transfer, and presenting hemoglobin. Basic demographics including age, gender, and comorbidities were collected. Patients were divided into several groups according to transfer status and type of repair (EVAR or open). The groups included patients presenting to and treated at community hospitals, patients presenting to community hospitals and transferred to the tertiary medical center, and patients presenting to and treated at the medical center. Primary outcomes included 30-day perioperative mortality and perioperative morbidity.

The main results of the upstate experience over 13 years are as follows:

- A total of 451 patients with rAAA were treated at 12 hospitals from January 2002 to September 2015.
    - Most patients (71%) presented initially to a community hospital.
    - Of these patients, 133 (41%) were treated at the community hospital and 188 (59%) were transferred to the academic medical center. The mean time interval of patient transfer to the medical center was 1.2 hours.
- There was no statistically significant difference in the mean age, gender, or prevalence of comorbidities including hypertension, smoking, diabetes, coronary artery disease, chronic kidney disease, and chronic obstructive pulmonary disease among the patients presenting to the community hospital or tertiary care center.
- Patients were far more likely to undergo EVAR at the medical center.
    - 94% of patients treated at community hospitals underwent open repair.
    - 318 patients were either transferred to or presented to the medical center, and 38% underwent open repair, whereas 62% underwent EVAR.
- At the community hospitals, the 30-day mortality rate was 46%. Among the transferred patients, 30-day mortality was 27%. In patients presenting to and treated at the medical center, overall 30-day mortality was also 27%.
- At the medical center, EVAR was associated with a lower 30-day mortality rate compared with open repair (20% vs 37%; $P = .001$).
- Transfer did not influence the mortality of EVAR (20% in EVAR presenting to medical center vs 20% in EVAR transferred; $P>.2$). Furthermore, all rAAA mortality at the medical center was 20% lower than the community hospitals (27% vs 46%; $P<.001$).

The logistics of regionalization

Our experience highlights the importance of creating a regional network of vascular surgeons and coordinated hospital care to minimize rAAA patient mortality and morbidity. Several other published reports support this strategy. McPhee and colleagues [10] analyzed rAAA in the United States from 2001 to 2006, showing that EVAR had a lower mortality rate than open repair and high-volume hospitals improved the survival of these patients. Lesperance and coworkers [11] also demonstrated that in the setting of expanding use of emergency EVAR for rAAA, there are disparities in outcomes across regions: in Washington, EVAR had a significantly lower mortality than open repair, but mortality for EVAR was higher in nonteaching hospitals. This supports the concept that facilities and surgeons with infrastructure in place may be best suited to treat complex pathologies, such as ruptured aneurysms.

In Upstate New York, we receive patients from a 200-mile radius via ground and helicopter transport. We have developed an educational system to assist emergency room doctors in the rapid diagnosis of rAAA and setting up a "hub and spoke" system similar to a trauma network. This allows us to transfer patients safely and reduce mortality because of the expertise of the physicians, the excellent training of support staff and nurses, and the on-shelf availability of numerous devices to treat complex anatomy. Developing this system required negotiation with numerous hospitals, emergency departments, and emergency medical technicians (EMTs) to transfer these patients immediately because of the decreased survival of patients staying at community hospitals and the high cost to the local community hospitals for treating those patients that do survive. Also, because the same group of surgeons who worked in these 12 hospitals also worked at Albany Medical Center, we realized it was not the skill of the surgeon that was the problem; it was more the availability of the OR and comprehensive postoperative care. Many community hospitals do not have 24-hour anesthesia in-house, nor do they have ORs open 24 hours a day like a tertiary care medical center. The concept of "scoop and run" was developed to deliver these patients, stable and unstable, to the facility that could best treat them. At our center, we have previously documented that patients stable and unstable had equal survival rates when EVAR was performed for rAAA, and the long-term survival of these patients was statistically improved over those patients undergoing open repair [2]. Only around 75% of patients have anatomy amenable to EVAR using currently available devices, thus centers offering treatment for rAAA need to have vascular surgeons who feel comfortable with EVAR and open repair. Also, for open repair, because the blood loss is significantly higher, these hospitals need to have the infrastructure to mobilize large amounts of blood products; an adequately staffed intensive care unit by intensivists; highly skilled nurses; and the backup of general surgery, cardiology, and other supporting services who may be involved in the care of these critically ill patients.

There have been reports by Mell and coworkers [12] showing that in a large nationwide inpatient database experience, the survival advantage of EVAR for rAAA was eclipsed by the increased mortality of the transfer process. To help avoid this, we created a vascular network to focus on minimizing the amount of time these patients spend in diagnosis and waiting for transfer. Unlike California, in Upstate New York, we are the only academic facility in our region. Thus, all community hospitals have one number to call 24 hours a day to transfer patients and we have a no refuse policy in our system. This allows for a smooth, fast transfer of patients out of these community hospitals to the tertiary care center. Some patients lose their window of opportunity because the transferring hospital has to find an accepting physician and hospital. In prior analysis, we have found that the mean time interval of patient transfer to the medical center was 1.2 hours. Involving the community hospitals in our algorithms and simplifying the transfer process has created a comradery among these facilities in feeling that they are all working together to treat this highly lethal pathology. In our recent review, nearly 200 patients were transferred and the number of patients who died in transfer was small. There was almost no difference in lowest systolic blood pressure, the need for ACLS protocol, and arrival hemoglobin between transferred and nontransferred patients. Although there is an inherent selection bias based on the initial evaluation of every patient presenting from community hospitals with rAAA, there does not seem to be a major difference between patients transferred and those initially presenting to the tertiary care medical center.

One of the major tenets of our algorithm is to allow hypotensive hemostasis to occur. In looking at some of the older studies, especially the one by Kai Johansen [13] from Washington where he had a high mortality in patients, those patients mostly were resuscitated in the field, which may have precipitated a secondary rupture after the blood pressure was elevated. In our series we have taught the referring physicians to avoid crystalloid resuscitation if the patient is mentating and does not have any significant end organ dysfunction. By allowing this to happen, the aneurysm rupture tamponade may be more effective. We do not advocate giving the patient pharmacologic pressers or significant boluses with crystalloid, and if the patient needs volume, prefer to provide packed red blood cells in a one-to-one fashion. This, combined with the newer technology of endovascular repair and swift transfer, has allowed us to have a lower mortality in our tertiary care center than in the community hospitals.

Is widespread regionalization feasible?

One of the major issues our study raised was whether this system could be translatable to other parts of the country. Although we have the unique logistics that allow one surgical group to cover these 15 hospitals that were evaluated, we also cover numerous hospitals where there is no vascular surgery coverage who directly transfer patients to us for care of rAAA. To facilitate this, we communicated with these institutions to follow the same protocols that have been established within our personal vascular group network. We allowed these hospitals to access our network to transfer patients as soon as the diagnosis was made. We believe this allowed us access to more patients, and for those patients who are in an area that are underserved by vascular surgeons to have direct access to our tertiary care center.

Another concern is whether it was the repair of ruptured aneurysm by EVAR or the multidisciplinary approach and infrastructure set up that helped us reduce mortality. Our anecdotal bias is that those facilities with a secure infrastructure (ie, hybrid OR, shelf stock, blood bank access, cardiac anesthesiology, and 24-hour in-house intensivist and consultants) were better prepared for these complicated patients than hospitals of the same size or even larger who did not have the infrastructure. We believe that it is the combination of these systems in place at the tertiary care medical center that improves outcomes instead of one single factor alone. But we also noticed during the 13-year time period that our open mortality decreased and we believe that this was caused by the infrastructure; obviously, not the technical skills of the surgeons, because they were the same whether they were at the smaller outside community hospitals or the tertiary care center.

Another observation we found was that as time elapsed, patients were more likely to be transferred to the tertiary care center. In the first year of adopting this protocol approximately 50% were transferred, and toward the end more than 80% of patients were transferred. This happened even though our ability to perform EVAR was disseminated throughout some of the larger hospitals during that time period. Patients that remained at the community hospitals in the latter portion of the time period were those patients who presented during the daylight/work hours when ORs and appropriate support were available. Off-hours, most patients were transferred because of time constraints to adequately assemble staff in the outside hospitals. Again, this points to the infrastructure being more important than the newer technology. Although we have a consistent protocol at our tertiary care center, it was extremely ineffective from a cost standpoint to replicate this at each one of the outside hospitals, even the larger (>250 bed) hospitals.

We have continued to try to transfer most rAAA patients to the tertiary care medical center in the off-hours, because the tertiary medical center is better prepared to treat these patients and it may take the community hospitals an extended period of time to get the OR ready and get the technical staff who are needed for urgent EVAR. With that said, early diagnosis and early transfer for patients with rAAA is critical. Much of the mortality for rAAA comes from the delay in diagnosis, and a high index of suspicion by the emergency room physicians and the EMTs is important. However, this is more anecdotal data than it is hard science.

Lastly, the 30-day mortality for community hospitals was 46% compared with 27% and although one could explain this by patient selection, the choice of most of the physicians participating in these data are board-certified vascular surgeons who not only worked at the community hospitals but also were attendings at the tertiary care center. Early on in this experience, if patients were believed to be appropriate for a community hospital they were operated on there, but as we looked at our data and saw that the outcomes were better in transferring these patients, we all as a group became more aggressive about transferring even the unstable patients to Albany Medical Center for definitive care. Again, early on through evaluations of the operative notes, although we were concerned about transfer of patients that were hypotensive, we believed that this did not negatively impact their outcome and again were more aggressive in transferring these patients.

There are several limitations to our prior study. The increased mortality in the outside hospitals could be in part caused by selection bias; some patients not transferred were sicker than the patients that had been transferred, especially early in our experience. However, more recently we have instructed referring hospitals to transfer even the sickest patients who are hypotensive because our data have demonstrated that the greatest chance for survival is to get to the tertiary care center and have emergent surgery as quickly as possible.

Another major limitation was the paucity of documentation and data from the prehospital and emergency department setting for these patients. Because of the emergent nature of these cases, documentation was scant and only those patients with recorded data were analyzed for the comparison of patients transferred to the tertiary medical center with those initially presenting to the tertiary medical center. Finally, as resident work hours become shortened, trainees have less open experience and vascular surgeons perform virtually all open vascular cases, it may be unwise for general surgeons to perform emergent open aortic surgery. This is one of the reasons why we strongly believe that even with the small risk of mortality during transport, it is safer and better for all of these patients to be diagnosed quickly and transferred expeditiously to a tertiary care vascular center that can perform these operations any time of the day or night.

SUMMARY

The regionalization of high-risk vascular emergencies like rAAA is critically important to optimize patient outcomes and reduce mortality. Prior research has demonstrated improved survival after introduction of emergency protocols for rAAA and higher volume centers have better results with rAAA, especially with EVAR. In our experience, regionalization of rAAA repair to centers equipped for EVAR and open repair decreased overall mortality by approximately 20%. Patients tolerate transfer well because we found little difference in lowest blood pressure, the proportion of patients requiring ACLS protocol, and arrival hemoglobin between transferred and nontransferred patients. Transfer did not impact the low mortality of rEVAR at the tertiary care center. This highlights the importance of treatment algorithms and coordination with community hospitals and EMTs to encourage expeditious patient triage to specialized centers that offer 24/7 EVAR in addition to open surgery for rAAA. Nationally, there should be consideration of the development of standards and possible accreditation of centers capable of caring for rAAA.

References

[1] Mastracci TM, Garrido-Olivares L, Cina CS, et al. Endovascular repair of ruptured abdominal aortic aneurysms: a systematic review and meta-analysis. J Vasc Surg 2008;47(1): 214–21.

[2] Mehta M, Byrne J, Darling RC 3rd, et al. Endovascular repair of ruptured infrarenal abdominal aortic aneurysm is associated with lower 30-day mortality and better 5-year survival rates than open surgical repair. J Vasc Surg 2013;57(2):368–75.

[3] Starnes BW, Quiroga E, Hutter C, et al. Management of ruptured abdominal aortic aneurysm in the endovascular era. J Vasc Surg 2010;51(1):9–17 [discussion: 8].

[4] Moore R, Nutley M, Cina CS, et al. Improved survival after introduction of an emergency endovascular therapy protocol for ruptured abdominal aortic aneurysms. J Vasc Surg 2007;45(3):443–50.

[5] Mehta M, Taggert J, Darling RC 3rd, et al. Establishing a protocol for endovascular treatment of ruptured abdominal aortic aneurysms: outcomes of a prospective analysis. J Vasc Surg 2006;44(1):1–8 [discussion: 8].

[6] Mell MW, Schneider PA, Starnes BW. Variability in transfer criteria for patients with ruptured abdominal aortic aneurysm in the western United States. J Vasc Surg 2015;62(2):326–30.

[7] Holt PJ, Poloniecki JD, Gerrard D, et al. Meta-analysis and systematic review of the relationship between volume and outcome in abdominal aortic aneurysm surgery. British Journal of Surgery 2007;94(4):395–403.

[8] Veith FJ, Lachat M, Mayer D, et al. Collected world and single center experience with endovascular treatment of ruptured abdominal aortic aneurysms. Ann Surg 2009;250:818–24.

[9] Ullery BW, Tran K, Chandra V, et al. Association of an endovascular-first protocol for ruptured abdominal aortic aneurysms with survival and discharge disposition. JAMA Surg 2015. [Epub ahead of print].

[10] McPhee J, Eslami MH, Arous EJ, et al. Endovascular treatment of ruptured abdominal aortic aneurysms in the United States (2001-2006): a significant survival benefit over open repair is independently associated with increased institutional volume. J Vasc Surg 2009;49(4):817–26.

[11] Lesperance K, Andersen C, Singh N, et al. Expanding use of emergency endovascular repair for ruptured abdominal aortic aneurysms: disparities in outcomes from a nationwide perspective. J Vasc Surg 2008;47(6):1165–70 [discussion: 70–1].

[12] Mell MW, Wang NE, Morrison DE, et al. Interfacility transfer and mortality for patients with ruptured abdominal aortic aneurysm. J Vasc Surg 2014;60(3):553–7.

[13] Johansen K, Kohler TR, Nicholls SC, et al. Ruptured abdominal aortic aneurysm: the Harborview experience. J Vasc Surg 1991;13:240–5.

Advances in Surgery 52 (2018) 137–153

ADVANCES IN SURGERY

ELSEVIER
MOSBY

Diagnosis and Management of Hyperparathyroidism

Reema Mallick, MD, Herbert Chen, MD*

Department of Surgery, University of Alabama-Birmingham, 1808 7th Avenue South, Suite 502, Birmingham, AL 35233, USA

Keywords

- Hyperparathyroidism • Hypersecretion of parathyroid hormone
- Parathyroidectomy

Key points

- Hyperparathyroidism is a condition marked by hypersecretion of parathyroid hormone with often resultant calcium excess.
- There are several clinical consequences that may result secondary to underlying hyperparathyroidism.
- Surgical extirpation is the sole curative therapy, and today may be aided by various preoperative imaging modalities and intra-operative adjuncts.

INTRODUCTION

Hyperparathyroidism is a condition marked by hypersecretion of parathyroid hormone (PTH) with often resultant calcium excess. Although in the modern era it is frequently detected in the biochemical testing of otherwise asymptomatic individuals, there are several clinical consequences that may result secondary to underlying hyperparathyroidism. Failure to diagnose and treat these patients in an expeditious manner may amplify risk for renal, bone, and cardiovascular disease, diminish quality of life, and lead to overall increases in health care costs [1].

Surgical extirpation for this condition is a relatively novel endeavor, but is the sole curative therapy. It is only within the last 150 years that the anatomic and physiologic features along with the pathologic potential of the parathyroid glands have been elucidated [2–4], demonstrating these glands' central role in

Disclosure: The authors have nothing to disclose.

*Corresponding author. UAB Department of Surgery, 1808 7th Avenue South, Suite 502, Boshell Diabetes Building, Birmingham, AL 35233. E-mail address: herbchen@uab.edu

https://doi.org/10.1016/j.yasu.2018.03.006

calcium, phosphorus, and vitamin D homeostasis. Furthermore, it is only within the last several decades that operative techniques have been refined sufficiently to enable surgery for hyperparathyroidism to be a safe, generally outpatient procedure. Parathyroidectomy boasts cure rates exceeding 95% in the hands of experienced surgeons [1,5].

ANATOMY AND EMBRYOLOGY

A thorough understanding of the anatomy and embryology of the parathyroid glands is the foundation for successful operation. Although many of these can be identified at "typical" anatomic locations, knowledge of the embryologic pathways of the parathyroid glands can be particularly valuable in guiding surgeons when the position is ectopic.

The parathyroids arise from the endodermal pharyngeal pouches, the inferior from the third and the superior from the fourth, around weeks 5 to 6 of gestation. The superior glands undergo limited migration, leading to a relatively fixed position about 1 cm above the intersection of the recurrent laryngeal nerve and inferior thyroid artery. The inferior glands descend past the superior parathyroids, caudally and medially to lie along posterolateral surface of the inferior pole of the thyroid [6,7]. They are usually anterior and medial to the recurrent laryngeal nerve in contrast to the upper glands, which are generally posterior and lateral to the nerve. Given the extended migration, these inferior glands are more apt to be found in ectopic sites, ranging from within the capsule of the thymus (38% of inferior ectopic glands) to the retroesophageal space, carotid sheath, tracheoesophageal groove, submandibular region, and down into the mediastinum [8,9]. Rarely, these can also be found in an intrathyroidal location [10]. Although less likely to be variably located, common ectopic sites for superior glands similarly include the tracheoesophageal groove, posterior mediastinum, retroesophageal or retropharyngeal locations, and within the thyroid [11,12].

The glands can be challenging to differentiate from the amorphous adipose tissue in which they are embedded but are often a dull, yellow-tan hue, ovoid-shaped, and roughly 30 to 50 mg in weight. They are most commonly supplied by the inferior thyroidal artery, and about 70% to 80% of the time will demonstrate mirror-image symmetry in terms of the parathyroid glands found on the contralateral side [13]. Although most will have 4 glands, there has been up to a reported 13% incidence of supranumerary (5 or 6) parathyroids [14]. These glands can either be found adjacent to the normal parathyroids or in locations including the thymus or mediastinum and are associated with initial surgical failures [15].

PRIMARY HYPERPARATHYROIDISM

Primary hyperparathyroidism is the most common form of this disease encountered by surgeons, and overall, the most common cause of hypercalcemia in the outpatient setting. It impacts 1% of the population with nearly 100,000 new cases diagnosed annually [16]. The prevalence in elderly cohorts is thought to be even higher, up to 2% to 3% [17,18]. There is a female predominance with a ratio of 3:1 [19], and the condition most commonly arises in the fifth or sixth decade of life.

Although classic symptoms include nephrolithiasis, osteoporosis, gastrointestinal complaints, myalgias, arthralgias, and variable neuropsychiatric symptoms (Table 1) [20], asymptomatic identification of elevated calcium on serum chemistries can frequently be the first indicator (Ca >10.4 mg/dL) [21]. The diagnosis can then be confirmed by concomitant finding of an inappropriately high intact PTH. This finding, along with a comprehensive history, is important to exclude alternate causes of hypercalcemia, including granulomatous diseases such as sarcoidosis, other endocrinopathies, lithium- or thiazide-mediated imbalance, and either humeral malignancies such as multiple myeloma or the paraneoplastic syndromes of solid organ tumors. Additional useful laboratory studies in the workup include measurement of 25-hydroxyvitamin D_s levels, serum creatinine, phosphorus, and chloride, as well as alkaline phosphatase. Many patients with hyperparathyroidism will develop a characteristic hyperchloremic metabolic acidosis, and detection of concurrent vitamin D deficiency enables supplementation that may mitigate the osteoporosis experienced by some of these patients. Twenty-four hour urine calcium measurement can also be performed to rule out the possibility of benign familial hypocalciuric hypercalcemia.

Once the diagnosis is made, the specific causative pathologic condition must be clarified. Primary hyperparathyroidism may be secondary to benign parathyroid adenomas, multigland hyperplasia, or parathyroid carcinoma. Adenomas are the most common cause, affecting 85% of these patients. Most will have a single parathyroid adenoma, although about 5% to 10% will have two or more affected glands [22,23]. Hyperplasia is found in another 10% to 15% of cases and may be affiliated with familial endocrinopathies such as multiple endocrine neoplasia type I (MEN I) [24] or MEN IIa.

Finally, parathyroid carcinoma is a relatively rare entity found in less than 1% of these patients, and can be difficult to diagnose preoperatively. Features that may distinguish this from benign causes include relatively higher levels

Table 1
Prevalence of preoperative symptoms of primary hyperparathyroidism

Fatigue	97.4%	Headaches	72.9%
Muscle aches	93.0%	Polyuria	72.7%
Bone and joint pain	90.5%	Anxiety	72.4%
Concentration deficit	85.6%	Polydipsia	68.4%
Memory problems	84.7%	Dyspepsia	64.4%
Irritability	81.4%	Constipation	59.8%
Insomnia	81.4%	Abdominal pain	57.4%
Nocturia	78.5%	Urinary incontinence	53.9%
Depression	75.2%	Nausea/vomiting	46.2%

Data from Murray SE, Pathak PR, Pontes DS, et al. Timing of symptom improvement after parathyroidectomy for primary hyperparathyroidism. Surgery 2013;154(6):1466; with permission.

of serum calcium and intact PTH. Some present with palpable, fixed masses of the neck, and significant symptoms are more likely and may be more extreme presentations of those associated with hyperparathyroidism. Specifically, this may include increased instance of osteitis fibrosis cystica, pathologic fractures, and resultant renal insufficiency from recurrent nephrolithiasis [25]. It arises with relatively equal frequency between sexes, and certain hereditary disorders, such as hyperparathyroidism-jaw tumor syndrome, pose increased risk for this malignancy with a 15% incidence [26,27].

As a whole, surgery is the only curative therapy for primary hyperparathyroidism and is uniformly indicated for the symptomatic patient. Benefits of parathyroidectomy have been described as wide-ranging, with improved renal function and bone mineral density [28,29], resolution of insomnia [30], decreases in clinical dyspepsia [31], enhanced quality of life [32], and resolution of neuropsychiatric symptoms [33]. Many of these improvements are observed even in patients with only mild biochemical derangements [32].

Hyperparathyroidism has additionally been associated with increased risk for atherosclerotic disease and adverse cardiovascular events [34–36]. Parathyroidectomy appears to decrease these risks and prolong survival, with avoidance of the 10% increase in mortality that accompanies untreated disease [37]. In fact, only 1 year following surgery, relative risk of myocardial infarction declines from 2.5 to normal values [34]. Thus, the authors believe that all patients with primary hyperparathyroidism should be referred for surgical consultation.

For the asymptomatic patient, however, the 2014 Fourth International Workshop on the Management of Asymptomatic Primary Hyperparathyroidism has developed the most recent recommendations to aid in selection of those who should still be offered surgical resection [38]. These guidelines include patients with the following characteristics:

1. Age less than 50 years
2. Serum calcium greater than 1 mg/dL or greater than 0.25 mmol/L of the upper limit of the reference interval for total calcium and greater than 0.12 mmol/L for Ca^{2+}
3. T score ≤ -2.5 at the lumbar spine, femoral neck, the total hip, or the one-third radius for postmenopausal women or men older than 50 years. Significantly diminished bone mineral density or low-energy fracture is also considered an indication for surgery and requires imaging of the thoracic and lumbar spine or vertebral fracture assessment by dual-energy X-ray absorptiometry (DEXA)
4. Glomerular filtration rate of less than 60 mL/min. Patients should undergo renal imaging with radiograph, computed tomography (CT), or ultrasound to detect clinically occult nephrocalcinosis or nephrolithiasis. A complete urinary stone risk profile is requisite in patients whose urinary calcium excretion is greater than 400 mg/d.

For the patients who do not meet these criteria, an approach involving careful surveillance with annual or biannual calcium measurements as well as routine DEXA scan based on the individual patient risk factors is appropriate. Vertebral fracture assessment may be another useful monitoring adjunct for detection of subclinical disease. Vitamin D repletion should be offered to all patients pursuing observation given that levels greater than 30 ng/mL may enable modest reductions in PTH levels. Oral calcium intake does not need to be limited [38].

A less common presentation of primary hyperparathyroidism is the normocalcemic variant. Its natural history is less well defined [39], although it may simply be an early presentation of the classic form [40]. It is generally discovered after workup for nephrolithiasis, and like standard disease, should be treated aggressively. For asymptomatic patients, a similar algorithm as above can be used, with surgery reserved for those who become hypercalcemic or develop manifestations.

PREOPERATIVE LOCALIZATION STUDIES

Although imaging is not used for diagnostic purposes, in many cases, preoperative localization of a solitary adenoma will permit a targeted and minimally invasive approach to surgery. Several options exist, and algorithms of use depend predominantly on provider familiarity and institutional availability.

The classic imaging study for parathyroid disorders is nuclear imaging using Technetium (99mTc) sestamibi. The radiolabeled sestamibi is preferentially taken up by tissues with high mitochondrial content, including the thyroid, cardiac muscle, salivary glands, and the parathyroids. However, in comparison to the adjacent thyroid tissue, parathyroid adenomas will have continued sestamibi retention with slower washout, enabling identification of abnormal glands on delayed images [41]. This method has an up to 85% sensitivity in single adenoma disease, although utility drops precipitously in multigland hyperplasia [42,43].

A newer technique that supplements this traditional approach is single-photon emission computed tomography (SPECT) imaging, often further combined with conventional CT. The main advantage to this is the ability to acquire multiple two-dimensional images that can be merged to offer information on the spatial orientation of the gland of interest, including anterior-posterior positioning, to further improve surgical planning [44].

Ultrasonography is another potential adjunct and is a particularly appealing option given that it can be performed quickly and at relatively low cost by the treating surgeon. Although it may also be performed by radiologists or endocrinologists, accuracy in localization has been well demonstrated when completed by an experienced surgeon [45]. Parathyroid adenomas are identified sonographically by the characteristic appearance of hypoechoic extrathyroidal masses. This modality allows evaluation for adenomas in both traditional and ectopic locations [46] and also enables evaluation of the thyroid for nodules and identification of other concurrent pathologic conditions that may need to be addressed at the time of surgery [47]. Although most surgeons find ultrasound useful, there are studies that suggest that it may lead to unnecessary thyroid procedures [48]. In addition, ultrasound may facilitate image-guided fine needle aspiration (FNA) of the suspected lesion and confirmation of parathyroid tissue by quantification of PTH (noted to be more useful than cytologic confirmation [49,50]). Parathyroid FNA is NOT recommend for initial parathyroidectomy and reserved exclusively for reoperative cases when the target lesion is not clear. Sensitivity for ultrasound alone is around 76% [51], but it can be used as a complement to other forms of imaging [52].

Finally, one of the most recent additions to the surgeon's armamentarium of imaging modalities is 4dimensional (4D) CT [53]. Using this strategy, multiple images are obtained in different contrast and noncontrast phases, relying on the principle that adenomatous glands will demonstrate rapid uptake and washout of iodinated contrast. This method is particularly useful for smaller glands that may not be identified on other techniques and is not as user dependent as ultrasound. It is also more likely to accurately predict multigland disease [54,55]. A recent cost analysis proposes that surgeons preferentially use SPECT-CT combined with ultrasound as first-line studies, reserving the parathyroid-protocol CT for those glands that are still not able to be identified [56]. In the authors' practice, they reserve CT for reoperative cases.

Additional strategies used less often than those previously described include MRI, selective venous sampling, and parathyroid angiography. The value of MRI in the neck is limited by motion artifact secondary to respiration and deglutition [57], and selective venous sampling and angiography by the need for trained personnel and the invasive nature of these tests. Nevertheless, the procedures are still used in some specialized centers after failure of other imaging modalities. During selective venous sampling, the patient undergoes femoral venipuncture, and a baseline PTH is collected from the iliac vein. A catheter is then advanced to the superior vena cava to permit sampling from the neck and mediastinal veins for PTH levels. Gradients are then calculated between these samples and the control with a 50% increase in the PTH, suggesting drainage of the parathyroid adenoma into that vessel. This test has been found to be nearly 75% sensitive in those patients who have previously undergone nonlocalizing sestamibi [58]. Parathyroid angiography is another test that seeks to identify an abnormal gland by demonstration of the vascular blush of the adenoma after injection of the inferior thyroid artery; this test is mostly of historical value but has seen some renewed interest in its contemporary iteration of indocyanine-green angiography for intraoperative localization [59]. Overall, however, minimal experience with these procedures by most radiologists as well as the comparative time, expense, and risks associated when compared with noninvasive localization techniques have limited their routine use.

SURGICAL OPTIONS
Bilateral neck exploration
The gold-standard approach to surgical therapy for primary hyperparathyroidism has traditionally been bilateral neck exploration [60]. This technique requires the surgeon to pursue a full exploration of the neck with identification of all 4 glands and excision of the abnormal parathyroids. It is imperative for those patients in whom multigland disease is suspected, those who do

not successfully localize preoperatively, or patients affected by hereditary endocrinopathies [61]. The procedure is generally well tolerated, and risks include those inherent to procedures of the central neck, namely postoperative bleeding, recurrent laryngeal nerve injury, damage to the trachea or esophagus, transient or permanent hypocalcemia, and wound-related complications.

The patient is brought to the operating room and positioned supine with appropriate neck extension. Most frequently, this is performed under general anesthesia, with care taken to avoid neuromuscular blockade. The decision to use recurrent laryngeal nerve monitoring is based on surgeon preference but may require placement of an endotracheal tube enhanced with neuromonitoring electrodes. A curvilinear incision in made 1 to 2 cm below the cricoid cartilage and carried 2 to 4 cm in length between the medial borders of the sternocleidomastoid muscles, centered with the midline of the neck. A natural skin fold is selected whenever possible. Babcock clamps are used to grasp the sternohyoid and sternothyroid muscles and retract them laterally. Blunt dissection is used to elevate the muscles off the thyroid gland, and the thyroid is rotated medially to permit exposure of the tracheoesophageal groove. The superior gland is then localized by dissection on the posterolateral surface of the thyroid gland. Occasionally with adenomatous glands, the superior gland may fall behind the inferior artery toward the esophagus; the inferior gland may descend further as well, into the thyrothymic ligament or thymus itself. After both glands have been located, attention is turned to the contralateral side and the procedure is repeated. Once the abnormal gland or glands have been found, they are dissected away from the surrounding fat and ligated off of the vascular pedicle. Hemostasis is assured; the thyroid is returned to its anatomic location, and closure is performed of the strap muscles, platysma, and skin.

In the setting of 4-gland hyperplasia, a subtotal parathyroidectomy may be appropriate, entailing the excision of 3-and-one-half glands and retention of a 40 to 60 mg remnant gland with an intact vascular pedicle. Ideally, this gland is divided before excision of the other parathyroids to ensure continued viability throughout the case; an inferior gland is generally the best given the more anterior location if persistent disease develops and reoperation is needed. A clip with a 5-0 Prolene marking suture should be placed on the gland as an indicator to assist with future identification in this situation.

Overall, bilateral exploration is very effective, with the ability to fully survey all 4 glands and up to a 95% cure rate if performed by a high-volume surgeon [62]. In up to 16% of cases, however, the procedure will be made challenging because of ectopic positioning of one or more glands [63]. This problem can often be remedied by a thorough investigation of typical locations. For superior glands, the tracheoesophageal groove, retroesophageal space, posterior mediastinum, paraesophageal space, carotid sheath, and thyroid are the most common ectopic locations, in order of descending frequency. For the missing inferior gland, the thymus, anterior mediastinum, thyrothymic ligament, thyroid, carotid sheath, and the upper neck are the areas, in decreasing frequency, most commonly impacted by ectopic glands. The cervical removal of the thymic remnant is a potentially high-yield maneuver that can generally be used quickly and with impunity in the setting of the unidentified lower parathyroid. It can also be useful in suspected supernumerary glands [64]. Ectopic parathyroids embedded in the thyroid only impact 1% to 3% of patients [56], making this a comparatively rare situation.

Intraoperative adjuncts

A few techniques have been added to parathyroid surgery today to facilitate the successful operation. These techniques can be integrated into either standard or minimally invasive approaches.

The first is the use of intraoperative parathyroid hormone (IOPTH) monitoring, which capitalizes on the brief half-life of PTH, around 3 to 5 minutes. Venipuncture is performed preoperatively, during surgery, and within 5, 10, and 15 intervals following excision of the affected gland [65]. Either central draws from the internal jugular vein, made simple by its exposure in the surgical field, or peripheral collection from a large-bore intravenous line accessed by anesthesia is acceptable. These samples are sent for rapid parathyroid hormonal assay, and a 50% decline from preexcision value within 5 to 10 minutes postexcision is sufficient to predict cure in greater than 97% of patients [66,67]. Failure to drop as expected should alert the surgeon to the possibility of multigland disease [68].

Another potential intraoperative aid is use of radio-guided localization. Radio-guided localization harnesses the same concept as with the oft-used sestamibi scan. One to two hours before surgery, 10 mCl technetium 99m sestamibi is injected intravenously. Then, intraoperatively before incision, a background count will be acquired by placement of a gamma probe over the thyroid isthmus. During the exploration, the suspected adenoma is scanned in vivo; generally, the counts will be 50% greater than the background value. Following excision, ex vivo counts of the gland are taken. These counts should be equivalent to at least 20% of background and is an accurate marker for excision of either an adenoma or hyperplastic gland [69]. This technique has been demonstrated to be useful even in those patients who are found to have a nonlocalizing sestamibi study preoperatively [70] and to diminish operative times [71].

Ultrasound is one radiologic tool that can be used intraoperatively by the experienced operator. It has the distinct advantage of being able to be used preoperatively by the surgeon and then again during the course of the procedure to locate the previously identified gland.

Finally, less often used, but potentially quite useful, is localization of the parathyroid by venous sampling. This test requires bilateral internal jugular venous sampling with detection of a 10% differential as indicative of the affected side [72].

MINIMALLY INVASIVE PARATHYROIDECTOMY

Although bilateral neck exploration is the classic operative strategy, for the well-selected patient, a minimally invasive technique may be feasible. This enables a focused approach for single adenoma disease and results in shorter operative times, reduced morbidity, and higher rates of cure [5,73]. In fact, in those with a single adenoma, it is arguably the procedure of choice [74].

Minimally invasive parathyroidectomy is largely dependent on accurate preoperative localization and should be supplemented by intraoperative tools, including PTH monitoring and localization by radio-guidance. Commonly, this procedure can be performed both safely and comfortably under locoregional anesthesia [5,75].

Consistent principles as in standard parathyroidectomy apply. After the patient is placed in the supine position with gentle neck extension, a 2- to 3-cm incision is made 1 to 2 cm below the cricoid cartilage, generally centered in the midline. The strap muscles are separated in the midline. With anterolateral deflection of the sternothyroid and sternohyoid, the thyroid is bluntly dissected away from the muscles and mobilized medially. The target parathyroid and its associated pedicle are dissected out under direct vision. The gland is excised, hemostasis is assured, and cure is confirmed with intraoperative PTH testing. The suggestion of incomplete therapy should compel the surgeon to convert the operation to a bilateral neck exploration to look for multigland disease. Currently, around 10% of initial minimally invasive procedures will ultimately require conversion to a standard approach [76].

For those who successfully undergo this technique, however, these patients enjoy not only improved cosmesis but also shorter length of hospital stay (generally discharged home the same day) and lower cost of care [71].

Novel approaches to minimally invasive parathyroidectomy

More recently, several variations have been proposed that embrace but uniquely modify these original concepts of minimally invasive parathyroidectomy.

One approach is the focused lateral approach. This approach is best suited to the more posteriorly oriented parathyroid gland and avoids the typical initial steps of mobilization of the thyroid from the strap muscles, because they will instead be retracted in tandem [77]. A curvilinear incision is first created spanning 2 to 3 cm at the level of the adenoma (identified by radio-guidance or ultrasound). This incision will extend from the midline to the anterior border of the sternocleidomastoid. A plane is created between the sternocleidomastoid and the strap muscles. The former is retracted laterally, and the latter are retracted medially. The omohyoid is excluded, and the internal jugular vein comes into view. With care taken to avoid injury to the vagus nerve, the vein is retracted laterally, and the carotid is seen and dissected along the medial aspect to ultimately retract this laterally, as well. The edge of the thyroid capsule will then be rotated medially, permitting localization of an abnormal gland on the posterior surface and visualization of the tracheoesophageal groove. The parathyroid is excised deftly with assistance of intraoperative adjuncts, and the wound is closed in several layers. As with the anterior approach, positive preoperative localization is imperative for intraoperative success.

In addition to different open strategies, endoscopic and subsequent video-assisted approaches have been developed with the benefit of minimized pain and scarring and enhanced patient satisfaction. Endoscopic parathyroidectomy, first introduced by Gagner in 1996 [78], was one of the earliest such innovations. It requires access at the manubrium for a 5-mm camera with 2 or 3 lateral trocars for introduction of 2-mm needloscopic instruments. A plane is created below the platysma, and low-pressure continuous CO_2 insufflation (less than 8 mm Hg) along with external retractors is used to maintain the working space. Although this technique is not currently in widespread use, other endoscopic and remote access operations have since been established that hinge on this idea, including those from breast [79], axillary [80], and retroauricular [81] entry points. The introduction of robotic assistance has further revolutionized the execution of these operations. Their main advantage is excellent cosmesis, but new challenges arise, mostly owing to the need for extensive dissection to reach the target site, the protracted learning curve and potentially extended operative times, and risks related to excess CO_2 absorption.

Thus, an alternative that incorporates the benefit of video-assistance while using a more familiar point of entry has arisen, termed minimally invasive video-assisted parathyroidectomy. The most widely adopted iteration of this is the technique pioneered by Miccoli and colleagues [82]. A 1.5-cm incision is first created 2 cm above the sternal notch. A plane is developed between the thyroid and the strap muscles, and Farabeuf retractors are used to preserve the operative space. A 30° 5-mm endoscope and 2-mm surgical instruments are introduced directly into the incision. The procedure then progresses similarly to the previously described open minimally invasive approach. CO_2-mediated insufflation is unnecessary. Once identified, the parathyroid is usually dissected away bluntly using endoscopic visualization with spatulas and a small aspirator. The pedicle is clipped or ligated, and confirmation of a normalized IOPTH is sought. Although popular, there is still a long learning curve to mastery, with failure rates as high as 43% [83]. Some surgeons have chosen to simply use the camera alone in their execution of a minimally invasive parathyroidectomy, taking advantage of the enhanced videoscopic magnification.

EN BLOC RESECTION OF PARATHYROID CANCER

Although an uncommon variant of primary disease, parathyroid malignancy, if suspected preoperatively, requires diligent surgical planning to ensure the initial operation is oncologically sound. The tumor should be removed en bloc with the ipsilateral thyroid gland and potentially with a central compartment lymphadenectomy. This latter stipulation is controversial, because some argue that although lymph node metastases are infrequent, a potential source of disease may be left untreated and acts as a later source of local recurrence and distant spread should this step be obviated. It is important to recognize that there has been no evident improvement in survival demonstrated by this maneuver but a certain increase in risk for complications [84].

All preoperative imaging should be scrutinized for the possibility of aerodigestive tract involvement with suspicion of parathyroid cancer because it may be necessary to resect either a sliver or a segment of the trachea or esophagus if involved. Intraoperatively, a wide margin of normal tissue must be excised with the specimen, including the thymus if needed. It is critical that the gland's capsule not be disturbed to avoid the pitfall of malignant parathyromatosis and early recurrence. If the recurrent laryngeal nerve is found to be adherent to the tumor, this should be sacrificed.

In the case that a cancer be suspected intraoperatively based on dense adherence to surrounding structures, it is important to excise the gland en bloc just as those that have been diagnosed preoperatively. A frozen section biopsy need not be used; it is generally not useful, and when performed before excision, risks seeding the surgical bed.

Recurrence for these tumors will generally be within 2 to 5 years and may be secondary to incomplete excision or glandular disruption at the time of the index procedure. Repeat surgical therapy is used for palliative relief of the symptoms of hormonal excess.

SECONDARY AND TERTIARY HYPERPARATHYROIDISM

Although primary hyperparathyroidism is the form most typically treated surgically, it is important to also understand the role of surgical intervention in those with secondary and tertiary manifestations of the disease.

The secondary form of hyperparathyroidism commonly occurs in patients suffering from chronic kidney disease. It develops from renally mediated decreases in phosphate excretion and 1α-hydroxylase enzyme activity, which results in lower levels of functional 1,25-dihydroxyvitamin D3. These changes lead to hyperphosphatemia and diminished intestinal calcium absorption, producing the hypocalcemia that drives excess PTH secretion. The metabolic acidosis accompanying chronic kidney disease appears to have an additional individual impact on increasing intact PTH levels. Medical therapy is the mainstay for these patients, with phosphate binders, calcitriol, and calcium supplementation [85]. Dialysis is useful, and renal transplantation is definitive. Calcimimetic drugs like cinacalcet are a recently introduced pharmacologic option now available for refractory patients [86]. They operate by increasing the sensitivity of the calcium-sensing receptor to effectively lower PTH and can limit need for surgical therapy, but are not curative. Parathyroidectomy is generally reserved for severe or otherwise uncontrolled disease.

Tertiary hyperparathyroidism is the result of development of autonomous, unregulated glands following a long-standing period of secondary hyperparathyroidism. These patients are generally renal-transplant recipients with a prevalence of up to 30% with comorbid hyperparathyroidism in this population [87]. In contrast to the secondary form, surgery is the treatment of choice, although recent reports suggest that most of these patients never receive appropriate therapy.

Generally, the prescribed operation for these patients is the subtotal or 3-and-one-half gland parathyroidectomy, as previously outlined above, in order to adequately address all hyperplastic disease. An additional surgical option, but one less favored for first-time exploration, includes total parathyroidectomy with autotransplantation [88]. In this, the retained 40 to 50 mg parathyroid fragment is explanted and sectioned into $1 \times 1 \times 3$ mm segments. These segments are then placed into individual compartments within the brachioradialis muscle of the nondominant arm to engraft.

Despite subtotal and total excision as the classic surgical therapies for tertiary disease, some do still call for a more restrained operative approach. Single- or double-gland adenoma in these patients has previously been demonstrated in 20% to 28% [87,89,90], and these surgeons contend that, for these patients, a bilateral exploration with selective resection will still be curative.

PERSISTENT OR RECURRENT DISEASE

Reoperative surgery may need to be considered for the 5% to 10% of patients that display either persistent disease, that is, failure to achieve a euhormonal state with 6 months of surgery, or recurrent disease, which describes those with delayed development of refractory hypercalcemia following 6 months of normal levels. Recidivist disease may result secondary to inadequate localization of the adenoma at the initial operation, missed adenomas or multigland hyperplasia, truly recurrent adenomas or hyperplasia, or, more rarely, improperly managed parathyroid adenocarcinoma [23,91–94]. Some data support that those with a PTH $\geq$40 at the end of initial parathyroidectomy should be followed more closely, with increased risk of persistent disease or recurrence at 2 years [95].

Reoperative patients are generally best managed by experienced endocrine surgeons [96] because these surgeries are generally more challenging and pose greater risk for significant complications, including recurrent laryngeal nerve injury and permanent hypocalcemia. Decision to proceed with surgery should be a careful risk/benefit analysis given the increased morbidity, including, if a repeat exploration appears to be indicated, review of previous operative and pathology results. Biochemical panels should be rechecked, and imaging modalities, even if negative previously, should be repeated. A 4D CT scan may be especially useful and is highly sensitive, even in this remedial situation [91]. In the operating room, adjuncts like radio-guidance should be used to localize the gland if possible and limit dissection. Some champion a lateral approach to avoid the previously violated planes in the last operation, but no matter which surgical technique is used, it is imperative to exercise caution and limit unnecessary manipulation.

Most missed parathyroid glands will be found to be in relatively eutopic locations [92] but the surgeon should be prepared to explore common ectopic locations as previously described. Some glands will be determined to be in the mediastinum, for which both open approaches to excision or video-assisted thoracoscopic approaches may be feasible [97].

SUMMARY

Hyperparathyroidism is a common endocrine condition with a measurable impact on quality of life and overall health. It has the benefit of a very effective surgical treatment. Thus, it is essential that the surgeon be well versed in appropriate diagnostics, which can identify the causative abnormality, and the protean surgical strategies, which can be tailored to optimize patient outcomes.

References

[1] Wilhelm SM, Wang TS, Ruan DT, et al. The American Association of Endocrine Surgeons guidelines for definitive management of primary hyperparathyroidism. JAMA Surg 2016;151(10):959–68.

[2] Maccallum WG, Voegtlin C. On the relation of tetany to the parathyroid glands and to calcium metabolism. J Exp Med 1909;11(1):118–51.

[3] Rolleston H. The history of endocrinology. Br Med J 1937;1(3984):1033–6.

[4] Luckhardt AB, Rosenbloom PJ. The control and cure of parathyroid tetany in normal and pregnant animals. Science 1922;56(1437):48–9.

[5] Udelsman R. Six hundred fifty-six consecutive explorations for primary hyperparathyroidism. Ann Surg 2002;235(5):665–70 [discussion: 70–2].

[6] Burke JF, Chen H, Gosain A. Parathyroid conditions in childhood. Semin Pediatr Surg 2014;23(2):66–70.

[7] Fancy T, Gallagher D 3rd, Hornig JD. Surgical anatomy of the thyroid and parathyroid glands. Otolaryngol Clin North Am 2010;43(2):221–7, vii.

[8] Thompson NW, Eckhauser FE, Harness JK. The anatomy of primary hyperparathyroidism. Surgery 1982;92(5):814–21.

[9] Bliss RD, Gauger PG, Delbridge LW. Surgeon's approach to the thyroid gland: surgical anatomy and the importance of technique. World J Surg 2000;24(8):891–7.

[10] Mazeh H, Kouniavsky G, Schneider DF, et al. Intrathyroidal parathyroid glands: small, but mighty (a Napoleon phenomenon). Surgery 2012;152(6):1193–200.

[11] Scharpf J, Randolph GW. Thyroid and parathyroid glands. In: Lee K, Chan Y, Goddard JC, editors. KJ Lee's Essential Otolaryngology. New York: McGraw-Hill Education; 2015. p. 606–40.

[12] Lew JI, Solorzano CC. Surgical management of primary hyperparathyroidism: state of the art. Surg Clin North Am 2009;89(5):1205–25.

[13] Akerstrom G, Malmaeus J, Bergstrom R. Surgical anatomy of human parathyroid glands. Surgery 1984;95(1):14–21.

[14] Pattou FN, Pellissier LC, Noel C, et al. Supernumerary parathyroid glands: frequency and surgical significance in treatment of renal hyperparathyroidism. World J Surg 2000;24(11): 1330–4.

[15] McIntyre CJ, Allen JL, Constantinides VA, et al. Patterns of disease in patients at a tertiary referral centre requiring reoperative parathyroidectomy. Ann R Coll Surg Engl 2015;97(8):598–602.

[16] Clark OH. Hyperparathyroidism. Surg Technol Int 1991;I:291–4.

[17] Chen H, Parkerson S, Udelsman R. Parathyroidectomy in the elderly: do the benefits outweigh the risks? World J Surg 1998;22(6):531–5 [discussion: 5–6].

[18] Uden P, Chan A, Duh QY, et al. Primary hyperparathyroidism in younger and older patients: symptoms and outcome of surgery. World J Surg 1992;16(4):791–7 [discussion: 8].

[19] Miller BS, Dimick J, Wainess R, et al. Age- and sex-related incidence of surgically treated primary hyperparathyroidism. World J Surg 2008;32(5):795–9.

[20] Murray SE, Pathak PR, Pontes DS, et al. Timing of symptom improvement after parathyroidectomy for primary hyperparathyroidism. Surgery 2013;154(6):1463–9.

[21] Mundy GR, Cove DH, Fisken R. Primary hyperparathyroidism: changes in the pattern of clinical presentation. Lancet 1980;1(8182):1317–20.

[22] Abboud B, Sleilaty G, Helou E, et al. Existence and anatomic distribution of double parathy-roid adenoma. Laryngoscope 2005;115(6):1128–31.

[23] Alhefdhi A, Schneider DF, Sippel R, et al. Recurrent and persistence primary hyperparathy-roidism occurs more frequently in patients with double adenomas. J Surg Res 2014;190(1): 198–202.

[24] Rizzoli R, Green J 3rd, Marx SJ. Primary hyperparathyroidism in familial multiple endocrine neoplasia type I. Long-term follow-up of serum calcium levels after parathyroidectomy. Am J Med 1985;78(3):467–74.

[25] Shane E. Parathyroid carcinoma. Curr Ther Endocrinol Metab 1997;6:565–8.

[26] Cetani F, Pardi E, Borsari S, et al. Genetic analyses of the HRPT2 gene in primary hyperpara-thyroidism: germline and somatic mutations in familial and sporadic parathyroid tumors. J Clin Endocrinol Metab 2004;89(11):5583–91.

[27] Sharretts JM, Kebebew E, Simonds WF. Parathyroid cancer. Semin Oncol 2010;37(6): 580–90.

[28] Silverberg SJ, Shane E, Jacobs TP, et al. A 10-year prospective study of primary hyperpara-thyroidism with or without parathyroid surgery. N Engl J Med 1999;341(17):1249–55.

[29] Tamura Y, Araki A, Chiba Y, et al. Remarkable increase in lumbar spine bone mineral density and amelioration in biochemical markers of bone turnover after parathyroidectomy in elderly patients with primary hyperparathyroidism: a 5-year follow-up study. J Bone Miner Metab 2007;25(4):226–31.

[30] Murray SE, Pathak PR, Schaefer SC, et al. Improvement of sleep disturbance and insomnia following parathyroidectomy for primary hyperparathyroidism. World J Surg 2014;38(3): 542–8.

[31] Reiher AE, Mazeh H, Schaefer S, et al. Symptoms of gastroesophageal reflux disease improve after parathyroidectomy. Surgery 2012;152(6):1232–7.

[32] Adler JT, Sippel RS, Schaefer S, et al. Surgery improves quality of life in patients with "mild" hyperparathyroidism. Am J Surg 2009;197(3):284–90.

[33] Weber T, Eberle J, Messelhauser U, et al. Parathyroidectomy, elevated depression scores, and suicidal ideation in patients with primary hyperparathyroidism: results of a prospective multicenter study. JAMA Surg 2013;148(2):109–15.

[34] Vestergaard P, Mollerup CL, Frokjaer VG, et al. Cardiovascular events before and after sur-gery for primary hyperparathyroidism. World J Surg 2003;27(2):216–22.

[35] Hedback G, Oden A. Death risk factor analysis in primary hyperparathyroidism. Eur J Clin Invest 1998;28(12):1011–8.

[36] Hedback G, Oden A. Increased risk of death from primary hyperparathyroidism—an up-date. Eur J Clin Invest 1998;28(4):271–6.

[37] Hagstrom E, Hellman P, Larsson TE, et al. Plasma parathyroid hormone and the risk of car-diovascular mortality in the community. Circulation 2009;119(21):2765–71.

[38] Bilezikian JP, Brandi ML, Eastell R, et al. Guidelines for the management of asymptomatic primary hyperparathyroidism: summary statement from the Fourth International Workshop. J Clin Endocrinol Metab 2014;99(10):3561–9.

[39] Silverberg SJ, Clarke BL, Peacock M, et al. Current issues in the presentation of asymptom-atic primary hyperparathyroidism: proceedings of the Fourth International Workshop. J Clin Endocrinol Metab 2014;99(10):3580–94.

[40] Yener Ozturk F, Erol S, Canat MM, et al. Patients with normocalcemic primary hyperpara-thyroidism may have similar metabolic profile as hypercalcemic patients. Endocr J 2016;63(2):111–8.

[41] Coakley AJ, Kettle AG, Wells CP, et al. 99Tcm sestamibi—a new agent for parathyroid imag-ing. Nucl Med Commun 1989;10(11):791–4.

[42] Ruda JM, Hollenbeak CS, Stack BC Jr. A systematic review of the diagnosis and treatment of primary hyperparathyroidism from 1995 to 2003. Otolaryngol Head Neck Surg 2005;132(3):359–72.

[43] Chang CW, Tsue TT, Hermreck AS, et al. Efficacy of preoperative dual-phase sestamibi scanning in hyperparathyroidism. Am J Otolaryngol 2000;21(6):355–9.

[44] Profanter C, Wetscher GJ, Gabriel M, et al. CT-MIBI image fusion: a new preoperative localization technique for primary, recurrent, and persistent hyperparathyroidism. Surgery 2004;135(2):157–62.

[45] Steward DL, Danielson GP, Afman CE, et al. Parathyroid adenoma localization: surgeon-performed ultrasound versus sestamibi. Laryngoscope 2006;116(8):1380–4.

[46] Roy M, Mazeh H, Chen H, et al. Incidence and localization of ectopic parathyroid adenomas in previously unexplored patients. World J Surg 2013;37(1):102–6.

[47] Ryan S, Courtney D, Moriariu J, et al. Surgical management of primary hyperparathyroidism. Eur Arch Otorhinolaryngol 2017;274(12):4225–32.

[48] Weiss DM, Chen H. Role of cervical ultrasound in detecting thyroid pathology in primary hyperparathyroidism. J Surg Res 2014;190(2):575–8.

[49] Owens CL, Rekhtman N, Sokoll L, et al. Parathyroid hormone assay in fine-needle aspirate is useful in differentiating inadvertently sampled parathyroid tissue from thyroid lesions. Diagn Cytopathol 2008;36(4):227–31.

[50] Triggiani V, Resta F, Giagulli VA, et al. Parathyroid hormone determination in ultrasound-guided fine needle aspirates allows the differentiation between thyroid and parathyroid lesions: our experience and review of the literature. Endocr Metab Immune Disord Drug Targets 2013;13(4):351–8.

[51] Cheung K, Wang TS, Farrokhyar F, et al. A meta-analysis of preoperative localization techniques for patients with primary hyperparathyroidism. Ann Surg Oncol 2012;19(2): 577–83.

[52] Kutler DI, Moquete R, Kazam E, et al. Parathyroid localization with modified 4D-computed tomography and ultrasonography for patients with primary hyperparathyroidism. Laryngoscope 2011,121(6):1219 24.

[53] Rodgers SE, Hunter GJ, Hamberg LM, et al. Improved preoperative planning for directed parathyroidectomy with 4-dimensional computed tomography. Surgery 2006;140(6): 932–40 [discussion: 40–1].

[54] Starker LF, Mahajan A, Bjorklund P, et al. 4D parathyroid CT as the initial localization study for patients with de novo primary hyperparathyroidism. Ann Surg Oncol 2011;18(6): 1723–8.

[55] De Gregorio L, Lubitz CC, Hodin RA, et al. The truth about double adenomas: incidence, localization, and intraoperative parathyroid hormone. J Am Coll Surg 2016;222(6): 1044–52.

[56] Wang TS, Cheung K, Farrokhyar F, et al. Would scan, but which scan? A cost-utility analysis to optimize preoperative imaging for primary hyperparathyroidism. Surgery 2011;150(6): 1286–94.

[57] Stevens SK, Chang JM, Clark OH, et al. Detection of abnormal parathyroid glands in postoperative patients with recurrent hyperparathyroidism: sensitivity of MR imaging. AJR Am J Roentgenol 1993;160(3):607–12.

[58] Witteveen JE, Kievit J, van Erkel AR, et al. The role of selective venous sampling in the management of persistent hyperparathyroidism revisited. Eur J Endocrinol 2010;163(6): 945–52.

[59] Zaidi N, Bucak E, Okoh A, et al. The utility of indocyanine green near infrared fluorescent imaging in the identification of parathyroid glands during surgery for primary hyperparathyroidism. J Surg Oncol 2016;113(7):771–4.

[60] Laird AM, Libutti SK. Minimally invasive parathyroidectomy versus bilateral neck exploration for primary hyperparathyroidism. Surg Oncol Clin N Am 2016;25(1):103–18.

[61] Shah-Becker S, Goldenberg D. Surgical exploration for hyperparathyroidism. Operative techniques in otolaryngology-head and neck surgery 2016;27(3):129–35.

[62] Gunasekaran S, Wallace H, Snowden C, et al. Parathyroid ectopia: development of a surgical algorithm based on operative findings. J Laryngol Otol 2015;129(11):1115–20.

[63] Phitayakorn R, McHenry CR. Incidence and location of ectopic abnormal parathyroid glands. Am J Surg 2006;191(3):418–23.

[64] Scharpf J, Kyriazidis N, Randolph GW. Anatomy and embryology of the parathyroid gland. Operative techniques in otolaryngology 2016;27(3):117–21.

[65] Irvin GL 3rd, Dembrow VD, Prudhomme DL. Operative monitoring of parathyroid gland hyperfunction. Am J Surg 1991;162(4):299–302.

[66] Chen H, Mack E, Starling JR. A comprehensive evaluation of perioperative adjuncts during minimally invasive parathyroidectomy: which is most reliable? Ann Surg 2005;242(3): 375–80 [discussion: 80–3].

[67] Barczynski M, Konturek A, Cichon S, et al. Intraoperative parathyroid hormone assay improves outcomes of minimally invasive parathyroidectomy mainly in patients with a presumed solitary parathyroid adenoma and missing concordance of preoperative imaging. Clin Endocrinol (Oxf) 2007;66(6):878–85.

[68] Lee S, Ryu H, Morris LF, et al. Operative failure in minimally invasive parathyroidectomy utilizing an intraoperative parathyroid hormone assay. Ann Surg Oncol 2014;21(6): 1878–83.

[69] Murphy C, Norman J. The 20% rule: a simple, instantaneous radioactivity measurement defines cure and allows elimination of frozen sections and hormone assays during parathyroidectomy. Surgery 1999;126(6):1023–8 [discussion: 8–9].

[70] Chen H, Sippel RS, Schaefer S. The effectiveness of radioguided parathyroidectomy in patients with negative technetium tc 99m-sestamibi scans. Arch Surg 2009;144(7):643–8.

[71] Goldstein RE, Blevins L, Delbeke D, et al. Effect of minimally invasive radioguided parathyroidectomy on efficacy, length of stay, and costs in the management of primary hyperparathyroidism. Ann Surg 2000;231(5):732–42.

[72] Ito F, Sippel R, Lederman J, et al. The utility of intraoperative bilateral internal jugular venous sampling with rapid parathyroid hormone testing. Ann Surg 2007;245(6):959–63.

[73] Bergenfelz A, Lindblom P, Tibblin S, et al. Unilateral versus bilateral neck exploration for primary hyperparathyroidism: a prospective randomized controlled trial. Ann Surg 2002;236(5):543–51.

[74] Adler JT, Sippel RS, Chen H. The influence of surgical approach on quality of life after parathyroid surgery. Ann Surg Oncol 2008;15(6):1559–65.

[75] Chen H, Sokoll LJ, Udelsman R. Outpatient minimally invasive parathyroidectomy: a combination of sestamibi-SPECT localization, cervical block anesthesia, and intraoperative parathyroid hormone assay. Surgery 1999;126(6):1016–21 [discussion: 21–2].

[76] Hughes DT, Miller BS, Park PB, et al. Factors in conversion from minimally invasive parathyroidectomy to bilateral parathyroid exploration for primary hyperparathyroidism. Surgery 2013;154(6):1428–34 [discussion: 34–5].

[77] Shindo ML, Rosenthal JM. Minimal access parathyroidectomy using the focused lateral approach: technique, indication, and results. Arch Otolaryngol Head Neck Surg 2007;133(12):1227–34.

[78] Gagner M. Endoscopic subtotal parathyroidectomy in patients with primary hyperparathyroidism. Br J Surg 1996;83(6):875.

[79] Ohgami M, Ishii S, Arisawa Y, et al. Scarless endoscopic thyroidectomy: breast approach for better cosmesis. Surg Laparosc Endosc Percutan Tech 2000;10(1):1–4.

[80] Karagkounis G, Uzun DD, Mason DP, et al. Robotic surgery for primary hyperparathyroidism. Surg Endosc 2014;28(9):2702–7.

[81] Lee JM, Byeon HK, Choi EC, et al. Robotic excision of a huge parathyroid adenoma via a retroauricular approach. J Craniofac Surg 2015;26(1):e55–8.

[82] Miccoli P, Pinchera A, Cecchini G, et al. Minimally invasive, video-assisted parathyroid surgery for primary hyperparathyroidism. J Endocrinol Invest 1997;20(7):429–30.

[83] Hessman O, Westerdahl J, Al-Suliman N, et al. Randomized clinical trial comparing open with video-assisted minimally invasive parathyroid surgery for primary hyperparathyroidism. Br J Surg 2010;97(2):177–84.

[84] Hsu KT, Sippel RS, Chen H, et al. Is central lymph node dissection necessary for parathyroid carcinoma? Surgery 2014;156(6):1336–41 [discussion: 41].

[85] Gale SC, Demeure MJ. Secondary and tertiary hyperparathyroidism. In: Cameron JL, editor. Current surgical therapy. 8th edition. Philadelphia: Elsevier Mosby; 2005. p. 610–4.

[86] Ballinger AE, Palmer SC, Nistor I, et al. Calcimimetics for secondary hyperparathyroidism in chronic kidney disease patients. Cochrane Database Syst Rev 2014;(12):CD006254.

[87] Lou I, Schneider DF, Leverson G, et al. Parathyroidectomy is underused in patients with tertiary hyperparathyroidism after renal transplantation. Surgery 2016;159(1):172–9.

[88] Shepet K, Alhefdhi A, Usedom R, et al. Parathyroid cryopreservation after parathyroidectomy: a worthwhile practice? Ann Surg Oncol 2013;20(7):2256–60.

[89] Nichol PF, Starling JR, Mack E, et al. Long-term follow-up of patients with tertiary hyperparathyroidism treated by resection of a single or double adenoma. Ann Surg 2002;235(5): 673–8 [discussion: 78–80].

[90] Kilgo MS, Pirsch JD, Warner TF, et al. Tertiary hyperparathyroidism after renal transplantation: surgical strategy. Surgery 1998;124(4):677–83 [discussion: 83–4].

[91] Mortenson MM, Evans DB, Lee JE, et al. Parathyroid exploration in the reoperative neck: improved preoperative localization with 4D-computed tomography. J Am Coll Surg 2008;206(5):888–95 [discussion: 95–6].

[92] Akerstrom G, Rudberg C, Grimelius L, et al. Causes of failed primary exploration and technical aspects of re-operation in primary hyperparathyroidism. World J Surg 1992;16(4): 562–8 [discussion: 8–9].

[93] Mariette C, Pellissier L, Combemale F, et al. Reoperation for persistent or recurrent primary hyperparathyroidism. Langenbecks Arch Surg 1998;383(2):174–9.

[94] Shen W, Duren M, Morita E, et al. Reoperation for persistent or recurrent primary hyperparathyroidism. Arch Surg 1996;131(8):861–7 [discussion: 7–9].

[95] Rajaei MH, Bentz AM, Schneider DF, et al. Justified follow-up: a final intraoperative parathyroid hormone (ioPTH) over 40 pg/mL is associated with an increased risk of persistence and recurrence in primary hyperparathyroidism. Ann Surg Oncol 2015;22(2):454–9.

[96] Chen H, Wang TS, Yen TW, et al. Operative failures after parathyroidectomy for hyperparathyroidism: the influence of surgical volume. Ann Surg 2010;252(4):691–5.

[97] Weigel TL, Murphy J, Kabbani L, et al. Radioguided thoracoscopic mediastinal parathyroidectomy with intraoperative parathyroid hormone testing. Ann Thorac Surg 2005;80(4): 1262–5.

Advances in Surgery 52 (2018) 155–177

ADVANCES IN SURGERY

ELSEVIER
MOSBY

Management of Aortoenteric Fistula

Jayer Chung, MD, MSc

Division of Vascular Surgery and Endovascular Therapy, Michael E. DeBakey Department of Surgery, Baylor College of Medicine, One Baylor Plaza, MS 390, Houston, TX 77030, USA

Keywords

- Antibiotic impregnated Dacron • Aortoenteric fistula • Aortoenteric erosion
- Aortic graft infection • Axillobifemoral bypass • Cryopreserved allograft
- Neoaortoiliac surgery

Key points

- Aortoenteric fistulas are one of the most fatal conditions that a surgeon may face, with a postoperative mortality that approaches 50%.
- Although axillobifemoral bypass, removal of the infection, and repair of the enteric defect has been the traditional gold standard, multiple in situ reconstructions have evolved to overcome the disadvantages of axillobifemoral bypass.
- Aortoenteric fistulas complicating endograft placement represents an especially technically difficult repair.
- Most gastrointestinal complications after aortoenteric fistula repair result in mortality.

INTRODUCTION

Aortoenteric fistulae (AEF) represent the most lethal subset of aortic infections. AEF remain rare, despite the innumerable episodes of bacteremia that people experience in their lifetime. Patients' presentation range from those with an occult anemia, to those with catastrophic gastrointestinal (GI) hemorrhage and sepsis. Technical challenges include scarring from the infection and often, reoperative fields. The increased prevalence of endovascular aortic aneurysm repair (EVAR) mandates that modern surgeons need to be cognizant of the

Disclosure: The author has nothing to disclose.

E-mail address: Jayer.Chung@bcm.edu

https://doi.org/10.1016/j.yasu.2018.03.007

Abbreviations

AAA	Abdominal aortic aneurysm
AEE	Aortoenteric erosion
AEF	Aortoenteric fistula
CTA	Computed tomographic angiography
EGD	Esophagogastroduodenoscopy
EVAR	Endovascular aortic aneurysm repair
GI	Gastrointestinal
NAIS	Neoaortoiliac surgery

technical challenges associated with infected EVAR removal. The patients themselves are challenging, owing the presence of multiple comorbidities that render them relatively nutritionally and immunocompromised.

Cryopreserved allografts and endovascular stent grafts provide modern surgeons with alternative nuances to manage AEF. However, the foundation of therapy remains accurate and timely diagnosis, antibiotic therapy, resuscitation, surgical resection and debridement, and arterial and enteric reconstruction. The surgeon must balance the need to remove the infectious nidus, correct the bleeding source, and restore arterial and intestinal continuity against the ability of the patient to survive the physiologic insult of the surgery. To do so, surgeons must become familiar with the various options for arterial and enteric reconstruction to best tailor care for their patients.

DEFINITIONS AND EPIDEMIOLOGY

Primary AEF are defined as a spontaneous communication between the native aorta and any portion of the GI tract [1,2]. Primary AEF was first described by Sir Ashley Cooper in 1822 [3]. Primary AEF are infrequent. Since the initial description, collective experience in the world literature remains limited to less than 300 case reports [1,2]. The incidence of primary AEF varies depending on the study base, with Voorhoeve and colleagues [4] describing an incidence of 0.04% to 0.07% among patients who died of massive GI hemorrhage. The incidence is higher among patients with abdominal aortic aneurysms (AAAs), ranging from 0.69% to 2.36% [5,6].

Secondary AEF occur when there is a false communication between an enteric structure and a previous aortic graft. The incidence has been reported to be 1.6% after open AAA repair in the 36-year experience from the Mayo Clinic [7]. These occurred after a median follow-up of 4.3 years [7]. The reported rate of AEF is somewhat higher than expected, because the overall rate of all graft infections after open aortic surgery within randomized controlled trials and large retrospective registries ranges similarly between 0.19% to 2.0% [8,9]. Ascertainment and referral bias may be inflating the observed rate of AEF in the Mayo Clinic series [7]. The limited sample sizes of some of the largest single center experiences with AEF ratify the fact that the true rate of AEF after open aortic reconstruction may be lower than is reported in the Mayo experience. EVAR decreases the incidence of AEF to the range of 0.02% to 0.46% after AAA repair [10,11]. However, when EVAR is performed to repair an aortic pseudoaneurysm, the rate of AEF is significantly higher at 3.9% [10]. The median time to the development of AEF after EVAR has been reported to be 32 months, which seems to be shorter compared with the time to develop an AEF after open aortic surgery.

Secondary AEF are further classified as an aortoenteric erosion (AEE), and true AEF. AEE occur when there is an abnormal communication between the mucosa of the GI tract that involves the prosthetic graft, but not the surgical anastomosis between the graft and the aorta (Fig. 1). Bleeding from AEE occurs secondary to mucosal irritation. In contrast, an AEF is defined as an abnormal communication between the mucosa of the GI tract and the anastomosis of the graft and the aorta. Although AEF tend to present with more catastrophic bleeding, the distinction is largely academic, because the management of either entity is similar, without significant differences in outcomes. Hence, many studies group the 2 entities together [12]. Therefore, for the purposes of this article, the term AEF is used to include patients with AEE.

PATHOPHYSIOLOGY

The precise etiology of primary AEF formation is unclear, but it is most likely a combination of infection, degeneration of the aorta and enteric structure, and chronic mechanical pulsatile trauma resulting in erosion and fistula formation over time (Fig. 2) [1–6]. AAA is discovered in 83% of subjects with a primary AEF, indicating that the repetitive mechanical stress of repeated pulsation of the aneurysm coupled with the weakening of the aorta and GI tract are necessary features of primary AEF [13]. Primary AEF tends to occur in older patients, with a mean age of 64 years. Men are afflicted more frequently than women, likely owing to the increased prevalence of AAA in males [13]. Infection seems to be central to the development of primary AEF, with *Klebsiella* and *Salmonella* species most frequently implicated. Other reported etiologies include radiation damage, foreign bodies, cancer, radiotherapy, tuberculosis, and syphilis [1–6,13].

Pooled results show there that 80% of secondary AEF patients are male, again reflecting the male prevalence of AAA as well as atherosclerotic disease. Secondary AEF tends to afflict older patients; the median age has been reported to be 70 years. Infection seems to be central to the formation of secondary AEF. The proposed mechanism consists of infection resulting in inflammation, which subsequently degrades the aortic graft anastomosis, resulting in pseudoaneurysm formation. The added mechanical stress coupled with the inflammatory response results ultimately in an AEF. The central role of infection has been confirmed with animal models, particularly with virulent organisms like *S aureus* [14]. The results from animal models highlight the need for stringent adherence to surgical antiseptic technique, as well as perioperative antibiotics to prevent seeding of the aortic prosthesis at the time of initial surgery. Gentle

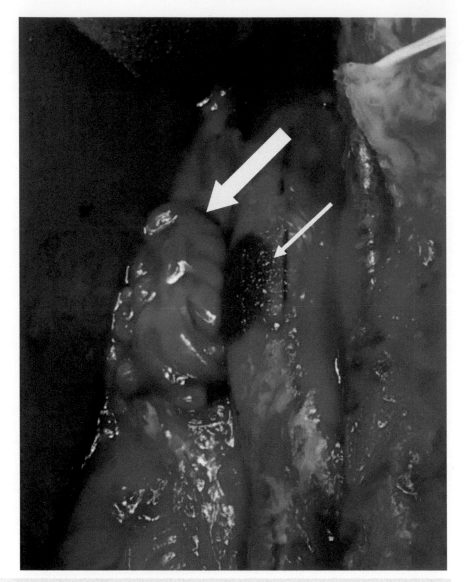

Fig. 1. Aortoenteric erosion (AEE) involving the body of a previously placed aortobifemoral bypass graft, and the fourth portion of the duodenum. Note the dark stain on the graft (*thin yellow arrow*), indicative of chronic exposure to bile. The adjacent bowel defect (*large yellow arrow*) was managed with resection and reanastomosis.

handling of the bowel is also critical to limit inadvertent retraction injury, thermal injury from electrocautery, or sharp injury (see Fig. 2).

The underlying original indication for the aortic procedure does not seem to predict whether the patient ultimately develops a secondary AEF. The most

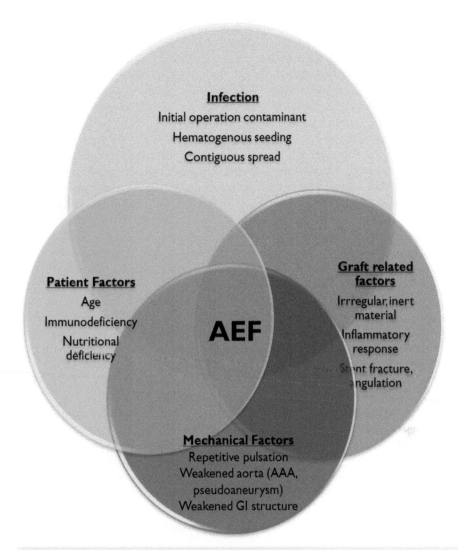

Fig. 2. Pathophysiology of aortoenteric fistulas (AEF) formation. Primary and secondary AEF occur via similar mechanisms, with the exception of the presence of the aortic prosthesis. The microorganisms responsible for the AEF are also somewhat different between primary and secondary AEF. Infection seems to be the main underlying cause of AEF. AAA, abdominal aortic aneurysm; GI, gastrointestinal.

common original procedures are open aneurysm repair (36%) and bypass grafting for aortoiliac occlusive disease (30%) [10,15]. It is unclear whether an end-to-end reconstruction versus and end-to-side anastomosis potentiates further pulsatile pressure on the adjacent bowel. Intuitively, it seems that end-to-side anastomoses may project anteriorly more than end-to-end anastomosis, resulting in greater transmission of repetitive pressure between the aortic graft and the adjacent bowel. Regardless, assiduous coverage of the graft with well-vascularized retroperitoneal tissue after aortic reconstructions is necessary to cushion the graft from the enteric structures. The most common site of primary and secondary AEF formation is the duodenum (62%) followed by the jejunum and ileum (12%), and then colon (5%). Pooled analyses shows that AEF occur somewhat more frequently than AEE [10,13,15], although some of the series show that AEE occurred more frequently [12].

The series describing AEF after EVAR are small. Hence, determining the risk factors for AEF after EVAR specifically are difficult to discern from those that predispose to EVAR infection without AEF. Urgent indications for the original EVAR seem to predispose to infection. Bergqvist and colleagues [16] reported on 16 cases of AEF after EVAR, and found that more than 37% were related to endoleak and/or persistent sac expansion. More than 30% of EVAR-related AEF were related to a defect in the aortic stents themselves (fracture, erosion of the stent, or angulation of the stent) [16]. These factors suggest that mechanical factors are critical to the pathogenesis of EVAR-related AEF. Infection contributes as well, given that patients receive multiple procedures for endoleaks and sac expansion, each with an iterative risk of seeding the graft (see Fig. 2) [11,16]. The median time to developing an AEF after EVAR is shorter than for open surgery. The author surmises that his results from more frequent surveillance of EVAR patients relative to open aortic surgical patients.

MICROBIOLOGY OF AORTOENTERIC FISTULA
Understanding the microbiology is critical to determining empiric antibiotic regimens. Primary AEF, as mentioned previously have been associated most frequently with *Salmonella* or *Klebsiella* species. However, multiple other organisms have been isolated, such as tuberculosis, syphilis, *Staphylococcus, Streptococcus, Escherichia coli, Enterococcus faecalis, Clostridium septicum,* and *Lactobacillus.* [2,4,5,13] Unfortunately, data are limited, because many authors did not describe collecting cultures at the time of operation [13]. The data suggest, however, the infections responsible for the development of AEF differ between primary and secondary AEF.

Secondary AEF after open aortic reconstructions are polymicrobial in two-thirds of patients [12,15]. Other species also cultured from the aorta are *Staphylococcus epidermidis, Klebsiella, Veillonella, Staphylococcus hominis,* and group B *Streptococcus* [15]. Other series report a predominance of gram-negative organisms [17]. The variability likely results from shear heterogeneity of microorganisms that can be present in the GI tract. One common theme, however, is the prevalence of *Candida* species, which appear in two-thirds of secondary AEF [10–13,15,17]. Although the cultured microorganisms after AEF have developed are heterogeneous, the actual organism(s) responsible for initiating the perigraft inflammation and subsequent fistula are frequently unable to be determined.

With respect to AEF after EVAR, the microbial isolates were similar to those derived from secondary AEF after open aortic reconstructions. Approximately

20% of the cultured isolates were polymicrobial. The most frequent organisms isolated included *S aureus,* and *E coli.* Other organisms include *Enterococcus, S epidermidis, Klebsiella, Pseudomonas aeruginosa, Bacteroides fragilis, Fusobacterium,* and *Haemophyilis* species [10,11]. Again, the inciting infection is difficult to ascertain once the AEF has developed, because bowel contamination likely overwhelms the infection that may have incited the AEF. Similar to AEF after open aortic reconstructions, *Candida* infections occur frequently [10–13,15,17].

DIAGNOSIS OF AORTOENTERIC FISTULA

Delays in diagnosis can be particularly disastrous in the setting of AEF. Delays persist owing to lack of knowledge regarding common clinical presentations, as well as the appropriate role of diagnostic testing. AEF occurs less frequently than other etiologies of upper GI bleeding and is, therefore, often overlooked. Physicians must maintain a high index of suspicion, because the presentation of AEF does not always fit within common clinical patterns. Unfortunately, each of the diagnostic modalities imperfectly diagnose AEF. Because of the difficulties accurately diagnosing AEF, and catastrophic consequences of inappropriate delay, it behooves surgeons to understand the strengths and weaknesses of different diagnostic modalities to expedite patient care.

Common clinical presentations

For primary AEF, the classic triad of GI hemorrhage, abdominal pain, and pulsatile abdominal mass was initially described by Sir Ashley Cooper in his seminal work [3]. With the exception of a history of prior aortic surgery, the presentation of primary and secondary AEF are similar. GI bleeding is the most frequent symptoms in primary AEF, affecting up to 94% of patients, with abdominal pain occurring in 48% and shock in 33% [13].

Similarly, GI bleeding is the most commonly reported symptom from the 3 largest single-center retrospective series on secondary AEF, with a cumulative reported prevalence of 48% [12,13,15,17,18]. Patients frequently present with a "herald bleed," where the bleeding temporarily ceases before the recurrence of life-threatening hemorrhage hours to days later [12]. The cumulative incidence of abdominal pain was present in 40%, with shock (hemorrhagic or septic) described in 23%. Other presenting symptoms include graft thrombosis with acute limb ischemia, peripheral abscess, nonspecific malaise with leukocytosis, and bacteremia. A pulsatile mass is inconsistently reported, so it is unclear whether the classic triad is truly valid. Some authors consider the combination of all 3 facets of the triad to occur rarely [13]. Publication bias likely exaggerates the significance of dramatic symptoms (ie, bleeding and shock), and underestimates the more subtle presentations of AEF (nonspecific malaise and leukocytosis). This bias likely explains the variability in the reported presentations. Regardless of the reason, the clinical presentations of AEF are not consistent, and mandates heightened suspicion on the part of the physician, especially in the setting of prior aortic surgery. One must assume that upper GI bleeding with a history of prior aortic surgery is an AEF until proven otherwise.

Computed tomographic angiography to diagnosis aortoenteric fistula

Computed tomographic angiography (CTA) is the mainstay of diagnosis [19,20]. The data describing the benefits of CTA lag behind the advances in hardware, software, and interpretation of CTA in practice. CTAs are reliable, widely available, quick to perform, relatively easy to interpret, and can help to rule out other pathologies that have symptoms overlap with AEF, but have a higher prevalence than AEF. These features are particularly useful in the setting of a hemodynamically unstable patient where the physician has a high index of suspicion of AEF. Effacement of distinct soft tissue planes between the enteric structure and the aorta/aortic graft, with thickening of the soft tissue between the GI tract and the aorta/aortic graft is frequently found [19,20]. Ectopic air within the aortic sac, or surrounding the aortic graft is highly suggestive of infection. Less frequently, fluid collections can also be found either within the aortic sac, or adjacent to it [19,20]. Extravasation of contrast into the bowel lumen is rarely found, but pathognomonic of an AEF. If one plans to perform endovascular procedures, however, one should avoid using oral contrast, because overlying contrast-filled loops of bowel obscure visualization of the vasculature.

The difficulty lies with small AEF, with minimal contamination. These AEF do not necessarily result in significant soft tissue thickening or air (Fig. 3). Moreover, not all AEF are associated with virulent organisms; hence, they do not incite a significant inflammatory response. With less virulent organisms, soft tissue thickening and effacement of soft tissue planes are less pronounced.

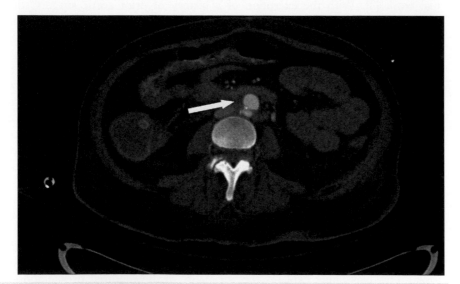

Fig. 3. The computed tomography angiogram shows subtle findings suggestive of aortoenteric fistula. There is effacement of the fat plane between the aortic graft and the overlying fourth portion of the duodenum, with mild soft tissue thickening surrounding the graft (*large yellow arrow*).

Clinical symptoms may be milder with less virulent organisms [19,20]. Early aortic graft infections and secondary AEF are difficult to discern from normal findings. Air is normal after open aortic reconstructions for 3 months [21]. Similarly, 58% of patients after EVAR have air seen within 3 days [22]. CTA is also requires iodinated contrast, which is nephrotoxic, and is concerning in patients presenting with azotemia. This author considers the risk of nephrotoxicity to be outweighed by the need for rapid diagnosis and acquisition of anatomic details for appropriate case planning.

Adjuncts for detecting aortoenteric fistula

Esophagogastroduodenoscopy (EGD) is performed frequently in the setting of upper GI bleeding. EGD has been reported to directly visualize an AEF, and sometimes underlying aortic graft material (Fig. 4). EGD may also show active bleeding, as well as an adherent clot within the bowel [17]. Unfortunately,

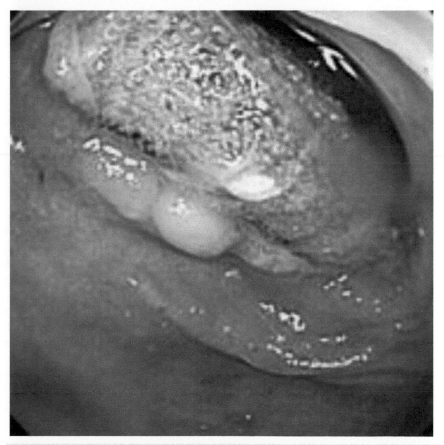

Fig. 4. Endoscopy revealing graft material visualized within the lumen of enteric structure. Although pathognomonic for an aortoenteric fistula, graft material is rarely visualized on endoscopy.

EGD remains an imperfect examination, with only 25% to 50% of AEF discovered by EGD, and performing worse for primary AEF [17,23]. The limitations include inability to visualize fistulae that occur beyond the duodenum, where a significant minority of AEF form. Pediatric colonoscopes are sometimes used to surmount this problem, although even these may not be long enough. Logistical difficulties may result in catastrophic delays in treatment, therefore limiting the usefulness of EGD in hemodynamically unstable patients. Finally, EGD may disturb the clot that had been preventing catastrophic hemorrhage from the AEF. Because of the risk of provoking emergent bleeding, some authors recommend performing endoscopy in the operating theater. The author limits the use of EGD in patients that are hemodynamically stable, with other imaging suggestive of an occult AEF.

Digital subtraction arteriography and duplex ultrasound examination have limited the usefulness in the setting of AEF. Digital subtraction arteriography may help to delineate anatomy, although with the advent of multidetector CTA and modern software rendering programs, the marginal benefit of arteriography has diminished. Rarely, the AEF may be demonstrated as extravasation from the aorta/aortic graft into the adjacent enteric structure [24]. Similarly, there are rare reports of duplex ultrasound examination identifying AEF [25]. Skilled duplex ultrasound technologists are not always available, especially in emergent situations. Moreover, overlying bowel and body habitus can hinder necessary visualization of the aortic graft. This author does not use ultrasound examination to attempt to identify AEF. This author performs digital subtraction arteriography only if a hybrid or endovascular procedure is being considered for the management of AEF.

Other diagnostic modalities

Tagged white blood cell scans, PET scanning with fluorodeoxyglucose, and single-photon emission computed tomography have all been used to diagnose occult aortic graft infections [26–28]. In the setting of AEF, these modalities are limited to those that are hemodynamically stable, because they are labor intensive, with prolonged examination times. Similarly magnetic resonance angiography may be used to diagnose AEF; however, magnetic resonance angiography suffers the same limitations of CTA when attempting to diagnose AEF from less virulent organisms, or early after an aortic graft placement. In addition, magnetic resonance angiography is time consuming, and more uncomfortable for the patient [29]. This author rarely performs these examinations in the setting of suspected AEF.

SURGICAL MANAGEMENT OF AORTOENTERIC FISTULA

When the diagnosis of AEF is suspected, expeditious surgical management can be life saving. There are multiple surgical strategies to maintain perfusion while extirpating the infection and restoring intestinal continuity. The method of repair for primary and secondary AEF are without significant differences. Procedures are loosely grouped into in situ reconstructions, versus extraanatomic bypass with aortic ligation. The latter represents the historical gold standard. In recent decades, however, in situ methods of maintaining arterial perfusion have gained popularity, in light of modest outcomes after axillobifemoral bypass and aortic stump ligation.

General preoperative considerations

An AEF presenting with hemorrhagic and/or septic shock requires resuscitation. An AEF is similar to a rupture mycotic aneurysm. Although resuscitation is critical, overresuscitation should be avoided. This is especially true in patients with herald bleeds, where the bleeding spontaneously ceases briefly. In these settings, the patients were able to temporize the AEF briefly with a tenuous thrombus, which may be dislodged with aggressive resuscitation. This author aims for a goal systolic blood pressure greater than 70 mm Hg, and less than 100 mm Hg for this reason, similar to the management in the setting of other ruptured AAAs [30].

In addition to hemodynamic resuscitation, appropriate broad-spectrum antibiotics should be administered after cultures are drawn. When AEF is suspected, broad spectrum antibiotics are instituted to cover gram-positive, gram-negative, and anaerobic organisms. Moreover, because yeast are frequently present in AEF, antifungal coverage should also be instituted. Individual institutions vary, and there is no specific regimen that will cover all AEF. This author favors vancomycin, piperacillin/tazobactam, and fluconazole for empiric therapy of primary and secondary AEF. This combination provides activity against all of the predominant organisms found frequently in the setting of AEF, until sensitivities and specificities can be obtained to tailor a narrower spectrum of antimicrobial activity.

For patients that are not en extremis, physicians may consider further diagnostic evaluations to assess cardiac and pulmonary risk before surgery. For these patients, upper endoscopy may also aid in the diagnosis to maximize diagnostic certainty before laparotomy. Although this information is unlikely to alter the operative plan, these data may help when discussing the risks and benefits of the operation with the patients and their caregivers.

For all patients, the value of a thorough discussion with the patient and/or caregivers cannot be overemphasized. The mortality of AEF is high, approaching 50% at 60 days from AEF repair and, in some series, morbidity exceeds 70% [12]. The series describing AEF repair are relatively small, and are often from centers of excellence, resulting in significant publication bias, and without nonoperative control arms, which may overestimate the benefits of repair [12,18]. Moreover, there are few data regarding functional outcomes after AEF repair.

General intraoperative considerations for open repair

AEF repair represents a significant technical challenge, regardless of the experience level of the surgeon. Anesthesiologists must be prepared to resuscitate aggressively in the face of life-threatening exsanguination. Simultaneously, they must also weigh the need to restrict fluid resuscitation against patient comorbidities, such as congestive heart failure and chronic pulmonary obstructive disease. The extensive exposures often required for AEF require consideration of the patient's temperature as well. The anesthesiologist must also be prepared to manage coagulopathy that often ensues in the setting of systemic heparin administration and prolonged aortic procedures. This author recommends a heated air pad that lies beneath the patient, as well as close communication with the anesthesiologist throughout the procedure regarding blood loss, resuscitation, and timing of aortic clamp application and release [31].

Obtaining proximal and distal control

The operative approach to primary or secondary AEF repair is the same, except for the need to manage an infected aortic prosthesis. One can obtain control in an open, or endovascular fashion. With respect to open control, supraceliac control is favored, as it provides proximal control before entrance to the AEF, when life-threatening hemorrhage can occur.

- Perform a midline laparotomy incision, and incise the gastrohepatic ligament.
- Incise the triangular ligament of the liver and retract the left lobe of the liver laterally.
- Palpate the esophagus with the aid of an orogastric or nasogastric tube, and encircle it with blunt dissection of the areolar tissues surrounding the distal esophagus. Retract the esophagus toward the left upper quadrant with a large Penrose drain.
- Divide the diaphragmatic crura. The aorta should be easily palpable here, with exposure continuing along the anterior surface until the aorta is exposed for a distance of 3 to 4 cm.
- Perform blunt finger dissection along either side of the aorta until the vertebrae can be palpated posteriorly [31].

Alternatively, intraaortic balloon control may be obtained. Balloon control does require additional team members, and equipment that does add to the complexity of the case in an urgent setting. The advantage, however, is that this may be performed with the patient awake, which provides the surgeon the luxury of proximal control without the added hemodynamic effects of anesthetic agents. This author recommends the use of balloon control in experienced centers.

- Obtain high exposure of the brachial artery (just distal to the axillary hair line) or axillary artery for a distance of 3 to 4 cm.
- Insert a 12-F sheath. The brachial exposure affords the ability to avoid either groin, which is often densely scarred in the setting of secondary AEF.
- Select the descending thoracic aorta, and position the molding aortic balloon under fluoroscopic guidance to the level of the supraceliac aorta, and inflate until the balloon opposes the aortic wall on either side.

Distal control depends on the extent of the infection. In the setting of prior femoral exposure and involvement of the femoral artery, this author recommends a lateral approach to the profunda and common femoral arteries [31]. This technique avoids a reoperative field, which can simplify control of the profunda and superficial femoral arteries. This technique can also be combined with a more traditional vertical incision overlying the common femoral artery should the surgeon find it necessary [31].

Resection and debridement of the infected aorta/aortic graft

After proximal and distal control, extirpation of the infection ensues, with dissection of the tethered bowel off of the aorta/aortic graft. Some authors recommend removing a small portion of the graft around where the bowel defect exists to minimize contamination of the field with enteric contents [18]. Others recommend temporarily closing the defect with several stitches in the bowel until the revascularization is complete [12]. Once the bowel is dissected free of the aorta/aortic graft, the proximal clamp can then be moved more distally, to either the suprarenal or infrarenal position. For primary AEF, the size of the defect in the aorta is typically small, but requires debridement back to healthy aorta. For secondary AEF, removal of the entire graft ensues, and the tissue surrounding the graft aggressively debrided and irrigated to remove as much of the infection as possible.

The safe removal of infected aortic endografts merits special mention. The difficulty lies in removing the active fixation elements on the graft, which are designed to prevent removal of the endograft without damaging the aortic neck. Moreover, they are sharp and represent a hazard to the surgeons attempting to remove it manually. The endograft must also be removed expeditiously, owing to backbleeding from the lumbar arteries, which can be prolific, and difficult to ligate with the endograft obstructing the view. Multiple methods have been advocated by multiple authors, with no clear champion.

- Obtain supraceliac control proximally, and distal control beyond the iliac limbs of the endograft. The supraceliac clamping provides room within the aorta to gently remove the suprarenal struts.
- After entering the sac, ligate any bleeding lumbar arteries posterior to the graft. The graft may be bisected if necessary to visualize the lumbar vessels.
- Analogous to methods used to reconstrain an endograft during fenestrated EVAR, have an assistant loop the endograft with an umbilical tape, thereby constraining the endograft.
- Pass another umbilical tape adjacent to the assistant's umbilical tape, and tie the umbilical tape.
- The process continues sequentially proximally until the endograft has been reconstrained.
- Next, the endograft can then be moved proximally slightly until the active fixation elements release from the aorta. The proximal portion can then be removed gently, and the proximal aortic clamp moved to a more distal location [12].
- The iliac limbs usually can simply be pulled gently free, because the active fixation elements prevent caudal migration, not caudad removal [12].

Axillobifemoral bypass with aortic stump ligation

Axillobifemoral bypass with aortic stump ligation is the conventional answer to the management of AEF. The advantage is that vascular surgeons are well-versed in the procedure. It is rapid and effective at maintaining lower extremity perfusion while removing the nidus of infection [32–34]. Axillobifemoral bypass can be performed in a staged fashion if the patient is hemodynamically stable, before explantation and debridement of the aorta/aortic graft, and aortic stump ligation. The optimal interval between the bypass and intraabdominal portion of the procedure is unknown. Because of competitive flow between the newly placed bypass and the native circulation, the interval between stages should be minimized, with the patient systemically heparinized between stages [32].

Unfortunately, axillobifemoral bypass is plagued by poor patency, high major amputation rates, and high reinfection rates [32–34]. Mortality ranges between 18% and 43% [32–34], with the lower rates cited in the staged procedures [32]. The risk of aortic stump rupture remains, occurring in up to 32% of patients at 3 months after the initial operation [32,35]. Aortic stump ligation requires 2 layers of 2-0 monofilament closure, which may not be available depending on the location of the AEF. Patency ranges between 64% and 80% at 5 years, with reinfection rates as high as 22% at 5 years (Fig. 5) [32–34].

In situ methods of arterial reconstruction

Owing to suboptimal outcomes with axillobifemoral bypass, surgeons have returned to in situ methods repairing AEF. Over the past 20 years, each of these methods have been preferred by individual institutions, each espousing advantages of their conduit of choice. The data are confounded by publication bias, ascertainment bias, referral bias, and small sample sizes. The only study to

A   **B**

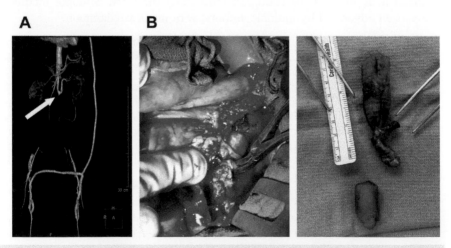

Fig. 5. A) This patient suffered a recurrent aortoenteric fistula after attempted aortic stump ligation. The patient originally underwent aortobifemoral bypass with a side branch to the left renal artery (*yellow arrow*). (B) With the first presentation, the patient underwent axillobifemoral bypass, with ligation of the aortic graft. The patient could not have the entire graft removed at the time of the initial operation. The recurrence highlights the need to remove as much graft as possible to prevent recurrence. The patient was treated with a spleno–left renal bypass with greater saphenous vein, and resection of the remaining graft.

directly compare axillobifemoral bypass with in situ reconstructions did not show superiority of either [17]. Taken as a whole, however, retrospective single-center series endorse the concept that in situ reconstruction is a superior alternative to extraanatomic bypass and aortic stump ligation (Table 1). No individual conduit for in situ reconstruction is clearly superior [13]. Each modality has unique advantages and disadvantages that are important to understand so that surgeons can tailor their repair to each individual case presentation.

RIFAMPIN-SOAKED AND SILVER-IMPREGNATED DACRON

This author favors rifampin-soaked Dacron grafts in the setting of emergent AEF repair. Rifampin has excellent activity against S epidermidis and moderate activity against S aureus. [40] It has been used as an agent to soak aortic grafts [18,40], owing to its affinity for collagen and gelatin coatings on grafts with stable bonding [40]. Dacron grafts are soaked in 600 mg of rifampin mixed with 250 mL of normal saline for at least 30 minutes [18]. The advantages include the ready availability, and relatively low cost compared with alternative conduits.

Rifampin-soaked grafts have been used with omental wrapping in the setting of AEF with excellent outcomes [18]. The marginal benefit of the omental wrapping is difficult to distinguish from the rifampin-soaked Dacron alone. Oderich and colleagues [18] described outcomes from the Mayo clinic, and represent the largest single-center series describing AEF repair, in which rifampin-soaked Dacron was used. At 5 years, the survival was 59%, and graft patency, 97%. Theoretically, synthetic grafts have a higher risk of reinfection compared with other conduits; however, in this series, the reinfection rate was laudable at 4%.

Silver-impregnated Dacron exerts its antimicrobial effects via disruption of bacterial cell membranes, which prevents cell division and DNA replication. Silver ions also disrupt bacterial protein transcription of messenger RNA. It has been found to be particularly active against methicillin-resistant S aureus infections [40]. Develva and colleagues [37] evaluated the French experience with silver-impregnated Dacron for the repair of AEF. Over 4 years, no patient required reintervention for anastomotic disruption. Thirty-nine percent of patients died in hospital, with 55% deceased at 1 year, highlighting the highly lethal nature of AEF repair. The 1-year patency rates were suboptimal, with primary patency of only 60.5%, but with a reasonable secondary patency of 89%. Four patients (22%) of their series had a reinfection.

There were several differences between the series by Oderich and colleagues [18] and the Develva and colleagues series. The experience with rifampin-soaked Dacron is significantly greater, such that infrequent events may be magnified in the experience with silver-impregnated Dacron. Rifampin should not be more effective at preventing recurrent infection, as shown by in vitro studies of rifampin versus silver [41]. Although rifampin may have improved activity versus silver against gram-positive organisms, gram-negative organism reinfections seem to plague rifampin-soaked Dacron reconstructions in animal

Table 1
Summary of retrospective trials describing results of extraanatomic versus in situ arterial reconstructions in aortoenteric fistula repair

Procedure	30-day mortality	Survival	Patency	Limb salvage	Persistent/ recurrent infection	Pros	Cons
Extraanatomic bypass and aortic stump ligation [32–34]	18%–43%	At 5 y: 57%	At 5 y: 63%–80%	At 5 y: 80%–83%	4%–22%	No extra training. Expeditious.	Aortic stump blowout. High reinfection, poor limb salvage and patency.
Rifampin-soaked Dacron with omental wrap [36]	9%	At 5 y: 59%	At 5 y: 97%	At 5 y: 100%	4%	Expeditious, available, lowest reinfection, durable.	Omentum not always available. Rifampin limited spectrum.
Silver-impregnated Dacron [37]	22%	At 1 y: 55%	At 1 y: primary patency, 61%; secondary patency, 89%	At 1 y: 72%	22%	Expeditious, durable, theoretically better antibiotic spectrum.	High reinfection rates, lower patency and limb salvage.
Cryopreserved allograft [38,39]	25%	At 5 y: 66%	At 5 y: primary patency, 97%	At 5 y: 93%	9%–14%	Durable, theoretically more resistant to infection.	Expensive, delays in availability, inconsistent quality of graft.
Neo-aorto iliac surgery [12,31]	24%	54% at 60 d, 18% at 5 y	At 5 y: primary patency, 81%; primary-assisted patency, 91%	At 5 y: 89%	4%	Durable, inexpensive, lowest reinfection rate, shorter postoperative antibiotics required.	Prolongs procedure, associated with higher mortality, surgeon unfamiliarity and fatigue.

studies [40]. Omental wrapping was performed in the Mayo Clinic series, which may partly explain why outcomes seem to be superior to silver-impregnated Dacron. Omental wrapping is not always feasible, however, especially in reoperative abdomens. Finally, partial graft excision was performed in several of the patients in the experience reported by Develva and colleagues [37], which may explain their higher graft reinfection rates.

CRYOPRESERVED ALLOGRAFT

Cryopreserved allograft is another viable alternative conduit for use in AEF repair (Fig. 6). Harlander-Locke and associates [38] reported a multicenter experience of in situ reconstructions for aortic graft infections using cryopreserved allograft, 33 of which were for AEF. AEF was not independently associated with complications in their cohort. Patency was excellent, with 98% patent at 1 year, and 97% remaining patent at 5 years. Results for the entire cohort suggest that reinfection is not necessarily obviated with cryopreserved allograft, with 2 patients requiring explantation of the allograft for recurrent sepsis (1%). If one assumes that persistent sepsis, recurrent infection, and AEF recurrence all represent persistent/recurrent infection, then the rate of persistent infection/reinfection with cryopreserved allograft is 14% [38].

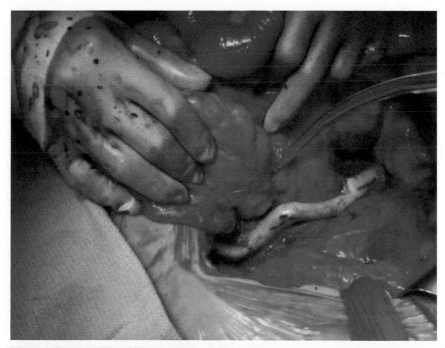

Fig. 6. Aortoiliac segment of cryopreserved allograft used to perform an aortouniiliac bypass for infection after debridement of a heavily contaminated retroperitoneal tunnel. Cryopreserved allograft was chosen, because omentum was unable to be mobilized sufficiently to this heavily soiled area. The contralateral limb was divided, and the stump oversewn.

Batt and colleagues [17] examined their experience with 37 AEF reconstructions, of which 8 used cryopreserved allograft. Three of the 8 allograft they used became reinfected. Despite improved preservation techniques, inconsistencies in the product remain. Both series describe rare episodes of graft rupture. Late graft degeneration and dilation is less of a problem, although may occur, with late pseudoaneurysm occurring in 3%. Allografts are not readily available, requiring ABO blood antigen matching and shipment. Finally, allografts are costly, with aortoiliac reconstructions costing approximately US$18,000 in 2011 [18].

NEOAORTOILIAC SURGICAL RECONSTRUCTION

Over the last 25 years, femoral veins have been increasingly used to manage aortic graft infections, although the expertise remains localized to several centers. When looking at all aortic graft infections, reconstructions with neoaortoiliac surgery (NAIS) using autogenous femoral veins to recreate the aorto-iliac system have the lowest reinfection rates, and have comparable durability to other in situ methods (Fig. 7) [15,17,42]. Kakkos and colleagues [15] found that, with respect to AEF, NAIS reconstructions had superior freedom from AEF-related mortality compared with other methods of in situ reconstruction. Chopra and colleagues [12] reported on the second largest single-center experiences of AEF repair from the University of Texas Southwestern, and the largest to use predominantly NAIS reconstructions. Most patients (72%) suffered in-hospital complications, with a 50% mortality at 60 days from the operation.

Owing to the limitations of small, single-center, retrospective series, the true relationship between the method of in situ arterial reconstruction and mortality is impossible to ascertain. The prolonged harvest time precludes the use of the femoral vein in emergent cases. The increased mortality rates noted in the series compared with the Mayo Clinic experience, however, are concerning, especially because mortality was not associated with emergent status or preoperative sepsis. Although NAIS seems to be beneficial in aortic graft infections, in the subset of AEF, the femoral vein harvest may add marginal morbidity, which can be avoided with other in situ methods of reconstruction [12]. This author reserves NAIS for patients who are hemodynamically stable, with sufficient physiologic reserve to tolerate a longer procedure.

ENDOVASCULAR THERAPY AS AN ADJUNCT OR DESTINATION THERAPY

Stent grafts, coils, and plugs may all be used to temporize bleeding, thereby converting an AEF repair to a more elective procedure [15,43]. Intuitively, temporizing an emergent problem should improve outcomes, by permitting time to resuscitate the patient, and optimize other concurrent medical conditions. Moreover, temporizing the patient also permits time for more thorough, informed discussions with patient and their caregivers. Pooled analyses of EVAR for AEF suggest that there is an early survival benefit of using

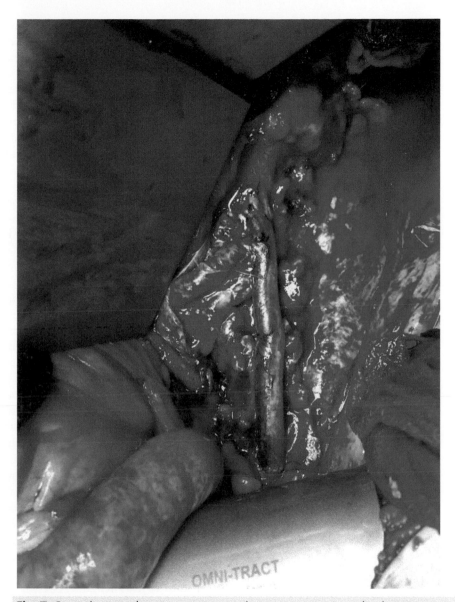

Fig. 7. Femoral vein used to manage a primary iliac mycotic aneurysm with colonic aortoenteric fistula.

EVAR over early in situ repair for AEF, which is lost in late follow-up [15]. The authors suggest that the temporary survival benefit implies that EVAR with planned subsequent explantation and definitive in situ repair may provide improved overall survival benefit relative to in situ reconstructions without endovascular temporization [15]. Given the difficulty with EVAR explantation, it is also conceivable that initial EVAR may worsen outcomes by increasing the marginal difficulty of the subsequent definitive in situ reconstruction. Moreover, given the location of the AEF, placement of an endograft without fenestrations or snorkels may be impossible.

As destination therapy, however, endovascular techniques are not durable. Recurrent hemorrhage after endograft exclusion of the AEF can occur as early as 1 month after endograft placement [44,45]. Pooled analysis revealed that recurrent/persistent infection or hemorrhage occurred in 44% of patients treated with an EVAR for AEF at a median of 13 months [45]. This finding corroborates what is already intuitive to most surgeons, namely that EVAR neither removes the infectious nidus nor corrects the enteric defect. There may be rare occasions where small enteric defects with minimal contamination can be managed with antibiotics and endovascular exclusion. For patients who are otherwise reasonable surgical candidates, open surgical repair of AEF should be offered.

Importance of repair of the intestinal defect

Multiple authors have highlighted the importance of appropriately managing the enteric defect in AEF [12,17,39]. GI complications independently predicted mortality by more than 3-fold. Batt and colleagues [17] found that reinfection resulted in 100% mortality, with all cases of reinfection owing to a failed duodenorraphy. Hence, for Batt and colleagues [17], recurrent infection resulted in 2 out of 3 deaths, the leading cause of mortality in their cohort.

The impact of GI complications is significant because enteric outcomes and the associated morbidity and mortality are potentially modifiable. Chopra and colleagues [12] described the changes that occurred at the University of Texas Southwestern after the outcomes describing the detrimental effect of GI complications after AEF repair was described [46]. Two members of the general surgery department were recruited to perform the enteric repairs. Strict attention was placed on general surgical principles of reapproximating well-vascularized, tension-free bowel edges after aggressive and wide debridement. Attention was also placed on early intervention for mesenteric ischemic complications. Fewer repairs were simple direct, 2-layer repairs of the enteric defect, with more complex repair (resection and reanastomosis, pyloric exclusions) performed over time. This process resulted ultimately in a statistically significant decrease in 60-day mortality over time, from 53% before 2007 to 8% after 2007. No patient with a complex enteric repair suffered an enteric leak postoperatively.

It is unclear whether complex GI reconstructions are necessary in all cases of AEF repair. Schoell and colleagues [39] examined 32 consecutive AEF repairs with cryopreserved allograft. Sixteen patients had the enteric defect repaired primarily, whereas the remainder had a more complex repair (resection with reanastomosis, Hartman's procedure). In their series, there were 3 recurrent AEF, 2 after complex enteric reconstruction. Moreover, most of the enteric defects repaired primarily in the University of Texas Southwestern experience did not leak [12]. Hence, performing larger, more complex GI reconstructions for all patients is unnecessary. The author surmises that centralizing the cases of enteric repair with a small cadre of experienced general surgeons most significantly decreased GI complications and mortality over time [12]. Further prospective multicenter cohorts will be required to quantify the association between the experience of the general surgeon and enteric outcomes during AEF repair.

SUMMARY

AEF are life-threatening conditions, with delays in diagnosis resulting in catastrophic hemorrhage, morbidity, and mortality. CTA remains the diagnostic procedure of choice, owing to the wide availability, interpretability, and high sensitivity and specificity. Further research is required to identify diagnostic tests for AEF with small enteric defects with less virulent organisms. Axillobifemoral bypass, with aortic stump ligation remains an acceptable option for repair, although mortality, limb salvage, and reinfection rates are suboptimal. In situ arterial reconstructions overcome many of the limitations of axillobifemoral bypass. Rifampin-soaked Dacron with omental wrapping has had the best published results, with less efficacy reported for silver-impregnated Dacron, cryopreserved allograft, and NAIS. However, these results are subject to significant publication bias, small sample sizes, and referral bias. Future appropriately powered multicenter registries should overcome the limitations that plague the single-center retrospective registries. The author favors rifampin-soaked Dacron with omental wrapping in emergent settings. NAIS is the most resistant to reinfection, but the most laborious; hence, this author reserves NAIS for those patients with smaller enteric defects, more indolent infections, and sufficient physiologic reserve to withstand the marginal increase in operative duration.

Among the many remaining challenges, management of AEF in the setting of prior EVAR is prescient owing to the increased prevalence of endograft use. Moreover, fenestrated endografts and snorkels have become more widely used, increasing the technical difficulty of endograft removal. Safe EVAR removal will require further refinement of technique, patient selection, and evaluation of prospectively obtained, multicenter outcomes. Second, the optimal management of the enteric defect also continues to defy surgeons. It is clear that mismanagement of the GI defect dramatically worsens morbidity and mortality. Similarly, it is clear that a boilerplate approach fails to accommodate the heterogeneity of enteric defects that occur with AEF. Other remaining challenges include the inclusion of nonoperative control arms within future studies. The nonoperative arms will be critical to optimize patient selection in the future.

References

[1] Keunen B, Houthoofd S, Daenens K, et al. Case of primary aortoenteric fistula: review of therapeutic challenges. Ann Vasc Surg 2016;33:230.e5-13.

[2] Ranasinghe W, Loa J, Allaf N, et al. Primary aortoenteric fistulae: the challenges in diagnosis and review of treatment. Ann Vasc Surg 2011;25:386.e1-5.

[3] Cooper A. Lectures on principles and practice of surgery with additional notes and cases by tyrrell. 5th edition. Philadelphia: Haswell; 1839 Barrington: Haswell.

[4] Voorhoeve R, Moll FL, de Letter JA, et al. Primary aortoenteric fistula. Report of eight new cases and review of the literature. Ann Vasc Surg 1996;10:40–8.

[5] Duncan JR, Renwick AA, Mackenzie I, et al. Primary aortoenteric fistula: pitfalls in the diagnosis of a rare condition. Ann Vasc Surg 2002;16:242–5.

[6] Skourtis G, Gerasimos P, Sotirios M, et al. Primary aortoenteric fistula due to septic aortitis. Ann Vasc Surg 2010;24:825, e7–11.

[7] Hallett JW, Marschall DM, Petterson TM, et al. Graft-related complications after abdominal aortic aneurysm repair: reassurance from a 36-years population-based experience. J Vasc Surg 1997;25:277–84.

[8] United Kingdom Small Aneurysm Trial Participants. Long-term outcomes of immediate repair compared with surveillance of small abdominal aortic aneurysms. N Engl J Med 2002;346: 1445–52.

[9] Vogel TR, Symons R, Flum DR. The incidence and factors associated with graft infection after aortic aneurysm repair. J Vasc Surg 2008;47:264–9.

[10] Kahlberg A, Rinaldi E, Piffaretti G, et al. results from the multicenter study on aortoenteric fistulization after stent grafting of the abdominal aorta (MAEFISTO). J Vasc Surg 2016;64:313–20.

[11] Capoccia L, Speziale F, Menna D, et al. Preliminary results from a national enquiry of infection in abdominal aortic endovascular repair (registry of infection in EVAR-R.I.EVAR). Ann Vasc Surg 2016;30:198–204.

[12] Chopra A, Cieciura L, Modrall JG, et al. Twenty-year experience with aorto-enteric fistula repair: gastro-intestinal complications predict outcome. J Am Coll Surg 2017;225:9–18.

[13] Saers SJF, Scheltinga MRM. Primary aortoenteric fistula. Br J Surg 2005;92:143–52.

[14] Bussuttil RW, Rees W, Baker JD, et al. Pathogenesis of aortoduodenal fistula: experimental and clinical correlates. Surgery 1979;85:1–13.

[15] Kakkos SK, Bicknell CD, Tsolakis IA, et al, Hellenic Co-operative Group on Aortic Surgery. Editor's choice- management of secondary aorto-enteric and other abdominal arterio-enteric fistulas: a review and pooled data analysis. Eur J Vasc Endovasc Surg 2016;52(6):770–86.

[16] Bergqvist D, Bjorck M, Byman R. Secondary aortoenteric fistula after endovascular aortic interventions: a systematic literature review. J Vasc Interv Radiol 2008;19:163–5.

[17] Batt M, Jean-Baptiste E, O'Connor S, et al. Early and late results of contemporary management of 37 secondary aortoenteric fistulae. Eur J Vasc Endovasc Surg 2011;41:748–57.

[18] Oderich GS, Bower TC, Hofer J, et al. In situ rifampin-soaked grafts with omental coverage and antibiotic suppression are durable with low reinfection rates in patients with aortic graft enteric erosion or fistula. J Vasc Surg 2011;53:99–106.

[19] Raman SP, Kamaya A, Federle M, et al. Aortoenteric fistulas: spectrum of CT findings. Abdom Imaging 2013;38:367–75.

[20] Vu QDM, Menias CO, Bhalla S, et al. Aortoenteric fistulas: CT features and potential mimics. Radiographics 2009;29:197–209.

[21] O'Hara PJ, Borkowski GP, Hertzer NR, et al. Natural history of periprosthetic air on computerized axial tomographic examination of the abdomen following abdominal aortic aneurysm repair. J Vasc Surg 1984;1:429–33.

[22] Sawhney R, Kerlan RK, Wall SD, et al. Analysis of initial CT findings after endovascular repair of abdominal aortic aneurysm. Radiology 2001;220:157–60.

[23] Song Y, Liu Q, Shen H, et al. Diagnosis and management of primary aortoenteric fistulas-experience learned from eighteen patients. Surgery 2008;143:43–50.

[24] Thompson WM, Jackson DC, Johnsrude IS. Aortoenteric and paraprosthetic-enteric fistulas: radiologic findings. AJR Am J Roentgenol 1976;127:235–42.

[25] MacKenzie DC. Aortoenteric fistula identified by clinical ultrasound. J Emerg Med 2015;48:699–701.

[26] Ketai L, Hartshorne M. Potential uses of computed tomography-SPECT and computed tomography-coincidence fusion images of the chest. Clin Nucl Med 2001;26:433–41.

[27] Erba PA, Leo G, Sollini M, et al. Radiolabelled leucocyte scintigraphy versus conventional radiological imaging for the management of late, low-grade vascular prosthesis infections. Eur J Nucl Med Mol Imaging 2014;41:357–68.

[28] Fukuchi K, Ishida Y, Higashi M, et al. Detection of aortic graft infection by fluorodeoxyglucose positron emission tomography: comparison with computed tomographic findings. J Vasc Surg 2005;42:919–25.

[29] Olofsson PA, Auffermann W, Higgins CB, et al. Diagnosis of prosthetic aortic graft infection by magnetic resonance imaging. J Vasc Surg 1988;8:99–105.

[30] Hinchliffe RJ, Powell JT. Improving the outcomes from ruptured abdominal aortic aneurysm: interdisciplinary best guidelines. Ann R Coll Surg Engl 2013;95:96–7.

[31] Chung J, Clagett GP. Neoaortoiliac system (NAIS) procedure for the treatment of the infected aortic graft. Semin Vasc Surg 2011;24:220–6.

[32] Reilly LM, Stoney RJ, Goldstone J, et al. Improved management of aortic graft infection: the influence of operation sequence and staging. J Vasc Surg 1987;5:421–31.

[33] Seeger JM, Pretus HA, Welborn MB, et al. Long-term outcome after treatment of aortic graft infection with staged extra-anatomic bypass grafting and aortic graft removal. J Vasc Surg 2000;32:451–9.

[34] Yeager RA, Taylor LM Jr, Moneta GL, et al. Improved results with conventional management of infrarenal aortic infection. J Vasc Surg 1999;30:76–83.

[35] O'Hara PJ, Hertzer NR, Beven EG, et al. Surgical management of infected abdominal aortic grafts: review of a 25-year experience. J Vasc Surg 1986;3:725–31.

[36] Oderich GS, Farber MA, Sanchez LA. Urgent endovascular treatment of symptomatic or contained ruptured aneurysms with modified stent grafts. Perspect Vasc Surg Endovasc Ther 2011;23:186–94.

[37] Develva JC, Deglise S, Berard X, et al. In-situ revascularisation for secondary aorto-enteric fistulae: the success of silver-coated Dacron is closely linked to a suitable bowel repair. Eur J Vasc Endovasc Surg 2012;44:417–24.

[38] Harlander-Locke MP, Harmon LK, Lawrence PF, et al. The use of cryopreserved aortoiliac allograft for aortic reconstruction in the United States. J Vasc Surg 2014;59:669–74.

[39] Schoell T, Manceau G, Chiche L, et al. Surgery for secondary aorto-enteric fistula or erosion (SAEFE) complicating aortic graft surgery: a retrospective analysis of 32 patients with particular focus on digestive management. World J Surg 2015;39:283–91.

[40] Schneider F, O'Connor S, Becquemin JP. Efficacy of collagen silver-coated polyester and rifampin-soaked vascular grafts to resist infection from MRSA and Escherichia coli in a dog model. Ann Vasc Surg 2008;22:815–21.

[41] Hardmann S, Cope A, Swann A, et al. An in vitro model to compare the antimicrobial activity of silver-coated versus rifampin-soaked vascular grafts. Ann Vasc Surg 2008;18:308–13.

[42] O'Connor S, Andrew P, Batt M, et al. A systematic review and meta-analysis of treatments for aortic graft infection. J Vasc Surg 2006;44:38–45.

[43] Han K, Lee DY, Kim MD, et al. Hybrid treatment: expanding the armamentarium for infected infrarenal abdominal aortic and iliac aneurysms. J Vasc Interv Radiol 2017;28:564–9.

[44] Danneels MIL, Verhagen HJM, Teijink JAW, et al. Endovascular repair for aorto-enteric fistula: a bridge too far or a bridge to surgery? Eur J Vasc Endovasc Surg 2006;32:27–33.

[45] Antoniou GA, Koutsias S, Antoniou SA, et al. Outcome after endovascular stent graft repair of aortoenteric fistula: a systematic review. J Vasc Surg 2009;49:782–9.

[46] Valentine RJ, Timaran CH, Modrall JG, et al. Secondary aortoenteric fistulas versus paraprosthetic erosions: is bleeding associated with a worse outcome? J Am Coll Surg 2008;207:922–7.

Advances in Surgery 52 (2018) 179–204

ADVANCES IN SURGERY

Benign Anorectal Surgery
Management

Jan Rakinic, MD

Department of Surgery, Southern Illinois University School of Medicine, 701 North First Street, Suite D-333, Springfield, IL 62781-0001, USA

Keywords
- Benign anorectal complaints • Anorectal pathology • Primary fistulotomy
- Perianal/perirectal abscess • Hemorrhoids

Key points

- Surgical management of benign anorectal complaints make up most ambulatory anorectal problems.
- Anorectal pathology is increasingly seen in patients with medically induced immunosuppression.
- Simple fistulas involve a minimum of external sphincter muscle, and are preferentially treated by primary fistulotomy.

HEMORRHOIDS

Nonsurgical options (rubber banding, injection sclerotherapy, infrared coagulation) are generally used for symptomatic grade 1 and 2 hemorrhoids that do not respond to conservative management, and are well described elsewhere [1]. Surgical intervention is best used for grades 3 and 4 hemorrhoids (Table 1) in the following situations:

- Nonoperative management has failed
- Disease unlikely to respond to nonoperative techniques
- Patients with significant external hemorrhoidal component
- Coagulopathic patients requiring management of hemorrhoidal bleeding

Patient management is straightforward.

Disclosure Statement: The author has nothing to disclose.

E-mail address: jrakinic@siumed.edu

https://doi.org/10.1016/j.yasu.2018.04.004

Table 1
Grades of internal hemorrhoids

Grade 1	Prominent hemorrhoidal vessels
	No prolapse
Grade 2	Prolapse with Valsalva
	Spontaneous reduction
Grade 3	Prolapse with Valsalva
	Manual reduction needed
Grade 4	Chronically prolapsed
	Manual reduction unsuccessful
	Not strangulated

- A single enema is sufficient preparation; antibiotics are not required.
- Anesthesia and position vary with surgeon preference and patient comorbidities.
- Prone jack-knife position with buttocks taped apart is preferred by most American surgeons for optimal visualization.
- The vast majority of hemorrhoid procedures are performed as outpatient surgery
- Postoperative care: appropriate pain control with minimal opiates; avoidance of hard, dry stools.

Closed hemorrhoidectomy (Ferguson technique)
- Elliptical incision starting at perianal skin and continuing to anorectal ring, dissecting hemorrhoidal tissue away from the sphincter (Fig. 1).
- Pedicle is suture ligated and hemorrhoidal tissue amputated.
- Wound is closed with running absorbable suture, leaving a few millimeters open on skin for drainage.
- One to 3 columns may be excised; preserve bridges of viable skin and mucosa between excision sites to prevent stenosis.
- Send each hemorrhoid separately for pathology; while occult cancers found at hemorrhoidectomy are rare, the location is helpful in planning the least morbid treatment.

Open hemorrhoidectomy (Milligan-Morgan)
- More common in the United Kingdom
- Excision similar; after the suture ligation of the pedicle and amputation of the bundle, wounds are left open to granulate
- One to 3 columns can be excised, with the same concern regarding viable bridges of skin and mucosa

Outcomes
- Long-term results of excision are excellent, with low rates of recurrence requiring reoperation.
- Open and closed techniques have similar postoperative pain, need for analgesics, and complications.
- Open approaches are quicker; closed show faster healing, although not significantly so [2,3].

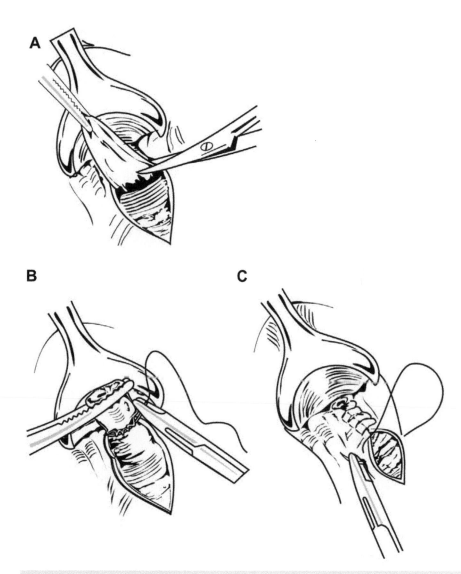

Fig. 1. Ferguson hemorrhoidectomy. (A) Elliptical incision starting at perianal skin and continuing to anorectal ring, dissecting hemorrhoidal tissue away from the sphincter. (B) Pedicle is suture ligated and hemorrhoidal tissue amputated. (C) Wound is closed with a running absorbable suture, leaving a few millimeters open on the skin for drainage. (*From* Rakinic J, Poola VP. Hemorrhoids and fistulas: new solutions to old problems. Curr Prob Surg 2014;51(3):98–137; with permission.)

Complications
- Bleeding: less than 5%, related to narrow male pelvis and surgeon; manage in operating room with direct ligation
- Urinary retention, fecal impaction: minimize opiates, avoid hard, dry stools

- Anal stenosis, disturbance in sensation/continence: minimize breadth of excised tissue
- Fistula: unusual, manage with primary fistulotomy
- Urinary tract infection: avoidance of retention

Stapled hemorrhoidopexy

- Excises circular strip of mucosa/submucosa well above hemorrhoids, elevating hemorrhoids to normal position
- Devascularization of hemorrhoids is not a goal
- Decreased pain because no skin incision
- Suitable for second-degree and third-degree hemorrhoids
- Not suitable: those with thrombosed internal hemorrhoids, significant external hemorrhoidal disease, fourth-degree hemorrhoids, patients who practice anal receptive sex

Familiarity with the stapler kit and steps of the procedure is integral to success. The technique has been described in detail elsewhere [1].
Correct placement of the purse string suture is critical.

- If placed too proximally, the hemorrhoids will not be lifted into their natural position.
- If too distally, the staple line will be too near the sensate region and will cause pain.

The depth of the purse string suture is also key.

- If too deep, full-thickness excision may result, with risk for pelvic abscess, fistula, or iatrogenic stapled rectovaginal fistula.
- The posterior vaginal wall must be assessed several times during purse string placement and before stapler firing to avoid the latter complication.

Outcomes
- Stapled hemorrhoidopexy (SH) causes less postoperative pain and less analgesic use than excision [4].
- SH has higher incidence of recurrence/need for additional operations.

Complications
Complications of SH are rare, but several complications must be specifically noted [5].

- Rectal obstruction and perforation
- Retroperitoneal sepsis and pelvic sepsis due to full-thickness excision
- Sphincter injury has occurred when muscle is incorporated into the stapler
- Iatrogenic stapled rectovaginal fistula
- Continued pain, bleeding, anal fissure, fecal urgency and frequency, due to improper purse string placement

Most of these will require reoperation, which is effective in treating pain and other symptoms, but a high rate of posttreatment bleeding and soiling remains.

Transanal hemorrhoidal dearterialization/mucopexy

- Nonexcisional technique
- Hypothesized to produce hemorrhoidal shrinkage

- Mucopexy was added to address continued postoperative bleeding/prolapse

A specialized anoscope containing a removable Doppler probe is required. The technique is well described elsewhere [1]. Key points:

- Suture ligation of all feeding hemorrhoidal arteries
- Mucopexy is performed in 2 to 4 positions in the anal canal, oversewing the redundant mucosa from proximal to distal, terminating the suture proximal to the dentate line, and tying the tails of the suture together to lift the hemorrhoid

Outcomes/complications
- Has its best outcome in grade 2 and possibly grade 3 hemorrhoids; however, other techniques provide superior durability [6].
- Almost 30% of patients will require a second operation for persistent prolapse.
- Continued bleeding and pain are reported by 10% of patients.

Thrombosed external hemorrhoids
- If edematous with no firm clot, or if clot has begun to soften/resorb, manage nonoperatively (Fig. 2).
- If thrombus is very firm, excision of the clot can be done with good pain relief, often in the clinic.
- The thrombus is a cluster of small clotted vessels, not one larger clot, so will not resolve with simple incision.

Excision of thrombosed external hemorrhoid (Fig. 3):

- Local anesthetic with epinephrine is used to produce a field block.
- An ellipse of skin overlying the thrombus is excised.
- Excise all the small clots that can be removed without excessive anodermal undermining.
- Bleeding should be minimal as feeding vessels are clotted; epinephrine in local anesthetic helps.
- Skin can be left open or closed per surgeon preference.
- Instruct patient to avoid hard stools and straining. Sitz baths provide comfort. Nonopiate pain medications are sufficient.

Hemorrhoidal skin tags and fibroepithelial polyps
- Firm fibroepithelial tags are more likely to cause symptoms of soiling and discomfort than more bland-appearing external skin tags (Fig. 4).
- Excision of these fibrous tags can be done safely in the outpatient operative setting.
- Potential complications include bleeding, infection, scarring that may alter stooling and sensation, and unresolved symptoms.

Special situations
Acute hemorrhoid crisis
- Internal hemorrhoids have prolapsed and become incarcerated due to internal sphincter spasm (Fig. 5).

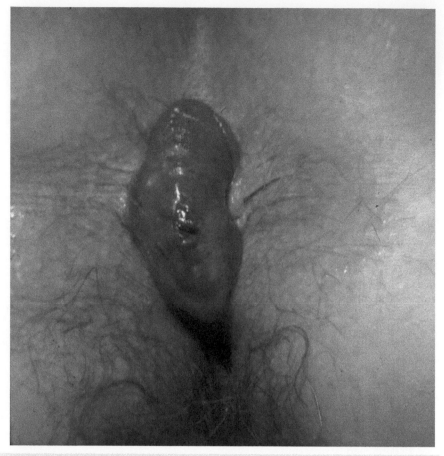

Fig. 2. Thrombosed external hemorrhoid. (*Courtesy of* American Society of Colon and Rectal Surgeons (ASCRS), Arlington Heights, IL; with permission.)

- The incarcerated internal hemorrhoids may be beefy red, or ulcerated and necrotic.
- Thrombosis of the external hemorrhoids often accompanies this.

The best option is expeditious excisional hemorrhoidectomy unless the patient is a prohibitive operative risk; in the presence of necrosis, excision is a necessity.

- Either an open or closed technique can be used; much of the edema resolves after anal block and sphincter relaxation.
- Excision is performed as described previously.
- Wounds may be closed or left open.
- Postoperative care is as usual after excisional hemorrhoidectomy; outcomes are good.

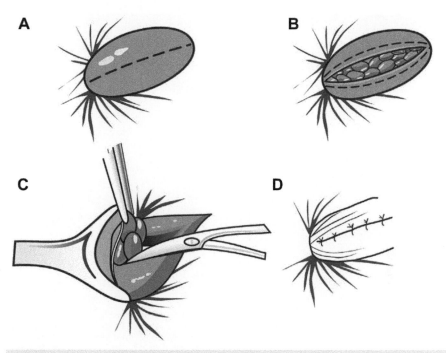

Fig. 3. Excision of thrombosed external hemorrhoid. (A) Incision made overlying clot. (B) Nest of small clots exposed. (C) Excision of clots with small scissor. (D) Wound may be closed or left open. (*From* Rakinic J, Poola VP. Hemorrhoids and fistulas: new solutions to old problems. Curr Prob Surg 2014;51(3):98–137; with permission.)

If not necrotic, nonexcisional management can be done.

- Circumferential injection of local anesthetic and reduction of the strangulated hemorrhoids, followed by bed rest
- Some surgeons follow this with banding of the internal component.
- A small older study found that only 15% of patients so treated went on to require excisional hemorrhoidectomy.
- Patients seem to prefer operative intervention in this setting.

Pregnancy
- Surgical intervention for hemorrhoids in pregnancy is reserved for strangulated hemorrhoids, or occasionally a very symptomatic external thrombosis.
- When necessary, operation should be done using local anesthesia with the patient positioned in the left lateral position to avoid compression of the inferior vena cava.

Rectal varices in portal hypertension
- Incidence of hemorrhoidal symptoms in portal hypertension is same as general population.
- Rectal varices and hemorrhoids are different.
- Rectal varices bleed much less commonly than esophageal varices.

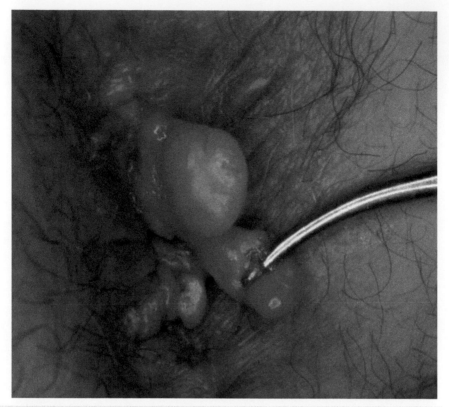

Fig. 4. Fibrotic external tags. (*Courtesy of* American Society of Colon and Rectal Surgeons (ASCRS), Arlington Heights, IL; with permission.)

In the rare instance of bleeding rectal varices, multidisciplinary treatment should be pursued.

- Medical management of portal hypertension
- Direct control methods, such as sclerotherapy and suture ligation, when necessary
- Transjugular intrahepatic portosystemic shunt
- Surgical portosystemic shunts

The immunocompromised patient
Anorectal pathology is increasingly seen in patients with medically induced immunosuppression, such as solid organ transplant recipients and patients on steroids or chemotherapy, as well as those with disease-induced immunosuppression, including human immunodeficiency virus (HIV). If immunocompromise can be expected to improve, conservative management should be pursued until immunity is normal or nearly so, as these patients may become eligible for operative management. Rubber band ligation and

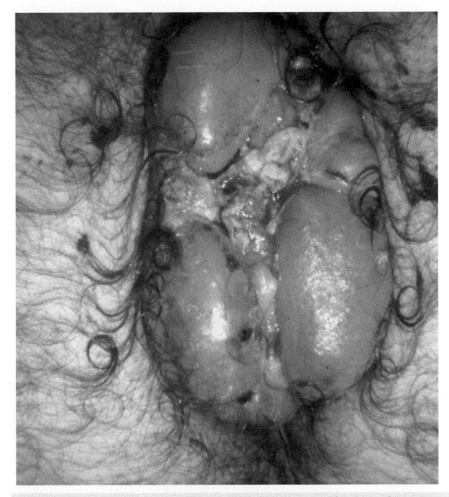

Fig. 5. Acute hemorrhoidal crisis. (*Courtesy of* American Society of Colon and Rectal Surgeons (ASCRS), Arlington Heights, IL; with permission.)

excisional hemorrhoidectomy are safe in HIV-positive patients on antiretroviral therapy with acceptable CD4 counts. For patients with ongoing immunocompromise, medical management should be pursued, reserving surgical intervention for medical failure, and with careful consideration of the implications of complications in this population.

PERIANAL/PERIRECTAL ABSCESS
- Most often due to cryptoglandular disease; other etiologies are unusual (Box 1).
- Methicillin-resistant *Staphylococcus aureus* (MRSA) gluteal abscess is most commonly misidentified lesion (Fig. 6, Table 2).

Box 1: Etiology of anorectal abscess

Cryptoglandular
Inflammatory bowel disease
  Crohn disease
Infectious
  Tuberculosis
  Actinomycosis
  Lymphogranuloma venereum
Traumatic
  Impaling injury, foreign body trauma
  Surgery, including episiotomy, hemorrhoidectomy, prostatectomy
Malignancy
  Carcinoma, leukemia, lymphoma
Radiation

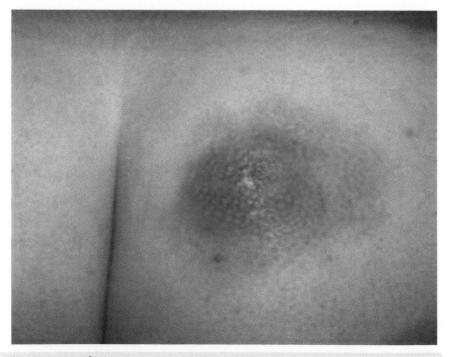

Fig. 6. MRSA infection.

Table 2
Differential diagnosis of anorectal abscess

Differentiation	Management
Pilonidal disease	5% of pilonidal sinuses track caudally
Inspect gluteal cleft for pits	Treat the originating pit; surgical management planned as for any pilonidal
Furuncle of skin/skin structures Often multiple	
Usually more lateral/distant from anus	Often respond to antibiotics directed toward skin flora; drain if unresponsive
Methicillin-resistant *Staphylococcus aureus* infection Often on crest of buttock	
Large area of induration/cellulitis surrounding a tiny central pus pocket	Primarily medical treatment (Bactrim or Vancomycin); do not debride cellulitis!

- Most abscesses can be drained in the clinic or emergency department without the need for drains or setons.
- Antibiotics are indicated only in immunocompromised patients, including diabetic patients; antibiotics are NOT a replacement for adequate drainage.
- Imaging, such as computed tomography or MRI, is indicated only in recurrent or complex presentations, such as supralevator or extralevator abscesses.

Abscesses should be drained at the point of maximal fluctuance, and as close to the anal opening as possible. Location of the abscess is key to correct management (Fig. 7). Perianal and ischioanal abscesses should be drained through the skin. Submucosal abscesses should be drained into the rectum to avoid causing an extrasphincteric abscess (Fig. 8). The approach to supralevator or extralevator abscesses may be dependent on the etiology, including Crohn disease or diverticulitis, and is beyond the scope of this article.

- Recurrence occurs in approximately 13% overall, usually if drainage is inadequate.
- Patients with horseshoe abscesses recur up to 50% of the time.
- Abscess results in anal fistula in 30% to 50% of cases [7].

Postanal space abscess
- Postanal space abscesses, both superficial and deep, present with dull rectal or "tailbone" pain.
- External erythema is rare.
- Fluctuance or fullness in the postanal space is palpable on digital rectal examination.
- Drain into the rectum by either internal sphincterotomy or an intersphincteric incision into the space in the posterior midline.
- Although superficial postanal abscesses may be drained through the skin, the rate of fistula is higher.

Horseshoe abscess
- Horseshoe abscesses arise from a deep postanal space abscess that extends to one or both ischiorectal fossae (Fig. 9).

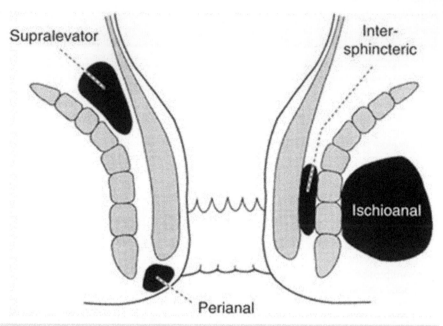

Fig. 7. Location of perianal abscesses. (*From* Davis BR, Kasten KR. Anorectal abscess and fistula. In: Steele SR, Hull TL, Read T, et al, editors. ASCRS textbook of colon and rectal surgery. 3rd edition. New York: Springer; 2016. p. 215–44; with permission.)

- These complex abscesses are managed by the modified Hanley procedure, first draining the deep postanal space, as noted previously.
- Lateral extension(s) are then drained with counterincisions.
- Loose setons may be placed for drainage, and removed as healing progresses.
- Recurrence is as high as 50%.

FISTULA IN ANO

Fistula in ano may be described using the Park classification (Fig. 10, Table 3) or by complexity (Box 2). Goals of management are preservation of sphincter function and prevention of recurrence. Identification of the primary and secondary openings is integral to choosing the proper operative approach. The external opening is commonly readily apparent, but identification of the internal opening can be more challenging. The Goodsall rule (Fig. 11) is often used to predict the location of the internal (primary) opening from the location of the external (secondary) opening; however, this is correct in only approximately 50% of cases.

- Examination under anesthesia may identify the internal opening; a probe can then be passed carefully through to the external opening, defining the track. This direction, from internal to external, is preferred as less likely to cause a false track.

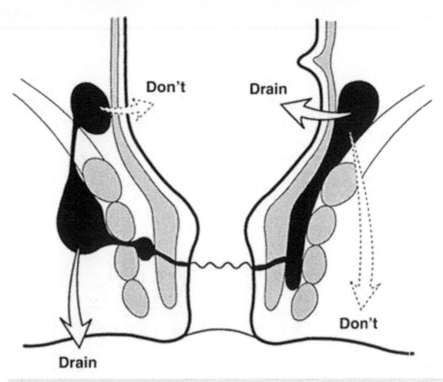

Fig. 8. Location of abscess drainage. (*From* Rakinic J, Poola VP. Hemorrhoids and fistulas: new solutions to old problems. Curr Prob Surg 2014;51(3):98–137; with permission.)

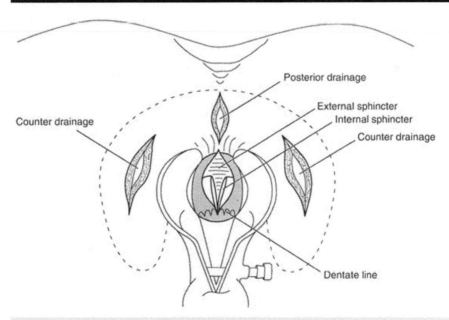

Fig. 9. Modified Hanley procedure. (*From* Davis BR, Kasten KR. Anorectal abscess and fistula. In: Steele SR, Hull TL, Read T, et al, editors. ASCRS textbook of colon and rectal surgery. 3rd edition. New York: Springer; 2016. p. 215–44; with permission.)

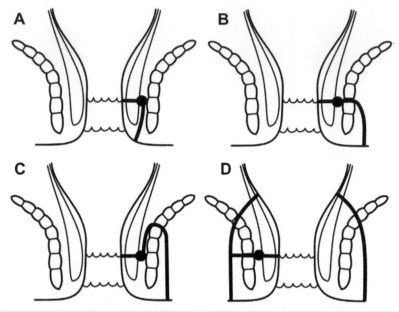

Fig. 10. Fistula locations. (*A*) Intersphincteric. (*B*) Transsphincteric. (*C*) Suprasphincteric. (*D*) Extrasphincteric. (*From* Rakinic J, Poola VP. Hemorrhoids and fistulas: new solutions to old problems. Curr Prob Surg 2014;51(3):98–137; with permission.)

Table 3
Park classification of fistula in ano

Intersphincteric	70% of all fistulas
	Arise from perianal abscess
	Variable amount of internal sphincter involved; no external sphincter involved
	May track cranially to above the levator
Transsphincteric	25% of fistulas
	Arise from ischioanal abscess
	Traverses portions of internal and external sphincters
	May extend through levator into pelvis
Suprasphincteric	5% or fewer of all fistulas
	Results from supralevator abscess
	Arises in intersphincteric space, tracks cranially above puborectalis into ischioanal fossa to perianal skin
Extrasphincteric	Rarest type of fistula
	Common causes: iatrogenic, penetrating rectal/perineal injury, Crohn disease, or cancer and cancer treatment
	Track passes from rectum above levator, through ischioanal fossa to perianal skin

Box 2: Simple and complex anal fistulas

Simple

Intersphincteric

Low-lying transsphincteric

Complex

Suprasphincteric

Extrasphincteric

Fistulas involving more than 30% of the external sphincter

Fistulas with multiple tracks

Anterior fistula in a woman

Rectovaginal fistulas

Fistulas in a patient with impaired continence

Recurrent fistula

Fistulas secondary to inflammatory bowel disease; infectious diseases including tuberculosis; human immunodeficiency virus (HIV); radiation; or neoplasm.

- If internal opening is not apparent, a probe may be passed carefully from the external opening toward the area thought to harbor the internal opening.
- Substances such as methylene blue, hydrogen peroxide, or milk can be injected into the external opening and sought at the dentate line.
- Following the granulation tissue present in the fistula track will help identify the internal opening, although this requires tissue division before the internal opening is identified.
- Grasping the track and noting the puckering of the anal crypt when traction is placed on the fistula track is useful in simple fistulas, but openings may be missed in complex fistula disease.

Low, simple fistula

Simple fistulas involve a minimum of external sphincter muscle, and are preferentially treated by primary fistulotomy.

- A probe is inserted into the track; tissue overlying the probe is divided and track curetted of epithelial and granulation tissue.
- Curettings can be sent for pathologic evaluation if there is concern for neoplasia.
- The wound is generally too saucerlike to pack; it is allowed to heal by secondary intention.
- Recurrence rate up to 7% is expected.
- Continence alteration (Table 4) is associated with female gender, high fistula, and prior fistula surgery.
- Patients with previous fistula surgery are at highest risk for continence disturbance.

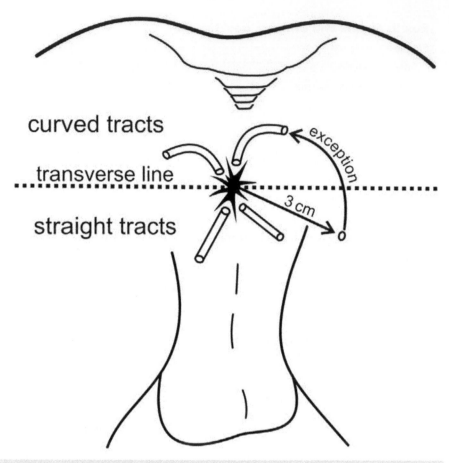

curved tracts

transverse line

straight tracts

exception

3 cm

Fig. 11. Goodsall rule. (*From* Rakinic J, Poola VP. Hemorrhoids and fistulas: new solutions to old problems. Curr Prob Surg 2014;51(3):98–137; with permission.)

High or complex fistula

Healing and preserved continence are often inversely related for complex or recurrent fistula disease, which makes these situations particularly challenging. Several alternatives are used to manage these types of fistula.

Setons/staged procedures

A seton is a nonabsorbable loop passed through the track to allow for drainage or a staged approach to complex fistulas. Using a silk suture as a seton

Table 4	
Expected continence alteration after fistulotomy	
Minor soiling	5%–40%
Incontinence to flatus	Up to 20%
Incontinence to liquid stool	Up to 3%

Box 3: Indications for seton use

A. Identification/promotion of fibrosis at complex fistula encircling all or much of sphincter mechanism

B. Mark fistula track in setting of extensive sepsis with distortion of normal anatomy

C. Anterior transsphincteric fistula in female patient

D. High transsphincteric fistula in patient with expected poor healing (HIV, Crohn disease, other immunosuppression)

E. Promote drainage/prevent abscess in anorectal Crohn disease

F. Other situations with concern that sphincter division would result in incontinence: previous anorectal procedures involving sphincters, multiple fistulas, elderly patients

From Rakinic J, Poola VP. Hemorrhoids and fistulas: new solutions to old problems. Curr Prob Surg 2014;51(3):98–137; with permission.

promotes inflammation and fibrosis, with the goal of allowing a second-stage fistulotomy to divide the remaining sphincter muscle when the divided ends will be kept in close proximity by the fibrosis [8]. A seton used as a drain and/or to prevent abscess collection should be nonreactive, such as a silastic vessel loop. Situations considered for seton use are shown in Box 3.

- The external and internal openings of the fistula track are identified.
- Skin, anal mucosa, and other nonmuscle tissues are divided to expose the sphincter, and the seton is passed through the track and secured.
- Silk setons are tied to themselves; other materials can be secured with 2 silk sutures.
- Sufficient room is left between the knot and the tissues to allow manipulation of the seton via the long knot.

Tying the seton tightly about the tissues to promote tissue ischemia and allow the seton to "cut through" the tissue is painful, and has been associated with a high rate of incontinence; with minor incontinence rate of 35% to 65% and major incontinence of up to 26%.

Horseshoe fistulas. Horseshoe fistulas are suprasphincteric fistulas with complete sphincter involvement, and often multiple external openings that arc at a significant distance from the internal opening. Treatment requires identification of the internal opening and proper drainage of the postanal space. This is classically done with the modified Hanley procedure, as described previously (see Fig. 9).

- The postanal space is unroofed, and any lateral extensions drained with counterincisions.
- Tracks are curetted; soft drains may be placed through the lateral extensions for several days.
- With the inciting cryptoglandular source obliterated, the lateral tracks should heal secondarily.

- Recurrence is as high as 18%.
- Disturbance in continence in up to 40%.

Anterior horseshoe fistulas. Anterior horseshoe fistulas are very uncommon and can be difficult to manage.

- There is no puborectalis muscle anteriorly; therefore, immediate fistulotomy would guarantee incontinence.
- The abscess or fistula track may lie deep to the transverse perinei muscle.
- Drain with division of the inferior half of the internal sphincter, or intersphincteric entry into the abscess, and seton placement.
- Counterincisions are done for any lateral tracks.

Continence-preserving approaches
Fibrin glue. Fibrin glue is appealing for use in fistula disease because of its simplicity and avoidance of continence disturbance. If it fails, the procedure can be repeated with very low risk, and failure does not preclude the patient from receiving other methods of treatment.

- Thirty percent to 60% success is achieved in properly selected patients.
- Both the internal and external openings of the fistula track must be clearly identified, and the track curetted to remove debris.
- A commercially available preloaded double-barrel syringe is introduced into the track via the external opening until the tip is seen through the internal opening.
- The syringe is emptied slowly and steadily, allowing the glue components to mix while steadily withdrawing the syringe to fill the fistula track from the internal opening out, avoiding any gaps in filling the track.
- Injection is followed by a 10-minute wait to allow the clot to stabilize.
- Adding intra-adhesive antibiotic or closing the internal opening does not improve outcomes.
- Fibrin glue in patients with Crohn fistulas showed a remission rate of 38% compared with 16% in the group that did not receive fibrin glue [9,10].

Fistula plug. The anal fistula plug (Box 4) is intended to be passed through the track and fixed into place, allowing ingrowth of normal tissues to obliterate the track. The details of placement vary according to manufacturer and also

---

Box 4: Anal fistula plug options

Biologic
   Surgisis Anal Fistula Plug, Cook Surgical (Bloomington, IN)
   Porcine small intestine
Synthetic
   Gore Bio-A Fistula Plug, WL Gore and Associates (Newark, DE)
   Polyglycolic acid-trimethylene carbonate bioabsorbable polymer

experience published in the literature. Healing rates are variable, and postoperative sepsis remains a concern [11].

- The plug has appeal similar to fibrin glue in its simplicity and preservation of continence.
- Mechanical bowel preparation and intravenous (IV) antibiotics are preferred.
- Use of a seton is suggested to allow sepsis to resolve, as well as make the wall of the track more fibrotic, which facilitates the procedure by identifying the fistula anatomy.
- Healing ranges between 24% and 62%.
- Failure is associated with more external sphincter involvement, shorter tracks, posterior fistula, tobacco smoking, diabetes, and previous failed attempts at repair.
- Postprocedural sepsis occurs in 5% to 30%.
- Plug dislodgment occurs in 3% to 10%.
- The data for plug treatment of anal fistulas in Crohn disease is sparse, with widely variable success reported (9%–80%).

Endorectal or dermal advancement flap. Advancement flap procedures obliterate the internal opening while avoiding any sphincter division (Fig. 12). Recurrence ranges from 23% to 40%; thicker flaps are associated with lower recurrence, and separate closure of the internal opening does not improve healing [12]. Reasonable success can be expected for advancement flaps in Crohn disease if there is no active rectal inflammation, although recurrence tends to be higher. Studies comparing fibrin glue and fistula plug with flap closure show superior outcomes after the flap procedure [13].

- Mechanical bowel preparation and IV antibiotics are used.
- Both internal and external openings and the track must be identified.
- External opening is saucerized to allow curettage of debris and irrigation.
- Any fibrous tissue at the internal opening that would hamper healing is excised.
- A flap of well-vascularized tissue is raised; mucosa, submucosa, and some muscle for endorectal flaps; skin and subcutaneous tissue for dermal flaps.
- If the internal opening is above the dentate line, an endorectal flap is used.
- If the internal opening is at the dentate line, a dermal flap is preferred to avoid a mucosal ectropion.
- The flap base should be twice the width of the tip to maintain good blood supply, and of length sufficient to allow tension-free coverage of the internal opening.
- The track and external opening are left open for drainage, and close by secondary intention.

Ligation of intersphincteric tract. The ligation of intersphincteric tract (LIFT) procedure is a sphincter-sparing approach (Fig. 13). Placement of a seton for a few weeks before operation is recommended to allow the track to mature. Failure is higher in anterior and longer fistulas, but repeat procedures remain feasible.

- A curvilinear incision is made in the intersphincteric groove; the fistula track is identified and dissected out with a soft probe in the track.

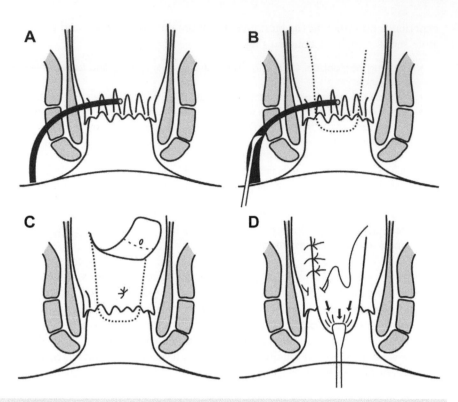

Fig. 12. Endorectal advancement flap. (A) Anatomy of track. (B) Track curettage. (C) Endorectal flap raised. (D) Flap advancement and securing; distal tip harboring fistula opening has been excised. (*From* Rakinic J, Poola VP. Hemorrhoids and fistulas: new solutions to old problems. Curr Prob Surg 2014;51(3):98–137; with permission.)

- Track in the intersphincteric groove is suture ligated with a 3-0 absorbable suture, first close to the internal sphincter, then again closer to external sphincter, leaving sufficient length of track to comfortably divide between the sutures. Probe is removed before suture ligation.
- The lateral portion of the track is curetted.
- Track division is confirmed by probing or injection.

Success rates are 40% to 90% when LIFT is done as the primary fistula procedure; 57% to 82% in recurrent fistulas. Most failures occur within 6 months of the procedure [14]. Types of failure, and the best methods for management, are described in Table 5. Combining LIFT and flap procedures does not improve results.

ANAL FISSURE

Anal fissures related to hypertonicity of the internal sphincter are most commonly located in the posterior midline, although approximately 20% of fissures in women are in the anterior midline. Examination of the anal canal at

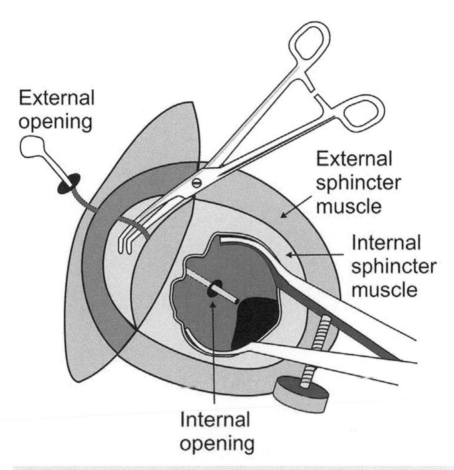

External
opening

External
sphincter
muscle

Internal
sphincter
muscle

Internal
opening

Fig. 13. LIFT procedure. (*From* Rakinic J, Poola VP. Hemorrhoids and fistulas: new solutions to old problems. Curr Prob Surg 2014;51(3):98–137; with permission.)

initial presentation is often limited due to pain. Although initial treatment is often begun without complete anorectal examination due to patient discomfort, it is imperative to perform digital examination and anoscopy within approximately 6 weeks of presentation to rule out other entities that may be causing

Table 5
Ligation of intersphincteric tract (LIFT) failure types

Type	Description	Management option(s)
1	Residual sinus track, no internal opening	Track curettage
2	Less complex intersphincteric fistula	Fistulotomy
3	Complete failure with track extending from original internal opening to 1 or more external openings	Fistulotomy Repeat LIFT, ± bioprosthetic interposition at intersphincteric site Flap closure

the anal pain. If abscess is considered, examination under anesthesia is indicated right away.

Fissure in the lateral position, painless fissure, delayed healing, or nonhealing despite adequate medical management heralds an atypical fissure. Most common causes are Crohn disease, HIV, sexually transmitted infection, and malignancy. Examination under anesthesia and biopsy is indicated to direct further treatment.

Most acute anal fissures of less than 6 weeks' duration heal with dietary modifications and supportive care. In chronic fissures with duration more than 6 weeks, further therapy is indicated.

Topical medications
- 0.2% glycerol trinitrate (GTN) ointment applied 3 times daily for 4 to 6 weeks heals 50% to 70% of fissures.
- 0.4% nitroglycerin (Rectiv) has a similar healing rate.
- The most concerning side effect, as with other nitrates, is dose-related headache.
- 2% diltiazem and 2% to 3% nifedipine are not approved by the Food and Drug Administration for treatment of anal fissure; however, they are used frequently as compounded topical medications in anal fissure; the same dosing is used.
- Healing rates are comparable to GTN with lower incidence of headache.

Botulinum toxin
Injection of botulinum toxin into the internal sphincter produces temporary paralysis that persists for 2 to 3 months, allowing fissure healing. Sustained changes in continence occur in approximately 7%. This approach is most often chosen when patients have failed topical therapy as described previously, and is favored in patients at higher risk for incontinence, such as women and the elderly [15].

- Avoid injection of local anesthetics before toxin injection, as the anesthetic decreases effectiveness of the toxin.
- The intersphincteric groove is palpated and botulinum toxin is injected into internal sphincter in 4 quadrants.
- Fissure location does not influence injection site.
- 100 units provides the best outcome.
- Most will have good symptom relief.
- Up to 40% will have symptom recurrence, but can be retreated with good results.

Lateral internal sphincterotomy
Lateral internal sphincterotomy (LIS) mechanically addresses the hypertonic internal sphincter by dividing a portion of it at one location, decreasing the tonicity. At one time the standard management for fissure, it is now reserved for nonresponse to medical management due to the relatively high rate of continence alterations.

Open technique

The anoderm is incised to expose the internal sphincter, usually in the right lateral position to avoid hemorrhoids. One-third to one-half of the muscle is sharply divided (Fig. 14).

Closed technique

An 11 or 15 blade is inserted into the intersphincteric groove and a portion of the internal sphincter is divided without incising the anal mucosa. The surgeon's finger provides counterpressure within the anal canal during muscle division. The authors prefer the open technique (Fig. 15).

More than 95% of fissures heal after LIS; however, fecal incontinence is reported as high as 30%. Fissure healing and risk of incontinence are related to extent of sphincterotomy: more muscle division produces higher healing, but also higher incontinence rate. Postoperative ultrasound has shown a higher than expected incidence of complete sphincterotomy after open technique [16]. This might argue for a more conservative approach.

Fissurectomy

Excision of the chronic anal fissure promotes faster healing as epithelized edges and scar tissue are excised. Fissurectomy in combination with botulinum toxin injection appears to have healing rates comparable to LIS with lower risk of fecal incontinence [17].

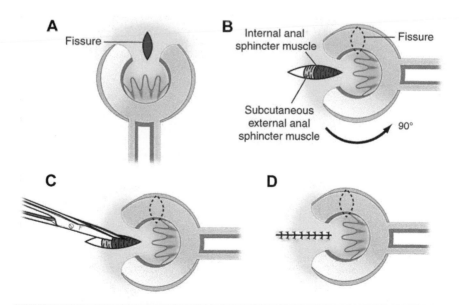

Fig. 14. Open LIS. (*From* Lu KC, Herzig DO. Anal fissure. In: Steele SR, Hull TL, Read T, et al, editors. ASCRS textbook of colon and rectal surgery. 3rd edition. New York: Springer; 2016. p. 205–14; with permission.)

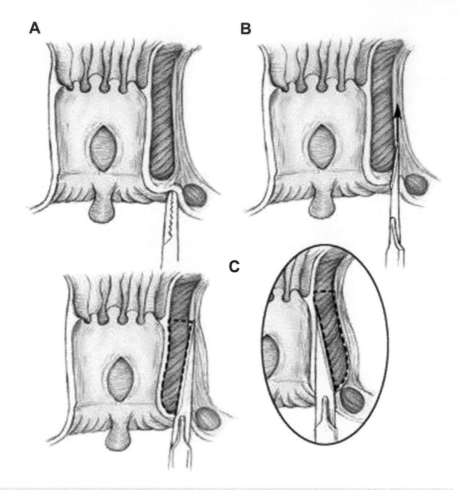

Fig. 15. Closed LIS. (*From* Lu KC, Herzig DO. Anal fissure. In: Steele SR, Hull TL, Read T, et al, editors. ASCRS textbook of colon and rectal surgery. 3rd edition. New York: Springer; 2016. p. 205–14; with permission.)

Special situations
Fissure without anal hypertonicity
- Medications directed toward relaxation of the anal sphincter are unlikely to provide benefit.
- Sphincterotomy is contraindicated.
- Fissurectomy with dermal advancement flap is the preferred approach, with near 100% healing rates and around 6% flap disruption [18].

Crohn disease
- Often in atypical location and deeper than the usual fissure
- May herald active Crohn disease in rectum or elsewhere
- Involvement of gastroenterologist for appropriate Crohn medical treatment is crucial

- Surgical intervention reserved for complications and performed with caution to avoid functional disruption of sphincter complex

CONDYLOMATA ACUMINATA

Condyloma acuminata are commonly encountered in the colorectal clinic. A significant number of patients will also have intra-anal lesions, hence anoscopy is mandatory. Lesions of the perineum, scrotum, vulva, and groins are not uncommon. HIV testing should be strongly considered in all patients presenting with anal warts, as treatment of previously undiagnosed HIV will result in resolution of many of the condylomatous lesions.

- Human papilloma virus serotypes 6 and 11 are typically encountered with benign condylomata.
- Serotypes 16 and 18 are associated with lesions with dysplasia or dysplastic potential, and invasive squamous cell carcinomas.

Smaller and less extensive lesions may be treated with topical modalities.

- Patient-applied 5% imiquimod cream and 0.5% podophyllotoxin solution produce clearance rates of 75% and 72%, respectively [19].
- 15% sinecatechins ointment, derived from green tea leaves, is reported to have 55% clearance rate when applied by patients for 6 weeks [20].
- Trichloroacetic acid, applied by the physician in the office setting, is inexpensive and effective in 55% to 80% of patients.
- Cryotherapy with liquid nitrogen, applied by physicians, has a 45% to 75% response.

Surgical excision is most beneficial for larger (>1 cm) and exophytic lesions; also provides specimen for pathology and subtype analysis.

- Excision is performed with sharp scissors, cautery, or laser, taking care to remove only the lesions and preserve surrounding normal tissue.
- Smaller lesions in perianal skin and within the anal canal are ablated with electrocautery.
- All members of the surgical team should be protected with masks, proper gloving, and smoke evacuation. The risk of live virus in the plume is controversial [11].

References

[1] Rakinic J, Poola VP. Hemorrhoids and fistulas: new solutions to old problems. Curr Prob Surg 2014;51(3):98–137.
[2] Ho YH, Buettner PG. Open compared with closed haemorrhoidectomy: meta-analysis of randomized controlled trials. Tech Coloproctol 2007;11:135–43.
[3] Altomare DF, Milito G, Andreoli F, et al, Ligasure for Hemorrhoids Study Group. Ligasure Precise vs. conventional diathermy for Milligan-Morgan hemorrhoidectomy: a prospective, randomized, multicenter trial. Dis Colon Rectum 2008;51:514–9.
[4] Giordano P, Gravante G, Sorge R, et al. Long-term outcomes of stapled hemorrhoidopexy vs conventional hemorrhoidectomy: a meta-analysis of randomized controlled trials. Arch Surg 2009;144:266–72.

[5] Sileri P, Stolfi VM, Franceschilli L, et al. Reinterventions for specific technique-related complications of stapled haemorrhoidopexy (SH): a critical appraisal. J Gastrointest Surg 2008;12:1866–72.

[6] Schuurman JP, Borel Rinkes IH, Go PM. Hemorrhoidal artery ligation procedure with or without Doppler transducer in grade II and III hemorrhoidal disease: a blinded randomized clinical trial. Ann Surg 2012;255:840–5.

[7] Van Koperen PJ, Wind J, Bemelman WA, et al. Long-term functional outcome and risk factors for recurrence after surgical treatment for low and high perianal fistulas of cryptoglandular origin. Dis Colon Rectum 2008;51:1475–81.

[8] Subhas G, Gupta A, Balaraman S, et al. Non-cutting setons for progressive migration of complex fistula tracts: a new spin on an old technique. Int J Colorectal Dis 2011;26:793–8.

[9] Grimaud JC, Munoz-Bongrand N, Siproudhis L, et al. Fibrin glue is effective healing perianal fistulas in patients with Crohn's disease. Gastroenterology 2010;138:2275–81.

[10] Cintron JR, Abcarian H, Chaudry V, et al. Treatment of fistula-in-ano using a porcine small intestinal submucosa anal fistula plug. Tech Coloproctol 2013;17:187–91.

[11] Gloster HM Jr, Roenig RK. Risk of acquiring human papillomavirus from the plume produced by the carbon dioxide laser in the treatment of warts. J Am Acad Dermatol 1995;32(3): 436–41.

[12] Khafagy W, Omar W, El Nakeeb A, et al. Treatment of anal fistulas by partial rectal wall advancement flap or mucosal advancement flap: a prospective study. Int J Surg 2010;8: 321–5.

[13] Van Koperen PJ, Bemelman WA, Gerhards MF, et al. The anal fistula plug treatment compared with the mucosal advancement flap for cryptoglandular high transsphincteric perianal fistula: a double-blinded multicenter randomized trial. Dis Colon Rectum 2011;54:387–93.

[14] Liu WY, Aboulian A, Kaji AH, et al. Long-term results of ligation of intersphincteric fistula tract (LIFT) for fistula–in-ano. Dis Colon Rectum 2013;56:343–7.

[15] Chen HL, Woo XB, Wang HS, et al. Botulinum toxin injection versus lateral internal sphincterotomy for chronic anal fissure: a meta-analysis of randomized controlled trials. Tech Coloproctol 2014;18(8):693–8.

[16] Garcia-Granero E, Sanahuja A, Garcia-Botello SA, et al. The ideal lateral internal sphincterotomy: clinical and endosonographic evaluation following open and closed internal sphincterotomy. Colorectal Dis 2009;11:502–7.

[17] Barnes TG, Zafrani Z, Abdelrazeq AS. Fissurectomy combined with high-dose botulinum toxin is a safe and effective treatment for chronic anal fissure and a promising alternative to surgical sphincterotomy. Dis Colon Rectum 2015;58(10):967–73.

[18] Giordano P, Gravante G, Grondona P, et al. Simple cutaneous advancement flap anoplasty for resistant chronic anal fissure: a prospective study. World J Surg 2009;33(5):1058–63.

[19] Komericki P, Akkilic-Materna M, Strimitzer T, et al. Efficacy and safety of imiquimod versus podophyllotoxin in the treatment of anogenital warts. Sex Transm Dis 2011;38(3):216–8.

[20] Tatti S, Stockfleth E, Beutner KR, et al. Polyphenon E: a new treatment for external anogenital warts. Br J Dermatol 2010;162(1):176–84.

Advances in Surgery 52 (2018) 205–222

ADVANCES IN SURGERY

Intraperitoneal Drainage and Pancreatic Resection

William E. Fisher, MD

Division of General Surgery, Michael E. DeBakey Department of Surgery, Elkins Pancreas Center, Baylor College of Medicine, 6620 Main Street, Suite 1425, Houston, TX 77030, USA

Keywords

- Pancreaticoduodenectomy • Distal pancreatectomy • Intraperitoneal drain
- Pancreatic fistula • Amylase

Key points

- Evidence regarding routine elimination of prophylactic intraoperative peritoneal drainage in all cases of pancreaticoduodenectomy strongly suggests that this approach will greatly increase mortality.
- Elimination of routine prophylactic intraperitoneal drainage during distal pancreatectomy does not appear to worsen or improve overall complications.
- This risk of increased morbidity and mortality with a selective drainage approach must be balanced against the risk of leaving a prophylactic drain in patients with a low risk of developing a pancreatic fistula.
- Drains in low-risk patients do in fact worsen outcomes if left in place too long, and early removal of drains in these patients improves outcomes.

EVOLUTION OF DRAINS IN PANCREAS SURGERY

The most important complication in pancreatic surgery is a postoperative pancreatic fistula. Numerous modifications in pancreatic surgery have been tried in an effort to prevent pancreatic fistula [1–11]. In pancreaticoduodenectomy, different anastomotic techniques (duct-to-mucosa, invaginated) and the use of pancreatic duct stents (internal and external) have been studied. In distal pancreatectomy, various transection methods (oversewing, stapling, stapling with mesh, transpapillary pancreatic duct stents) have been compared. In both types of resections, sealants, autologous tissue patches, and antisecretory

Disclosure: The author has no conflict of interest to declare.

E-mail address: wfisher@bcm.edu

https://doi.org/10.1016/j.yasu.2018.03.013

agents (octreotide, pasireotide) have been extensively studied. Despite all this effort, pancreatic fistula still occurs in about 10% of patients after pancreas resection and remains the most important unsolved problem in pancreatic surgery.

Abdominal drains have been the key mitigation strategy for pancreatic fistula since the origin of pancreatic resection in the early 1900s. Long before pancreas resection was possible, the writings of Hippocrates document the early use of drains to address infections and empyema [12]. These early drains were constructed of a wide range of materials and passively drained fluid collections. With the availability of rubber manufacturing, a soft rubber tube named after Dr Charles Bingham Penrose, a gynecologist, became popular [13]. In the early twentieth century, suction drainage, originally using devices with glass receptacles, became more widely used. Then, in the 1940s and 1950s, with the availability of plastics and other synthetic materials, surgeons began to use closed-suction drains. Later, modifications of drainage tubes in the 1970s were aimed at reducing collapse and/or clogging of the tube. Two neurosurgeons, Drs Fredrick E. Jackson and Richard A. Pratt, designed what is commonly referred to today as the "JP drain" [14]. The JP drain is a flat, rectangular silicone drain with multiple perforations and internal ridges to provide consistent drainage while preventing collapse when under suction. In addition, the "Blake drain" is a cylindrical silicone catheter with a solid crossed-shaped center and 4 open-fluted channels to prevent the plugging of draining perforations. Both the JP and Blake drains accomplish the task of closed-suction negative-pressure drainage, and the terms are frequently used interchangeably by surgeons. They remain patent under forces that can reach multiple atmospheres and are designed to avoid obstruction of drainage by body tissues (Fig. 1).

Two studies have compared Penrose drains to closed-suction drains in pancreas resection [15,16]. However, these studies were retrospectively conducted over a long period of time (17 years and 22 years, respectively); comparison of the drains was not the primary endpoint, and they yielded contradictory results. Still, the use of Penrose drains has almost universally fallen out of favor in pancreatic surgery because of concerns about retrograde infection and difficulties with keeping drainage fluid from coming in contact

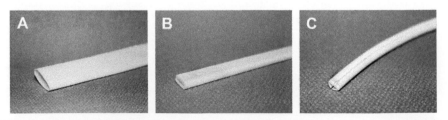

Fig. 1. Drains used in pancreas surgery: (A) Penrose, (B) Jackson-Pratt, (C) Blake.

with the skin. JP and Blake drains are very similar, and there is no literature comparing these drains in pancreatic surgery. Studies have been performed to objectively evaluate the pressure-generating capacities that different closed drainage reservoir systems can generate [17]. Maximal negative pressures (−71 to −175 mm Hg) were generated with the reservoirs empty of fluid, and less pressure was generated as drain reservoirs filled with fluid. Some surgeons warn against "stripping" of drains to maintain patency. Stripping involves gripping the drain near where it exits the abdomen to occlude the drain. Then, with the other hand, squeezing down the length of the tube, sliding the fingers toward the bulb suction end of the drain, before releasing. Stripping of drains was associated with increased negative pressure. In the United States, closed-suction drains are typically used in pancreas surgery, whereas in Europe, closed passive gravity drains are more common. A trial designed to compare the closed-suction drain versus the closed passive gravity drain in pancreatic resection has been proposed, but no results are available [18].

THEORETIC ADVANTAGES AND DISADVANTAGES OF DRAINS IN PANCREAS SURGERY

Until recently, it has been considered surgical dogma that drains must be placed at the time of pancreatic resection. Although the main purpose of drains in pancreatic surgery is to mitigate a pancreatic fistula, drains will also evacuate bile or lymphatic fluid that may accumulate in the operative bed and serve to herald hemorrhage after pancreatectomy. In most cases, drainage is the only treatment required when a pancreatic fistula develops. If the pancreatic secretions are controlled by prompt evacuation from the peritoneal cavity, the leak typically eventually seals, and the drainage stops without any further intervention. However, drains have been shown to be unnecessary or even detrimental in other operations, such as splenectomy, gastrectomy, and colectomy. In a recent global survey of experienced pancreatic surgeons, 14% never leave drains, 27% use drains selectively, and of those who place drains, 51% reported that they remove them early (postoperative day ≤3) [19]. This trend away from the use of drains in pancreatic surgery has been supported by recent literature and concern that drains may increase complications, particularly in patients without clinically significant postoperative pancreatic fistula.

Opponents of drains following pancreatectomy raise several theoretic concerns (Table 1). Some argue that the negative pressure generated by closed-suction drains, which can exceed 100 mm Hg, may actually cause some postoperative pancreatic fistulas by traumatizing or eroding into the pancreatic anastomosis or transection line, although no firm empiric evidence exists to endorse this supposition. For this reason, many surgeons were taught to place drains adjacent to but not directly on the anastomotic site or pancreatic transection line. Drains have also been proposed as a portal of entry for bacteria, which could lead to subsequent infection at the site of the anastomosis. This

Table 1
Potential advantages and disadvantages of prophylactic intraperitoneal drainage in pancreatectomy

Advantages	Disadvantages
Control pancreatic fistula	Traumatize anastomosis/cause fistula
Control bile leak	Portal of entry for bacteria, increase infection
Control lymphatic (chyle) leak	Often does not control fistula/abscess and percutaneous drain still required
Early warning of postoperative hemorrhage	Patient discomfort/anxiety/dissatisfaction

concern has not been proven with closed-suction drains. In fact, in most patients (92%) with pancreatic fistula and abdominal infection following pancreaticoduodenectomy, the organisms are enteric bacteria and can be demonstrated in peritoneal fluid as early as postoperative day 1 [20]. The bacteria likely responsible come from the gastrointestinal tract, possibly the bile, particularly in patients with preoperative biliary stenting, not by moving retrograde through peritoneal drains. Opponents of drains also deem that drains placed at the time of surgery are frequently ineffective in controlling pancreatic leak or abscess, and additional postoperative percutaneous drainage is frequently still required [21]. Some surgeons reason that an image-guided drain can be placed postoperatively if needed achieving the same result as a prophylactic drain placed at the time of resection. Data to support these concepts are limited.

The incidence of postoperative pancreatic fistula in earlier literature varied greatly depending on the definition applied at each surgical center. In 2005, the International Study Group on Pancreatic Fistula (ISGPF) published an objective and internationally accepted definition to allow comparison of different surgical experiences [22]. An all-inclusive definition is a drain output of any measurable volume of fluid on or after postoperative day 3 with amylase content greater than 3 times the serum amylase activity. Three different grades of postoperative pancreatic fistula (grades A, B, C) are defined according to the clinical impact on the patient's hospital course (Table 2). Grade A fistulas are completely asymptomatic, do not alter the postoperative course, and more recently have not been reported as complications is most surgical trials.

ELIMINATION OF ROUTINE PROPHYLACTIC PERITONEAL DRAINAGE IN PANCREATIC SURGERY

The need for routine placement of drains at the time of pancreatic resection was first questioned by Jeekel in 1992 [23]. Since then, multiple retrospective cohort studies and 3 randomized clinical trials have addressed this question [21,24–29]. Although retrospective cohort studies have shown either no difference or a decreased overall complication rate with elimination of routine drainage, these data points need to be interpreted with caution. These studies are retrospective, small, single-institution cohort studies, which are

Table 2
International Study Group on Pancreatic Fistula definition of postoperative pancreatic fistula

Grade	A[a]	B	C
Clinical conditions	Well	Often well	Ill, appearing bad
Specific treatment[a]	No	Yes/no	Yes
Ultrasound imaging/CT (if obtained)	Negative	Negative/positive	Positive
Drains left in place >3 wk or repositioned through endoscopic or percutaneous procedures	No	Yes	Yes
Reoperation or lead to single or multiple organ failure	No	No	Yes
Death related to postoperative pancreatic fistula	No	No	Possibly yes
Signs of infections	No	Yes	Yes
Sepsis	No	No	Yes
Readmission	No	Yes/no	Yes/no

[a]As of 2016, the "grade A postoperative pancreatic fistula" is now redefined and called a "biochemical leak," because it has no clinical importance and is no longer consider a true pancreatic fistula.
From Bassi C, Dervenis C, Butturini G, et al. Postoperative pancreatic fistula: an international study group (ISGPF) definition. Surgery 2005;138(1):11.

susceptible to multiple sources of bias. These studies do not control for changing institutional practices and the evolution of surgical techniques over time. Most importantly, these studies lack randomization, introducing a great deal of bias and potential confounding differences between the 2 treatment groups.

A randomized controlled trial by Conlon and colleagues [27] evaluated the use of drains in 179 patients (drain, n = 88 vs no drain, n = 91) at a single institution. The study included patients undergoing both pancreaticoduodenectomy and distal pancreatectomy. There was no significant difference in the number or type of complications between the 2 groups (drain, 63% vs no drain, 57%), and they noted no difference in mortality, which was followed to 30 days after surgery. The investigators reported an increased incidence of pancreatic fistula in the group randomized to drain placement. However, this study was conducted before the ISGPF definition of postoperative pancreatic fistula. The combination of different types of pancreatectomy complicates interpretation of these results. Also, as a single-center study, the results may not be universally applicable.

A multicenter randomized controlled trial by Van Buren and colleagues [28] studying the effect of elimination of routine prophylactic drainage in all patients undergoing pancreaticoduodenectomy had very different results. The absence of intraoperatively placed drains was associated with an increase in the number of patients that had at least one $\geq$ grade 2 complication (drain, 52% vs no drain, 68%; $P = .047$) and a higher complication severity ($P = .027$). This study was stopped by an independent data safety monitoring board because of an increase in mortality from 3% to 12% in the patients undergoing pancreaticoduodenectomy without intraperitoneal drain placement. Patients without intraoperatively placed drains who developed a pancreatic fistula were promptly treated with percutaneous drainage, but their outcomes were still inferior to patients who had a prophylactic drain placed at the time of resection. This study was conducted at 9 high-volume pancreas specialty sites, and patients were followed more rigorously: 60 days for morbidity and 90 days for mortality. A drain may not prevent the occurrence of a clinically relevant postoperative pancreatic fistula, but it mitigates the risk of morbidity and mortality when one occurs. This study revealed the danger of eliminating routine prophylactic drainage following pancreaticoduodenectomy.

In apparent contrast, a recent 2-center randomized controlled trial by Witzigmann and colleagues [29] evaluated 395 patients (drain, n = 202 vs no drain, n = 193) following pancreaticoduodenectomy and found no difference in overall in-hospital mortality (drain, 3% vs no drain, 3.1%; $P = .936$). However, the screening and randomization process in this study have been criticized because 3200 patients were eligible for enrollment at the 2 centers during the study period, suggesting a screening bias. Also, drains were placed in 21% of patients who were allocated to the no-drain group, suggesting surgeons liberally deviated from the protocol in higher-risk situations resulting in additional selection bias. Of note, 42 patients were not treated per protocol and underwent the intervention to which they had not been randomized (drain, n = 40 vs no drain, n = 2). The study was analyzed on an intent-to-treat basis. The investigators found a significant reduction in clinically relevant postoperative pancreatic fistula (drain, 11.9% vs no drain, 5.7%; $P = .03$) and fistula-associated complications (drain, 26.4% vs no drain, 13%; $P = .0008$) in the no-drain group. The latter complications included postoperative hemorrhage, intraabdominal abscess, and delayed gastric emptying. However, as expected, the 40 patients who were randomized to the no-drain group but deviated from protocol and received intraperitoneal drains due to surgeon concerns had worse outcomes. Specifically, they had a higher rate of fistula (crossover, 6 [15%] vs no drain, 5 [3.3%]; $P = .004$) and surgical morbidity (22 [55%] vs 57 [37.3%]; $P = .042$). The Van Buren study suggests that these patients would have had even greater morbidity and mortality if the surgeon had not deviated from the randomization and decided to leave a drain, despite the patient being randomized to the no-drain group.

It is important to acknowledge the difference between pancreaticoduodenectomy and distal pancreatectomy [30]. Studies that combine these 2 operations are difficult to interpret because the complication spectrum of the 2 operations is different. The downstream complications associated with a pancreatic fistula in a pancreaticoduodenectomy are further complicated by the presence of a biliary and enteric anastomosis, which is not present after distal pancreatectomy.

Several nonrandomized studies have examined the benefits of routine intraperitoneal drainage after distal pancreatectomy. In a retrospective review of 69 patients undergoing distal pancreatectomy over a 14-year period, including

30 patients without intraperitoneal drainage, there was no difference among groups in intra-abdominal complications or the need for therapeutic intervention [31]. Behrman and colleagues [32] recently used the American College of Surgeons National Surgical Quality Improvement Program (ACS-NSQIP) Pancreatectomy Demonstration Project to compare a propensity score matched cohort of patients undergoing distal pancreatectomy with and without intraperitoneal drainage. Among 761 patients, 606 received a prophylactic drain. Propensity score matching was possible in 116 patients. After matching, drain and no-drain groups were not different with respect to demographics or operative data. Pancreatic fistula (including grade A) was significantly more common in those who received a drain. However, there was no difference in clinically relevant (grade B/C) postoperative pancreatic fistula. Drain placement did not reduce intra-abdominal sepsis, the need for postoperative percutaneous drainage, or reoperation. The weakness of these retrospective studies is their lack of randomization resulting in potential differences between the groups and potential for bias.

One randomized prospective multicenter clinical trial has assessed the effect of eliminating routine drainage in all patients undergoing distal pancreatectomy [33]. When distal pancreatectomy was performed without routine prophylactic intraperitoneal drainage, there was no clinically significant increase or decrease in the rate of ≥ grade 2 complications compared with that in patients who had a drain placed at the time of resection. The study was powered to detect a 15% increase or decrease in the complication rate. Although distal pancreatectomy without routine intraperitoneal drainage was associated with a higher incidence of intra-abdominal fluid collection, there was no difference in clinically relevant postoperative pancreatic fistula, intra-abdominal abscess, postoperative imaging, percutaneous drain placement, readmission, reoperation, or quality-of-life scores.

Elimination of routine prophylactic intraperitoneal drainage during distal pancreatectomy does not appear to worsen or improve overall complications. However, the effect of intraperitoneal drainage on mortality after distal pancreatectomy must be analyzed with caution. The only randomized prospective trial available was not powered to detect a difference in mortality, which occurs very infrequently following distal pancreatectomy. Based on this study, one cannot with certainty state that omission of a drain in distal pancreatectomy will not affect mortality. Some surgeons may still conclude that routine drainage is prudent, particularly in high-risk patients who may not have the reserve to survive complications. In these patients, the risk of delayed drainage of a pancreatic fistula, should one occur, may outweigh the risk of a drain, which the study demonstrated does not increase overall complications.

Taken together, these data points indicate that the practice of never leaving a prophylactic drain at the time of pancreaticoduodenectomy is likely to result in worse outcomes, perhaps dramatically worse. Poor outcomes are likely due to the fact that even at high-volume pancreas centers with immediate availability of interventional radiology to perform percutaneous drainage, there is an unavoidable lag between the beginning of a pancreatic fistula, the clinical manifestations that alert the surgeon to the need for a drain, and the eventual placement of the drain. During this period of time, which may be as short as hours, some patients will develop increased harm because of altered pathophysiology leading to increased intra-abdominal infection, sepsis, and in some cases, multisystem organ failure and death. Distal pancreatectomy without intraperitoneal drainage may be an acceptable practice, particularly in low-risk patients. However, routinely placing a drain does not seem to worsen the outcomes. Therefore, unless patients can be selected as low risk with a high sensitivity, it may be prudent to place a drain.

SELECTIVE PROPHYLACTIC PERITONEAL DRAINAGE IN PANCREATIC SURGERY

Although it is clear that it is not safe to eliminate routine prophylactic drainage in all patients following pancreaticoduodenectomy, the next logical question is whether it is safe to eliminate routine prophylactic drainage in a subset of low-risk patients. Three case series have been published comparing outcomes of routine versus selective drainage. In the study by Mehta and colleagues [34], drains were placed "at the discretion of the attending surgeon," and the investigators did not clearly define the criteria used for selective drainage. As one might predict, patients deemed as high risk, and thus allocated to the drain group, had longer operative times, greater estimated blood loss, greater number of transfusions, and underwent more vein resections with reconstruction. There was no difference in duct size, and gland texture was not reported. A single-institution case-control study by Lim and colleagues [35] also assessed selective use of drains over 3 years, but the patient cohort was small (n = 14), and once again there were no defined criteria for routine versus selective drain use. A drain was placed if the pancreatic texture was soft or if the pancreatic duct was less than 3 mm. In patients with hard pancreatic texture and/or duct dilatation greater than 3 mm, drain placement was "left to the surgeon's discretion." The group that had no intraperitoneal drains placed had a lower incidence of postoperative pancreatic fistula and decreased length of stay.

In order to take a selective drainage approach, the surgeon needs to be able to reliably predict, at the time of surgery, which patients are at very low risk of developing a pancreatic fistula and therefore do not need a drain. A 10-point Fistula Risk Score has been proposed and validated [36]. It is based on the presence or absence of risk factors for clinically relevant postoperative pancreatic fistula, including soft/normal pancreatic parenchyma, high-risk disease pathologic condition (all pathologic conditions other than pancreatic adenocarcinoma or pancreatitis), small pancreatic duct diameter, and elevated intraoperative blood loss (Table 3). This novel tool offers a weighted approach that assigns quantitative values to the presence of the aforementioned risk factors. The aggregate of these values creates a score on a scale from 0 to 10 that can further segregate into one of 4 risk zones: (1) negligible risk, 0 points; (2) low risk, 1 to 2 points; (3) moderate risk, 3 to 6 points; (4) high risk,

Table 3

Fistula Risk Score: a validated metric for the prediction of the occurrence of a clinically relevant postoperative pancreatic fistula following pancreaticoduodenectomy

Risk factor	Parameter	Points[a]
Gland texture	Firm	0
	Soft	2
Pathology	Pancreatic adenocarcinoma or pancreatitis	0
	Ampullary, duodenal, cystic, islet cell	1
Pancreatic duct diameter, mm	≥5	0
	4	1
	3	2
	2	3
	≤1	4
Intraoperative blood loss, mL	≤400	0
	401–700	1
	701–1000	2
	>1000	3

[a]Total 0 to 10 points.

From Callery MP, Pratt WB, Kent TS, et al. A prospectively validated clinical risk score accurately predicts pancreatic fistula after pancreatoduodenectomy. J Am Coll Surg 2013;216:4; with permission.

7 to 10 points. The Fistula Risk Score is a valuable risk adjustment method that allows for objective assessments of clinical practice and fistula risk and mitigation strategies (Table 4).

The randomized controlled trial by Van Buren and colleagues, examining elimination of routine prophylactic abdominal drainage during pancreaticoduodenectomy, was reassessed by McMillan and colleagues using the Fistula Risk Score [37]. Patients with negligible/low risk of fistula were found to have a higher (although not statistically significant) rate of clinically relevant postoperative pancreatic fistula when intraperitoneal drains were used (14.8% vs 4%; $P = .352$), whereas patients with moderate to high risk had a significantly

Table 4

Postoperative pancreatic fistulas grouped by Fistula Risk Score zones

	Negligible risk (0 points)	Low risk (1–2 points)	Moderate risk (3–6 points)	High risk (7–10 points)
Patients, N (% total)	63 (10.6)	166 (27.9)	301 (50.7)	64 (10.8)
Clinically relevant postoperative pancreatic fistula, N (%)	—	11 (6.6)	39 (12.9)	18 (28.1)

Five hundred ninety-four pancreaticoduodenectomies were performed at 3 institutions. Postoperative pancreatic fistulas were graded by ISGPF standards. The Fistula Risk Score was calculated for each patient and were evaluated across the 4 discrete risk zones.

From Miller BC, Christein JD, Behrman SW, et al. A multi-institutional external validation of the fistula risk score for pancreatoduodenectomy. J Gastrointest Surg 2014;18(1):177; with permission.

reduced rate of fistula when drains were used (12.2% vs 29.5%; $P = .05$). When drains were used, there was a linear trend in mortality with escalating Fistula Risk Score. In the absence of drains, the probability of mortality increased exponentially with increasing Fistula Risk Score. These results support the concept that a drain mitigates the frequency and severity of complications in patients who are at risk for fistula. Whether there is a benefit to eliminating drains in low-risk patients is not entirely clear. The trend toward increased complications in low-risk patients who had drains in this study may be confounded by the timing of drain removal. Drains were not universally removed early in the Van Buren study; they were removed when drain amylase concentration was less than 350 U/L and/or output was less than 20 mL/d, on average, not until postoperative day 7.

A drain management protocol recently proposed by McMillan and colleagues [38] included selective drainage in negligible/low-risk patients based on the Fistula Risk Score. The investigators reported a clinically relevant postoperative pancreatic fistula rate of zero in the negligible/low-risk group. However, it must be pointed out that surgeons liberally deviated from this protocol when they had concerns based on their experience. This practice must be approached with great caution, particularly for pancreaticoduodenectomy, until further higher level evidence is available.

It is clear that some patients are at very low risk of developing a pancreatic fistula following pancreaticoduodenectomy. For example, in patients with a dilated pancreatic duct and firm pancreatic texture who undergo a straightforward operation with minimal blood loss, it seems logical, to some experienced pancreatic surgeons, that routine prophylactic intraperitoneal drainage may be safely eliminated in this subset. It is less clear which patients are at low risk of a pancreatic fistula following distal pancreatectomy because the Fistula Risk Score could not be validated for this procedure [39]. Pancreatic texture does not appear to correlate as directly with the incidence of pancreatic fistula following distal pancreatectomy. A firm pancreas theoretically holds sutures better and decreases the incidence of a pancreatic leak following pancreaticoduodenectomy. In contrast, firm pancreatic texture may impair the ability of stapling devices to seal the pancreatic transection margin during distal pancreatectomy. A preoperative or intraoperative test to predict which patients will not develop a postoperative pancreatic fistula with very high sensitivity is needed to use a selective drainage approach, particularly in pancreaticoduodenectomy, where the outcome is clearly worse if a pancreatic fistula develops in the absence of a prophylactic drain placed at the time of resection. The outcome of omitting a prophylactic intraoperative drain in a patient who is inaccurately predicted to not develop a postoperative pancreatic fistula could be death, although the outcome of leaving a prophylactic intraoperative drain in a patient who does not go on to develop a postoperative fistula is not likely to be compromised, particularly if the initial clinical course is routine and the drain is removed early.

EARLY DRAIN REMOVAL FOLLOWING PANCREATECTOMY

Although the value of a drain is clear in the setting of a pancreatic fistula, there is concern regarding the potential harm a drain could cause in patients undergoing pancreatic resection who will not develop a pancreatic fistula, which is the majority. The strategy of routine elimination of prophylactic intraoperative peritoneal drainage in all cases does not appear to be safe because it subjects the 10% who will go on to develop a leak to extreme risk. A strategy of selective drainage may be appropriate in a small subset of patients who we can confidently predict will not go on to develop a fistula. However, this strategy is complicated by lack of a sensitive test, particularly in distal pancreatectomy. An alternative strategy is to place a drain at the time of surgery but remove the drain early when the initial postoperative course indicates the patient will recover without developing a pancreatic fistula. This strategy may mitigate any potential disadvantages of routine prophylactic intraperitoneal drainage.

Kawai and colleagues [40] were the first to report on early drain removal after pancreatectomy. In this prospective cohort study, patients had drains removed on postoperative day 8 (n = 52) or early on postoperative day 4 (n = 52) regardless of drain amylase values. This study predated the ISGPF classification of pancreatic fistula, and the investigators defined postoperative pancreatic fistula as more than 50 mL of drainage fluid per day with a 3-fold serum amylase level on postoperative day 4. The rate of pancreatic fistula was significantly lower in the group assigned to early removal (3.6% vs 23%; $P = .004$). The incidence of intra-abdominal infection was also significantly reduced in the early removal group (7.7% vs 38%; $P = .0003$). Drain cultures in both groups were negative on postoperative day 4; however, 31% of cultures were positive by postoperative day 7, suggesting ascending bacterial infection as a potential mechanism for intra-abdominal infectious complications secondary to prolonged drain placement. It should be noted, Penrose drains were used in this study rather than closed-suction drains.

Adachi and colleagues [41] evaluated a total of 71 patients undergoing distal pancreatectomy: 41 in the early removal group (postoperative day 1) and 30 in the late removal group (> postoperative day 5). Closed-suction drains were removed on postoperative day 1 regardless of amylase values, and patients were treated with antibiotics, octreotide, and gabexate mesilate if drain amylase was greater than 10,000 U/L. Once again, early removal was favored with a 0% incidence of clinically relevant postoperative pancreatic fistula in the early removal group, compared with 16% in the late removal group.

Beane and colleagues [42] recently performed a retrospective analysis of the ACS-NSQIP database on outcomes for early versus delayed drain removal in patients undergoing pancreaticoduodenectomy. Patients with a postoperative day 1 drain fluid amylase concentration ≤5000 U/L were defined as low risk for subsequent pancreatic fistula, and early drain removal was defined as on or before postoperative day 3. Their analysis showed early drain removal in patients at low risk for pancreatic fistula was associated with a reduction in overall morbidity (35.3% vs 52.3%; $P = .01$), decreased length of stay (6 vs

8 days; $P<.01$), and a decreased incidence of clinically relevant postoperative pancreatic fistula (0.9% vs 7.9%; $P = .02$).

A recent *Cochrane Review* concluded that early drain removal in low-risk patients may be superior to late removal, but the quality of the evidence was low [43]. The available literature favors an early drain removal strategy to mitigate postoperative complications in patients at low risk of developing clinically relevant postoperative pancreatic fistula, but the data to guide surgeons in selecting low-risk patients are quite limited.

To use a strategy for early drain removal, a simple, sensitive, and objective method to predict in the early postoperative period, which patients are not likely to develop a clinically relevant postoperative pancreatic fistula, would be valuable. Drain amylase concentration has been proposed as a method to make this determination [44–47]. A meta-analysis done by Giglio and colleagues [48] included 13 studies (n = 4416 patients) with the aim of defining the accuracy of drain amylase concentrations in predicting postoperative pancreatic fistula. The investigators determined that the probability of developing a pancreatic fistula if postoperative day 1 drain amylase concentration is less than 100 U/L is 3%, and if greater than 5000 U/L, the probability is 70%. Unfortunately, only 34% of patients have a postoperative day 1 drain amylase less than 100 U/L, whereas 30% have a postoperative day 1 drain amylase greater than 5000 U/L. The investigators suggested that a cutoff value of 350 U/L, which was associated with an approximate 4% incidence of pancreatic fistula, may be more clinically useful because 50% of patients were found to have values in this range.

Only one randomized prospective trial, by Bassi and colleagues [49] from Italy in 2010, has examined the outcome of early drain removal in patients undergoing pancreatectomy. This single-center study combined patients undergoing pancreaticoduodenectomy and distal pancreatectomy. Penrose drains were used. Patients were randomized to early ($\leq$ postoperative day 5) drain removal if postoperative day 1 drain fluid amylase concentrations were $\leq$5000 U/L. Early drain removal was associated with a decreased rate of pancreatic fistula (1 [1.8%] vs 15 [26%]; $P = .0001$; odds ratio [OR] 20), abdominal complications (7 [12.2%] vs 30 [52.6%]; $P = .001$; OR 7.9), and pulmonary complications (15 [26.3%] vs 30 [52.6%]; $P = .007$). In the early removal group, median in-hospital stay was shorter (8.7 [SD $\pm$ 4.0] vs 11.3 [SD $\pm$ 7.2]; $P = .018$) and was significantly less costly (€10,071 [SD $\pm$ 2700] vs €12,140 [SD $\pm$ 6400]; $P = .020$). This evidence suggests that drains in low-risk patients do in fact worsen out-comes if left in place too long and that early removal of drains in these patients improves outcomes.

The management of drains by experienced pancreatic surgeons participating in a prospective pancreas surgery registry in the United States was recently assessed (Villafane-Ferriol N, McElhany A, Van Buren G II, et al. Submitted for publication). Among 244 patients with a postoperative day 1 drain, fluid amylase concentration $\leq$5000 U/L, only 90 (37%) had their drains removed early (before postoperative day 5). Patients in the late drain removal group had more complications (84 [55%] vs 30 [33%]; $P = .001$), including pancreatic fistula (55 [36%] vs 4 [4%]; $P<.0001$), delayed gastric emptying (27 [18%] vs 3 [3%]; $P = .002$), and longer length of stay (7 days vs 5 days; $P<.0001$). In subset analysis for procedure type, complications and pancreatic fistula remained significant for both pancreaticoduodenectomy and distal pancreatectomy.

Patients with a postoperative day 1 drain fluid amylase concentration greater than 5000 U/L have a 70% incidence of clinically relevant postoperative pancreatic fistula and clearly should not have their drains removed early. However, many experienced pancreatic surgeons are still reluctant to remove drains early when the postoperative day 1 drain fluid amylase concentration is ≤5000 U/L because this may not reliably predict the absence of a clinically relevant postoperative pancreatic fistula. Using a lower amylase concentration on postoperative day 1, such as ≤350 U/L, would more accurately predict the absence of a subsequent clinically relevant fistula, but only half of the patients will have values this low.

McMillan and colleagues [50] used the Fistula Risk Score to risk-stratify a subset of 106 patients undergoing pancreaticoduodenectomy that had previously been reported in the randomized prospective trial of early drain removal by Bassi. Patients with a moderate/high risk of fistula and a postoperative day 1 drain amylase less than 5000 U/L had significantly lower rates of clinically relevant postoperative pancreatic fistula when they were randomized to early (postoperative day 3) drain removal. These results indicate that even among patients at higher risk for fistula according to the Fistula Risk Score, the postoperative day 1 drain amylase is a more reliable predictor of subsequent clinically relevant postoperative pancreatic fistula and could be a more accurate and practical guide to postoperative drain management.

It is important to note that drains were not removed on postoperative day 1 in the only randomized prospective trial of early drain removal [49]. Further evaluation occurred in the early postoperative period, and drains were removed on postoperative days 3 to 5 if additional criteria were met. If the appearance of the drain fluid suggested a pancreatic fistula, early hemorrhage after pancreatectomy, or bile leak, the drain was left in place. In addition, abdominal ultrasound was performed on postoperative day 3 and, if this showed a fluid collection greater than 5 cm, the drain was left in place.

In addition to postoperative day 1, a second analysis of drain fluid amylase concentration later in the postoperative course may add additional useful data to predict an evolving or subsequent clinically relevant postoperative pancreatic fistula. Very few data points are available to guide surgeons in this approach. Partelli and colleagues [51] demonstrated that postoperative day 5 drain fluid amylase concentration greater than 200 U/L had a sensitivity of 90% and a specificity of 83% in predicting postoperative pancreatic fistula. Okano and colleagues [52] calculated drain amylase output as the product of drain fluid amylase concentration and the volume of drain fluid output. The ratio of postoperative day 3 and day 1 drain amylase output was lower in patients who did not develop a clinically relevant postoperative pancreatic fistula.

The value of postoperative day 3 drain fluid amylase concentration as a second screen to more accurately identify patients at risk for pancreatic fistula was evaluated in a retrospective cohort study [53]. Patients with a postoperative day 1 drain fluid amylase ≤5000 U/L were divided into 2 groups based on whether their postoperative day 3 drain fluid amylase concentration was greater than 350 U/L. Among patients with an initial postoperative day 1 drain fluid amylase ≤5000 U/L, overall morbidity was higher in patients who also had a postoperative day 3 drain fluid amylase concentration greater than 350 U/L. The rate of clinically relevant postoperative pancreatic fistula was higher (22% vs 4%; $P<.001$) in the higher risk group for patients undergoing pancreaticoduodenectomy but not distal pancreatectomy. The data suggests that patients with a drain fluid amylase concentration 5000 U/L on postoperative day 1, and 350 U/L when measured again on postoperative day 3, would be safe candidates for early drain removal. However, this retrospective data must be interpreted with caution. Drains were almost always removed late in the high-risk group (postoperative day 3 drain fluid amylase >350), so it is not clear if the prolonged presence of a drain in these patients contributed to the worse outcomes. In the low-risk group, only 46% of the patients had drains removed early (on or before postoperative day 5), and morbidity was greater in the late drain removal group (51 [50%] vs 124 [28%]; $P = .003$).

SUMMARY OF THE DATA, RESEARCH GAPS, AND RECOMMENDATIONS

A critical review and analysis of the world literature on the topic of drain placement and postoperative management following pancreatectomy allow some conclusions, but gaps in knowledge remain [54]. Evidence regarding routine elimination of prophylactic intraoperative peritoneal drainage in all cases of pancreaticoduodenectomy strongly suggests that this approach will greatly increase mortality. The only multicenter randomized controlled trial focused on pancreaticoduodenectomy, in which all eligible patients were randomized with strict protocol adherence, resulted in a 4-fold excess mortality in the no-drain group. This study included only pancreaticoduodenectomy patients and was conducted at multiple sites, and patients were followed rigorously for mortality up until 90 days. An increase in not only morbidity but also mortality from 3% to 12% indicates the risk of eliminating prophylactic abdominal drains in all patients undergoing pancreaticoduodenectomy is unacceptably high, and this approach is not advised. Patients without intraoperatively placed drains at the time of pancreaticoduodenectomy who go on to develop a pancreatic fistula are frequently not salvaged by percutaneous drainage and suffer increased morbidity and mortality. This study was performed by expert pancreatic surgeons in high-volume pancreatic referral centers offering state-of-the-art multidisciplinary 24-hour interventional radiology and intensive care. Outcomes in less equipped settings would certainly be even worse. Therefore, any strategy in which prophylactic drains are not placed at the time of pancreaticoduodenectomy deserves intense scrutiny.

The potential catastrophic outcome of omitting a prophylactic intraperitoneal drain at the time of pancreaticoduodenectomy in a patient who is erroneously predicted to not develop a fistula makes a selective drainage strategy perilous in the absence of an extremely sensitive predictor of fistula risk. The Fistula Risk Score may provide such a tool, but few patients are categorized into the negligible-risk category. Even among these negligible-risk patients, an occasional technical error that is not accounted for in the scoring system may result in a pancreatic fistula and a bad outcome in the absence of a prophylactic abdominal drain placed at the time of resection.

This risk of increased morbidity and mortality with a selective drainage approach must be balanced against the risk of leaving a prophylactic drain in low-risk patients. An accurate assessment of the disadvantage of leaving a drain in a setting where pancreatic fistula is less likely, such as cases with a firm pancreas and dilated pancreatic duct, is needed. Placement of a prophylactic abdominal drain at the time of pancreas resection is very unlikely to result in mortality. However, data do suggest that a drain left greater than 5 days in patients who are at low risk may increase complications. Selective use of drains in low-risk patients after pancreaticoduodenectomy has been promoted as a way to decrease risk caused by a drain. However, the potential increased risk of complications caused by prolonged drainage in patients who do not develop a postoperative pancreatic fistula would likely be minimized or eliminated by early removal when drain amylase concentrations and the patient's initial postoperative course support an uncomplicated recovery.

Based on the available data, the safest strategy seems to be routine prophylactic intra-abdominal drainage at the time of pancreaticoduodenectomy with early drain removal in most patients. If the drain fluid amylase concentration on postoperative day 1 is greater than 5000 U/L, the drain should be left in place because the risk of a pancreatic fistula is very high. Although further data from prospective randomized clinical trials are needed, a reasonable approach is to monitor the patient closely in the early postoperative period, and if the patient clinically appears well, and the drain amylase concentration is low, remove the drain early to mitigate any disadvantages of prolonged drain placement. Otherwise, the drain should be left in place, because it will mitigate the bad outcomes associated with a clinically relevant postoperative pancreatic fistula.

References

[1] Zhang S, Lan Z, Zhang J, et al. Duct-to-mucosa versus invagination pancreaticojejunostomy after pancreaticoduodenectomy: a meta-analysis. Oncotarget 2017;8:46449–60.

[2] Sachs TE, Pratt WB, Kent TS, et al. The pancreaticojejunal anastomotic stent: friend or foe? Surgery 2013;153:651–62.

[3] Poon RT, Fan ST, Lo CM, et al. External drainage of pancreatic duct with a stent to reduce leakage rate of pancreaticojejunostomy after pancreaticoduodenectomy: a prospective randomized trial. Ann Surg 2007;246:425–33.

[4] Pessaux P, Sauvanet A, Mariette C, et al. External pancreatic duct stent decreases pancreatic fistula rate after pancreaticoduodenectomy: prospective multicenter randomized trial. Ann Surg 2011;253:879–85.

[5] Winter JM, Cameron JL, Campbell KA, et al. Does pancreatic duct stenting decrease the rate of pancreatic fistula following pancreaticoduodenectomy? Results of a prospective randomized trial. J Gastrointest Surg 2006;10:1280–90.

[6] Lowy AM, Lee JE, Pisters PW, et al. Prospective, randomized trial of octreotide to prevent pancreatic fistula after pancreaticoduodenectomy for malignant disease. Ann Surg 1997;226:632–41.

[7] Allen PJ, Gönen M, Brennan MF, et al. Pasireotide for postoperative pancreatic fistula. N Engl J Med 2014;370:2014–22.

[8] Kitahata Y, Kawai M, Yamaue H. Clinical trials to reduce pancreatic fistula after pancreas surgery-review of randomized controlled trials. Transl Gastroenterol Hepatol 2016;1:4.

[9] Lillemoe KD, Cameron JL, Kim MP, et al. Does fibrin glue sealant decrease the rate of pancreatic fistula after pancreaticoduodenectomy? Results of a prospective randomized trial. J Gastrointest Surg 2004;8:766–72.

[10] Iannitti DA, Coburn NG, Somberg J, et al. Use of the round ligament of the liver to decrease pancreatic fistulas: a novel technique. J Am Coll Surg 2006;203:857–64.

[11] Hassenpflug M, Hartwig W, Strobel O, et al. Decrease in clinically relevant pancreatic fistula by coverage of the pancreatic remnant after distal pancreatectomy. Surgery 2012;152:S164–71.

[12] Meyerson JM. A brief history of two common surgical drains. Ann Plast Surg 2016;77:4–5.

[13] Romm S. The persons behind the name: Charles Bingham Penrose. Plast Reconstr Surg 1982;70(3):397–9, Baltimore. Williams and Wilkins.

[14] Jackson FE, Pratt RA. Technical report: a silicone rubber suction drain for drainage of subdural hematomas. Surgery 1971;70:578–9.

[15] Schmidt CM, Choi J, Powell ES, et al. Pancreatic fistula following pancreaticoduodenectomy: clinical predictors and patient outcomes. HPB Surg 2009;2009:404520.

[16] Yoshikawa K, Konishi M, Takahashi S, et al. Surgical management for the reduction of postoperative hospital stay following distal pancreatectomy. Hepatogastroenterology 2011;58:1389–93.

[17] Grobmyer SR, Fraham D, Brennan MF, et al. High-pressure gradients generated by closed-suction surgical drainage systems. Surg Infect (Larchmt) 2002;3:245–9.

[18] Čečka F, Loveček M, Jon B, et al. DRAPA trial-closed-suction drains versus closed gravity drains in pancreatic surgery: study protocol for a randomized controlled trial. Trials 2015;16:207.

[19] McMillan MT, Malleo G, Bassi C, et al. Defining the practice of pancreaticoduodenectomy around the world. HPB (Oxford) 2015;17:1145–54.

[20] Nagakawa Y, Matsudo T, Hijikata Y, et al. Bacterial contamination in ascitic fluid is associated with the development of clinically relevant pancreatic fistula after pancreatoduodenectomy. Pancreas 2013;42:701–6.

[21] Correa-Gallego C, Brennan MF, D'angelica M, et al. Operative drainage following pancreatic resection: analysis of 1122 patients resected over 5 years at a single institution. Ann Surg 2013;258:1051–8.

[22] Bassi C, Dervenis C, Butturini G, et al, International Study Group on Pancreatic Fistula Definition. Postoperative pancreatic fistula: an international study group (ISGPF) definition. Surgery 2005;138:8–13.

[23] Jeekel J. No abdominal drainage after Whipple's procedure. Br J Surg 1992;79:182.

[24] Heslin MJ, Harrison LE, Brooks AD, et al. Is intra-abdominal drainage necessary after pancreaticoduodenectomy? J Gastrointest Surg 1998;2:373–8.

[25] Fisher WE, Hodges SE, Silberfein EJ, et al. Pancreatic resection without routine intraperitoneal drainage. HPB (Oxford) 2011;13:503–10.

[26] Adham M, Chopin-Laly X, Lepilliez V, et al. Pancreatic resection: drain or no drain? Surgery 2013;154:1069–77.

[27] Conlon KC, Labow D, Leung D, et al. Prospective randomized clinical trial of the value of intraperitoneal drainage after pancreatic resection. Ann Surg 2001;234:487–93.

[28] Van Buren G, Bloomston M, Hughes SJ, et al. A randomized prospective multicenter trial of pancreaticoduodenectomy with and without routine intraperitoneal drainage. Ann Surg 2014;259:605–12.

[29] Witzigmann H, Diener MK, Kienkötter S, et al. No need for routine drainage after pancreatic head resection: the dual-center, randomized, controlled PANDRA trial. Ann Surg 2016;3:528–37.

[30] Pratt W, Maithel SK, Vanounou T, et al. Postoperative pancreatic fistulas are not equivalent after proximal, distal, and central pancreatectomy. J Gastrointest Surg 2006;10:1264–78.

[31] Paulus EM, Zarzaur BL, Behrman SW. Routine peritoneal drainage of the surgical bed after elective distal pancreatectomy: is it necessary? Am J Surg 2012;204:422–7.

[32] Behrman SW, Zarzaur BL, Parmar A, et al. Routine drainage of the operative bed following elective distal pancreatectomy does not reduce the occurrence of complications. J Gastrointest Surg 2015;19:72–9.

[33] Van Buren G, Bloomston M, Schmidt CR, et al. A prospective randomized multicenter trial of distal pancreatectomy with and without routine intraperitoneal drainage. Ann Surg 2017;266:421–31.

[34] Mehta V, Fisher S, Maithel S, et al. Is it time to abandon routine operative drain use? A single institution assessment of 709 consecutive pancreatioduodenectomies. J Am Coll Surg 2013;276:635–42.

[35] Lim C, Dokmak S, Cauchy F. Selective policy of no drain after pancreaticoduodenectomy is a valid option in patients at low risk of pancreatic fistula: a case-control analysis. World J Surg 2013;37:1021–7.

[36] Callery MP, Pratt WB, Kent TS, et al. A prospectively validated clinical risk score accurately predicts pancreatic fistula after pancreatoduodenectomy. J Am Coll Surg 2013;216:1–14.

[37] McMillan MT, Fisher WE, Van Buren G, et al. The value of drains as a fistula mitigation strategy for pancreatoduodenectomy: something for everyone? Results of a randomized prospective multi-institutional study. J Gastrointest Surg 2015;19:21–31.

[38] McMillan MT, Malleo G, Bassi C, et al. Multicenter, prospective trial of selective drain management for pancreatoduodenectomy using risk stratification. Ann Surg 2017;265(6):1209–18.

[39] Ecker BL, McMillan MT, Allegrini V, et al. Risk factors and mitigation strategies for pancreatic fistula after distal pancreatectomy: analysis of 2026 resections from the international, multi-institutional distal pancreatectomy study group. Ann Surg 2017; https://doi.org/10.1097/SLA.0000000000002491.

[40] Kawai M, Tani M, Terasawa H, et al. Early removal of prophylactic drains reduces the risk of intra-abdominal infections in patients with pancreatic head resection: prospective study for 104 consecutive patients. Ann Surg 2006;244:1–7.

[41] Adachi T, Kuroki T, Kitasato A, et al. Safety and efficacy of early drain removal and triple-drug therapy to prevent pancreatic fistula after distal pancreatectomy. Pancreatology 2015;15:411–6.

[42] Beane JD, House MG, Ceppa EP, et al. Variation in drain management after pancreatoduodenectomy: early versus delayed removal. Ann Surg 2017; https://doi.org/10.1097/SLA.0000000000002570.

[43] Cheng Y, Xia J, Lai M, et al. Prophylactic abdominal drainage for pancreatic surgery. Cochrane Database Syst Rev 2016;(10):CD010583.

[44] Ansorge C, Nordin JZ, Lundell L, et al. Diagnostic value of abdominal drainage in individual risk assessment of pancreatic fistula following pancreaticoduodenectomy. Br J Surg 2014;101:100–8.

[45] Ceroni M, Galindo J, Guerra JF, et al. Amylase level in drains after pancreatoduodenectomy as a predictor of clinically significant pancreatic fistula. Pancreas 2014;43:462–4.

[46] Hasselgren K, Benjaminsson-Nyberg P, Halldestam I, et al. The prognostic value of drain amylase on post-operative day one after the Whipple procedure. J Pancreas 2016;17: 213–8.

[47] Israel J, Rettamel R, Leverson G, et al. Does postoperative drain amylase predict pancreatic fistula after pancreatectomy? J Am Coll Surg 2014;218:978–87.

[48] Giglio M, Spalding D, Giakoustidis A, et al. Meta-analysis of drain amylase content on post-operative day 1 as a predictor of pancreatic fistula following pancreatic resection. Br J Surg 2016;103:328–36.

[49] Bassi C, Molinari E, Malleo G, et al. Early versus late drain removal after standard pancreatic resections: results of a prospective randomized trial. Ann Surg 2010;252:207–14.

[50] McMillan MT, Malleo G, Bassi C, et al. Drain management after pancreatoduodenectomy: reappraisal of a prospective randomized trial using risk stratification. J Am Coll Surg 2015;221:798–809.

[51] Partelli S, Tamburrino D, Crippa S, et al. Evaluation of a predictive model for pancreatic fistula based on amylase value in drains after pancreatic resection. Am J Surg 2014;208: 634–9.

[52] Okano K, Kakinoki K, Suto H, et al. Persisting ratio of total amylase output in drain fluid can predict postoperative clinical pancreatic fistula. J Hepatobiliary Pancreat Sci 2011;18: 815–20.

[53] Villafane-Ferriol N, Van Buren G II, Mendez-Reyes JE, et al. Sequential drain amylase to guide drain removal following pancreatectomy. HPB (Oxford) 2018. [Epub ahead of print].

[54] Villafane-Ferriol N, Shah RM, Mohammed S, et al. Evidence-based management of drains following pancreatic resection: a systematic review. Pancreas 2018;47:12–7.

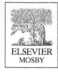

Advances in Surgery 52 (2018) 223–233

ADVANCES IN SURGERY

How Long Should Patients with Cystic Lesions of the Pancreas Be Followed?

Caitlin A. McIntyre, MD, Peter J. Allen, MD*

Department of Surgery, Hepatopancreatobiliary Service, Memorial Sloan Kettering Cancer Center, 1275 York Avenue, New York, NY 10065, USA

Keywords
• Pancreatic cyst • IPMN • Mucinous cystic neoplasm • Surveillance • Resection

Key points

- Pancreatic cystic neoplasms with a low risk for malignancy should undergo initial radiologic surveillance, and resection is indicated if high-risk features develop within the cyst.
- Surveillance should be continued indefinitely for patients with suspected mucinous neoplasms, as the risk of developing invasive carcinoma does not seem to decrease over time.
- Patients who undergo partial pancreatectomy for noninvasive intraductal papillary mucinous neoplasms are at an increased risk for both disease recurrence and pancreatic cancer in their pancreatic remnant; thus, long-term surveillance is recommended.
- Surgical resection for noninvasive mucinous cystic neoplasms is curative, and patients do not have a documented increase in risk in their pancreatic remnant.
- Patients with presumed serous cystadenoma should be monitored for local growth.

INTRODUCTION

Pancreatic cystic lesions have been increasingly identified on cross-sectional imaging studies and have been reported to be present in approximately 2.6% of patients who have undergone computed tomography (CT) imaging and up

Disclosures: The authors have nothing to disclose.

*Corresponding author. Department of Surgery, Hepatopancreatobiliary Service, Memorial Sloan Kettering Cancer Center, 1275 York Avenue, C-896, New York, NY 10065. E-mail address: allenp@mskcc.org

https://doi.org/10.1016/j.yasu.2018.03.014

to 13.5% of patients who have undergone MRI studies performed for reasons unrelated to the pancreas [1,2]. Many of these lesions will be precancerous in nature; because of this, there has been an increased focus on the management of asymptomatic pancreatic cysts. Pancreatic cystic neoplasms (PCNs) include malignant, premalignant, and benign lesions and are managed based on their presumed biological behavior. Premalignant pancreatic cysts are precursors to pancreatic cancer and include mucinous cystic neoplasms (MCNs) and intraductal papillary mucinous neoplasms (IPMNs). Benign lesions, such as serous cystadenoma (SCA), are presumed to have nil metastatic potential; however, even these may increase in size and cause local symptoms, such as biliary or gastric outlet obstruction.

MCNs are defined by ovarian-type stroma on pathologic evaluation and are, thus, almost exclusively seen in women. These neoplasms are most typically unilocular, present as a single lesion, and most commonly detected in the fifth decade of life [3]. Both MCNs and IPMNs produce mucin but differ with respect to their histopathologic appearance and in their connection with the pancreatic ductal system. MCNs do not typically have direct communication with the pancreatic duct. Up to 12% of resected MCNs harbor invasive carcinoma; the risk of malignancy has been reported to correlate with increased cyst size, age, and the presence of a nodule [4–6]. Patients with both noninvasive and microinvasive disease experience excellent long-term disease-specific outcomes, and surgical resection is curative in this subset of patients [4,7].

IPMNs are the most common cystic lesion of the pancreas accounting for approximately 35% of pancreatic cysts [8]. IPMNs are well-established precursors to pancreatic ductal adenocarcinoma. In contrast to MCN, these lesions are more commonly found in males and older patients and may be seen throughout the gland [3]. IPMNs may contain a spectrum of low-grade, moderate-grade or high-grade dysplasia and can progress to invasive carcinoma. Radiographically, these have been classified according to their involvement with the ductal system and are typically classified as main-duct IPMN (MD-IPMN), branch-duct IPMN (BD-IPMN), or mixed-duct IPMN based on whether the main pancreatic duct is dilated. The importance of this classification system is that the risk of high-grade dysplasia or invasive carcinoma differs based on main duct involvement. This risk is highest in those with MD-IPMN, with the risk of invasive disease being approximately 25% to 40%. In patients with BD-IPMN, this risk is between 15% and 20% in resected patients [9]. Patients with IPMN-associated carcinoma have been reported to experience significant heterogeneity in a long-term disease specific outcome. This outcome depends on the histopathologic form of carcinoma (tubular vs colloid) and the stage of disease at presentation [10,11].

Serous cystic neoplasms (SCNs) are predominantly benign cystic lesions of the pancreas most commonly seen in women and distributed uniformly throughout the pancreas [12]. They are characterized by a distinctive honeycomb pattern on CT and do not connect with the pancreatic duct. Most of these lesions have an indolent course; less than 30 cases of invasive serous cystadenocarcinomas have been reported [13]. SCNs have been shown to grow on average between 0.28 and 0.6 cm per year [14–16] and can cause symptoms as they increase in size. Resection is considered curative, however, given its benign nature, is generally only indicated if the cyst is symptomatic, large in size, or if there was a period of rapid growth.

Historically, routine resection was recommended for all cystic lesions of the pancreas; there was initial resistance to a more selective treatment approach [14]. Premalignant mucinous lesions pose a particular challenge as the risk of subjecting patients to the morbidity and mortality of a pancreatectomy must be weighed against the risk of an individual's lesion progressing to pancreatic cancer in their lifetime. When the risk of progression to malignancy is greater than the risk of the operation itself, resection may be deemed appropriate. Guidelines for resection were initially proposed by the International Association of Pancreatology in 2006 and have subsequently been revised as more is learned about the biology of IPMN [9,17,18]. In brief, patients who are presumed to harbor high-grade dysplasia or invasive disease are recommended for resection, whereas those with low-risk disease are typically recommended for radiographic surveillance. In 2015, the American Gastroenterological Association (AGA) proposed that surveillance be discontinued after 5 years if the cyst remained stable [19]. This recommendation has generated much controversy. In this article, the authors discuss the need for long-term surveillance in both unresected and resected cystic neoplasms of the pancreas and evaluate the risk of development of invasive carcinoma in these patients over time.

DIAGNOSIS OF PANCREATIC CYSTIC NEOPLASMS

Initial imaging studies for PCNs may include ultrasound, triple-phase CT scan of the pancreas, or MRI for detailed characterization of cyst features, including nodules, septations, and ductal involvement. Early studies have suggested that both CT and MRI are unable to reliably predict the degree of dysplasia, with both studies having a reported accuracy of 40% to 75% [20,21]. The addition of magnetic resonance cholangiopancreatography (MRCP) to MRI may improve diagnostic accuracy, particularly when attempting to differentiate BD-IPMN from MD-IPMN or MCN [22,23]. However, a recent study demonstrated that single solitary cystic lesions that could represent either MCN or BD-IPMN can be distinguished on preoperative imaging with an accuracy of only 67% [24].

Endoscopic ultrasound (EUS) is a useful adjunct to cross-sectional imaging; however, there is some risk associated with this procedure, and the information gained is highly operator-dependent. The ability of EUS to determine a connection with the pancreatic ductal system or the presence of malignancy is similar to that of MRI [25]. The greatest benefit of EUS is the ability to obtain cyst fluid through fine-needle aspiration, which allows for both cytologic and biochemical evaluation of the cyst. Cyst fluid carcinoembryonic antigen (CEA) is currently considered the most accurate test for the identification of mucinous cysts (sensitivity 73%, specificity 65%–84%) [26,27]. Although this test may allow differentiation of the mucinous subtype, it has not been shown to be helpful in defining the degree of dysplasia, as the level of cyst fluid CEA elevation has not been found to be predictive of malignancy [27]. Cytologic assessment of the cyst fluid has a low sensitivity, as many of these aspirates will be paucicellular; however, the specificity may be as high as 90% for the diagnosis of malignancy [28,29].

Combined, these modalities offer a noninvasive approach to assist in determining the cyst subtype and whether surgical resection is indicated, yet limitations exist when using these modalities alone. Preoperative studies are imprecise in differentiating mucinous versus nonmucinous cysts as well as predicting which patients with mucinous cysts have high-risk lesions. The overall preoperative diagnostic accuracy of PCN ranges from 47% to 78% [30–32], and mucinous versus nonmucinous cysts are correctly identified approximately 75% of the time [30]. Furthermore, although guidelines exist for predicting high-risk mucinous lesions, these can be inaccurate in a subset of patients. A recent study demonstrated that the Fukuoka guidelines and the AGA's guidelines have a similar ability to predict high-grade dysplasia or invasive carcinoma preoperatively, with sensitivities of 28% and 35% and specificities of 96% and 94%, respectively [33]. Given these diagnostic limitations, caution must be taken when radiographic surveillance is recommended and surveillance imaging should not be discontinued too early.

SURVEILLANCE OF UNRESECTED PANCREATIC CYSTIC NEOPLASMS

Patients with unresected pancreatic cysts should undergo routine radiographic surveillance. Not only are patients with mucinous cysts at an increased risk of developing pancreatic cancer but even patients with benign cysts, such as SCA, may experience growth and symptoms from their lesion. The AGA's 2015 guidelines stated that surveillance may be discontinued in patients with cysts that are radiographically stable at 5 years, as the risk of progression to malignancy is very low in this population [19]. However, many groups advocate that surveillance should be continued indefinitely, as there is a substantial risk of malignant progression in IPMN, even if the cyst remains stable on initial imaging studies.

The authors' group recently published a series of more than 3000 patients with IPMN, 2472 of whom were initially managed with radiographic surveillance [34]. In this cohort, 25% of patients experienced cyst growth, 11% underwent subsequent resection, and 3% developed invasive carcinoma (Fig. 1). Patients who were followed for 5 years or more had a significantly larger rate of cyst growth as compared with patients followed for less than 5 years (44% vs 20%). Patients who had stable cysts at 5 years had a similar rate of growth to those monitored for less than 5 years, yet those patients with stable cysts still had approximately 4 times the risk of developing pancreatic cancer as compared with the general population [34]. An additional study from Europe demonstrated that the 1-, 5-, and 10-year IPMN-specific survival in patients with unresected IPMN was significantly lower in patients with an indication

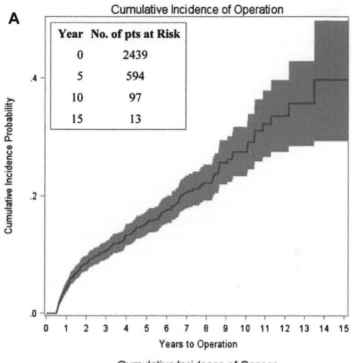

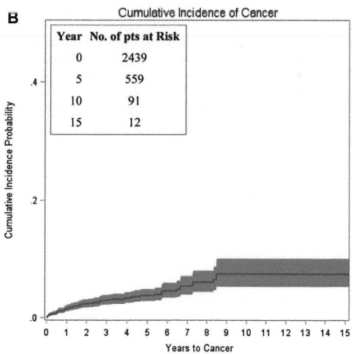

for operation as compared with those without an indication for resection (91%, 75%, and 75% vs 100%, 100%, and 94%) [35]. These findings suggest that the risk of progression of mucinous cysts does not decrease over time and that continued surveillance is warranted.

IPMNs share similar characteristics with other precancerous metaplastic and neoplastic processes, such as Barrett esophagus or ulcerative colitis. Patients have a known risk factor for malignancy and, hence, undergo screening to monitor for progression to an invasive cancer. For example, in Barrett esophagus, routine surveillance with upper endoscopy and biopsy is recommended to monitor for the development of high-grade dysplasia or carcinoma, at which point further endoscopic or operative therapy is indicated [36]. It is not presumed that the risk of progression to esophageal cancer is alleviated because of stability for a period of time. IPMNs are neoplastic processes with cancerous potential. A period of radiographic stability for patients with these lesions does not seem to predict a decreased future risk of malignancy. Because of our limited ability to define mucinous versus nonmucinous cysts and our inability to predict progression in those with mucinous lesions, the authors think that all fit patients with PCN undergo routine surveillance to monitor for disease progression.

The time over which a pancreatic cyst progresses to carcinoma and, hence, the interval at which follow-up should be continued has not been well established and differs based on guidelines and cyst characteristics [18,19,37]. Given the significant risk of progression at both the site of the primary cyst and elsewhere in the gland, the authors typically recommend that patients have a short interval study (3 to 6 months) after the initial diagnosis and annually thereafter if unchanged. More frequent imaging is suggested if there is an increased concern for change or the development of high-risk features. Additionally, the authors recommend that patients with SCA undergo radiographic surveillance annually to biannually to monitor for growth. However, in contrast to mucinous cysts, the frequency of imaging in patients with serous cysts may decrease over time with cyst stability.

INDICATIONS FOR RESECTION

Surgical resection is reserved for those patients who have an increased risk of malignancy. The benefits of resection must be weighed against the morbidity and mortality of a pancreatectomy. This decision depends on both cyst characteristics and the surgical fitness of the patients. The Fukuoka guidelines outline criteria for resection of both MCN and IPMN and aim to identify patients with

Fig. 1. Cumulative incidence of crossover to operation (A) and invasive carcinoma (B). pts, patients. (*From* Lawrence SA, Attiyeh MA, Seier K, et al. Should patients with cystic lesions of the pancreas undergo long-term radiographic surveillance?: results of 3024 patients evaluated at a single institution. Ann Surg 2017;266(3):540; with permission.)

an increased likelihood of invasive carcinoma or high-grade dysplasia on preoperative imaging [9,18]. It is well established that MCNs have an increased risk of malignancy and that surgical resection is curative given the unifocal nature of the disease and young age at presentation. Operative intervention is generally recommended for all patients with presumed MCN. Most patients with MD-IPMN will undergo resection secondary to the increased risk of malignancy; however, selected patients may be managed nonoperatively in the appropriate clinical setting [18]. A more selective approach can be taken in patients with BD-IPMN, as the risk of progression to malignancy is notably lower in these patients. Resection should be considered in any cyst associated with high-risk stigmata, including obstructive jaundice, a solid component, and main pancreatic duct (MPD) dilatation greater than 10 mm. IPMN with "worrisome features," such as size greater than 3 cm, small (<5 mm) enhancing mural nodule, thickened cyst walls, MPD 5 to 9 mm, or abrupt change in the caliber of the pancreatic duct, should undergo further workup and subsequently resection or close surveillance [9,18]. Progression of disease or development of one of the aforementioned features at any time would prompt operative intervention in patients undergoing surveillance. Resection may also be indicated in patients with benign pancreatic cysts (ie, SCA) if the lesion is symptomatic, large in size, or undergoes rapid growth [14,15].

SURVEILLANCE OF RESECTED PANCREATIC CYSTIC NEOPLASMS

Patients who undergo resection and are found to have pancreatic adenocarcinoma should undergo lifelong surveillance according to well-established oncologic guidelines. Greater controversy exists regarding the long-term surveillance of patients who undergo resection for noninvasive mucinous lesions. In patients who undergo resection of a pathologically confirmed noninvasive MCN, there is no indication for further radiologic surveillance [38]. In multiple series, patients who underwent resection for noninvasive MCN did not experience disease recurrence either in the remnant pancreas or at distant sites during follow-up and had a 5-year overall survival of 100% as compared with 57% in invasive MCN [4,5]. Because MCNs present as single lesions without risk for disease elsewhere in the gland, surgical resection is curative and these patients do not require long-term follow-up.

Following resection of noninvasive IPMNs, the authors currently recommend that patients undergo continued surveillance. In contrast to noninvasive MCNs, there is a substantial risk of remnant gland recurrence after resection. The authors, therefore, recommend that all patients who have had a partial pancreatectomy for noninvasive IPMNs undergo routine postoperative imaging, whereas those who have had a total pancreatectomy for noninvasive disease do not warrant further follow-up.

Multiple early studies demonstrated gland recurrence of IPMN multiple years after the initial resection [10,39], and more recent studies have shown a recurrence rate of 17% to 22% in patients with noninvasive disease

[40–42]. Patients who undergo resection for a noninvasive IPMN have a risk of developing a new IPMN and invasive pancreatic cancer and may require further operative management even greater than 10 years after resection [40]. The authors' group recently looked at IPMN progression after pancreatectomy for noninvasive or microinvasive disease, and it was noted that 22% of patients experienced progression within the pancreas with a median follow-up of 42 months. In this study, progression was defined as a new cystic lesion 1 cm in size, 50% growth of a residual lesion, or the development of local or metastatic cancer. Of note, 16% of these recurrences were invasive carcinoma, and 17% occurred greater than 5-years after resection [42].

Which patients will recur has not yet been well established; however, several factors are associated with an increased risk, including high-grade dysplasia in the resected specimen [43,44] and possibly patients who have undergone resection for distal lesions [42,45,46]. Although it is well known that IPMNs can involve the entire pancreatic duct, some studies have shown pancreatic margin status to be significant with respect to the risk of recurrence, whereas others have not [40,43,45,47]. Given the significant risk of recurrence and the inability to accurately predict which patients are at greatest risk for this event, the authors currently think that all patients should undergo postoperative surveillance. The authors recommend that patients who have a partial pancreatectomy for a noninvasive IPMN undergo annual cross-sectional imaging to evaluate the remnant pancreas for recurrent disease and that this surveillance be continued as long as they are fit for an operation.

SUMMARY

The authors recommend ongoing radiographic surveillance for patients with unresected pancreatic cystic neoplasms, particularly those thought to be mucinous in nature, as the timeline of progression to invasive carcinoma in these lesions is not yet well defined. It is necessary to monitor for the development of high-risk features concerning for malignant transformation that would prompt operative intervention. Patients who have undergone resection for a noninvasive MCN do not require long-term surveillance given the low risk of recurrence and excellent survival. However, patients who have undergone partial pancreatectomy for noninvasive IPMNs should be considered for long-term postoperative surveillance, as they are at an increased risk of recurrence and the development of pancreatic cancer.

References

[1] Laffan TA, Horton KM, Klein AP, et al. Prevalence of unsuspected pancreatic cysts on MDCT. AJR Am J Roentgenol 2008;191(3):802–7.
[2] Lee KS, Sekhar A, Rofsky NM, et al. Prevalence of incidental pancreatic cysts in the adult population on MR imaging. Am J Gastroenterol 2010;105(9):2079–84.
[3] Kloppel G, Kosmahl M. Cystic lesions and neoplasms of the pancreas. The features are becoming clearer. Pancreatology 2001;1(6):648–55.
[4] Crippa S, Salvia R, Warshaw AL, et al. Mucinous cystic neoplasm of the pancreas is not an aggressive entity: lessons from 163 resected patients. Ann Surg 2008;247(4):571–9.

[5] Reddy RP, Smyrk TC, Zapiach M, et al. Pancreatic mucinous cystic neoplasm defined by ovarian stroma: demographics, clinical features, and prevalence of cancer. Clin Gastroenterol Hepatol 2004;2(11):1026–31.

[6] Yamao K, Yanagisawa A, Takahashi K, et al. Clinicopathological features and prognosis of mucinous cystic neoplasm with ovarian-type stroma: a multi-institutional study of the Japan Pancreas Society. Pancreas 2011;40(1):67–71.

[7] Lewis GH, Wang H, Bellizzi AM, et al. Prognosis of minimally invasive carcinoma arising in mucinous cystic neoplasms of the pancreas. Am J Surg Pathol 2013;37(4):601–5.

[8] Gaujoux S, Brennan MF, Gonen M, et al. Cystic lesions of the pancreas: changes in the presentation and management of 1,424 patients at a single institution over a 15-year time period. J Am Coll Surg 2011;212(4):590–600 [discussion: 600–3].

[9] Tanaka M, Fernandez-del Castillo C, Adsay V, et al. International consensus guidelines 2012 for the management of IPMN and MCN of the pancreas. Pancreatology 2012;12(3):183–97.

[10] Sohn TA, Yeo CJ, Cameron JL, et al. Intraductal papillary mucinous neoplasms of the pancreas: an updated experience. Ann Surg 2004;239(6):788–97 [discussion: 797–9].

[11] Yopp AC, Katabi N, Janakos M, et al. Invasive carcinoma arising in intraductal papillary mucinous neoplasms of the pancreas: a matched control study with conventional pancreatic ductal adenocarcinoma. Ann Surg 2011;253(5):968–74.

[12] Galanis C, Zamani A, Cameron JL, et al. Resected serous cystic neoplasms of the pancreas: a review of 158 patients with recommendations for treatment. J Gastrointest Surg 2007;11(7):820–6.

[13] Bramis K, Petrou A, Papalambros A, et al. Serous cystadenocarcinoma of the pancreas: report of a case and management reflections. World J Surg Oncol 2012;10:51.

[14] Allen PJ, D'Angelica M, Gonen M, et al. A selective approach to the resection of cystic lesions of the pancreas: results from 539 consecutive patients. Ann Surg 2006;244(4):572–82.

[15] Malleo G, Bassi C, Rossini R, et al. Growth pattern of serous cystic neoplasms of the pancreas: observational study with long-term magnetic resonance surveillance and recommendations for treatment. Gut 2012;61(5):746–51.

[16] Tseng JF, Warshaw AL, Sahani DV, et al. Serous cystadenoma of the pancreas: tumor growth rates and recommendations for treatment. Ann Surg 2005;242(3):413–9 [discussion: 419–21].

[17] Tanaka M, Chari S, Adsay V, et al. International consensus guidelines for management of intraductal papillary mucinous neoplasms and mucinous cystic neoplasms of the pancreas. Pancreatology 2006;6(1–2):17–32.

[18] Tanaka M, Fernandez-Del Castillo C, Kamisawa T, et al. Revisions of international consensus Fukuoka guidelines for the management of IPMN of the pancreas. Pancreatology 2017;17(5):738–53.

[19] Vege SS, Ziring B, Jain R, et al. American Gastroenterological Association institute guideline on the diagnosis and management of asymptomatic neoplastic pancreatic cysts. Gastroenterology 2015;148(4):819–22 [quiz: 12–3].

[20] Visser BC, Yeh BM, Qayyum A, et al. Characterization of cystic pancreatic masses: relative accuracy of CT and MRI. AJR Am J Roentgenol 2007;189(3):648–56.

[21] Lee HJ, Kim MJ, Choi JY, et al. Relative accuracy of CT and MRI in the differentiation of benign from malignant pancreatic cystic lesions. Clin Radiol 2011;66(4):315–21.

[22] Waters JA, Schmidt CM, Pinchot JW, et al. CT vs MRCP: optimal classification of IPMN type and extent. J Gastrointest Surg 2008;12(1):101–9.

[23] Sahani DV, Kadavigere R, Blake M, et al. Intraductal papillary mucinous neoplasm of pancreas: multi-detector row CT with 2D curved reformations–correlation with MRCP. Radiology 2006;238(2):560–9.

[24] Roch AM, Bigelow K, Schmidt CM 2nd, et al. Management of undifferentiated solitary mucinous cystic lesion of the pancreas: a clinical dilemma. J Am Coll Surg 2017;224(4): 717–23.

[25] Kim JH, Eun HW, Park HJ, et al. Diagnostic performance of MRI and EUS in the differentiation of benign from malignant pancreatic cyst and cyst communication with the main duct. Eur J Radiol 2012;81(11):2927–35.

[26] Brugge WR, Lewandrowski K, Lee-Lewandrowski E, et al. Diagnosis of pancreatic cystic neoplasms: a report of the cooperative pancreatic cyst study. Gastroenterology 2004;126(5):1330–6.

[27] Nagula S, Kennedy T, Schattner MA, et al. Evaluation of cyst fluid CEA analysis in the diagnosis of mucinous cysts of the pancreas. J Gastrointest Surg 2010;14(12):1997–2003.

[28] Pitman MB, Yaeger KA, Brugge WR, et al. Prospective analysis of atypical epithelial cells as a high-risk cytologic feature for malignancy in pancreatic cysts. Cancer Cytopathol 2013;121(1):29–36.

[29] Genevay M, Mino-Kenudson M, Yaeger K, et al. Cytology adds value to imaging studies for risk assessment of malignancy in pancreatic mucinous cysts. Ann Surg 2011;254(6): 977–83.

[30] Cho CS, Russ AJ, Loeffler AG, et al. Preoperative classification of pancreatic cystic neoplasms: the clinical significance of diagnostic inaccuracy. Ann Surg Oncol 2013;20(9): 3112–9.

[31] Del Chiaro M, Segersvard R, Pozzi Mucelli R, et al. Comparison of preoperative conference-based diagnosis with histology of cystic tumors of the pancreas. Ann Surg Oncol 2014;21(5):1539–44.

[32] Salvia R, Malleo G, Marchegiani G, et al. Pancreatic resections for cystic neoplasms: from the surgeon's presumption to the pathologist's reality. Surgery 2012;152(3 Suppl 1): S135–42.

[33] Ma GK, Goldberg DS, Thiruvengadam N, et al. Comparing American Gastroenterological Association pancreatic cyst management guidelines with Fukuoka consensus guidelines as predictors of advanced neoplasia in patients with suspected pancreatic cystic neoplasms. J Am Coll Surg 2016;223(5):729–37.e1.

[34] Lawrence SA, Attiyeh MA, Seier K, et al. Should patients with cystic lesions of the pancreas undergo long-term radiographic surveillance?: results of 3024 patients evaluated at a single institution. Ann Surg 2017;266(3):536–44.

[35] Del Chiaro M, Ateeb Z, Hansson MR, et al. Survival analysis and risk for progression of intraductal papillary mucinous neoplasia of the pancreas (IPMN) under surveillance: a single-institution experience. Ann Surg Oncol 2017;24(4):1120–6.

[36] Shaheen NJ, Falk GW, Iyer PG, et al. ACG clinical guideline: diagnosis and management of Barrett's esophagus. Am J Gastroenterol 2016;111(1):30–50 [quiz: 51].

[37] Berland LL, Silverman SG, Gore RM, et al. Managing incidental findings on abdominal CT: white paper of the ACR incidental findings committee. J Am Coll Radiol 2010;7(10): 754–73.

[38] Xourafas D, Tavakkoli A, Clancy TE, et al. Noninvasive intraductal papillary mucinous neoplasms and mucinous cystic neoplasms: recurrence rates and postoperative imaging follow-up. Surgery 2015;157(3):473–83.

[39] White R, D'Angelica M, Katabi N, et al. Fate of the remnant pancreas after resection of noninvasive intraductal papillary mucinous neoplasm. J Am Coll Surg 2007;204(5): 987–93 [discussion: 993–5].

[40] He J, Cameron JL, Ahuja N, et al. Is it necessary to follow patients after resection of a benign pancreatic intraductal papillary mucinous neoplasm? J Am Coll Surg 2013;216(4): 657–65 [discussion: 665–7].

[41] Miller JR, Meyer JE, Waters JA, et al. Outcome of the pancreatic remnant following segmental pancreatectomy for non-invasive intraductal papillary mucinous neoplasm. HPB (Oxford) 2011;13(11):759–66.

[42] Al Efishat M, Attiyeh MA, Eaton AA, et al. Progression patterns in the remnant pancreas after resection of non-invasive or micro-invasive intraductal papillary mucinous neoplasms (IPMN). Ann Surg Oncol 2018;25(6):1752–9.

[43] Kang MJ, Jang JY, Lee KB, et al. Long-term prospective cohort study of patients undergoing pancreatectomy for intraductal papillary mucinous neoplasm of the pancreas: implications for postoperative surveillance. Ann Surg 2014;260(2):356–63.

[44] Rezaee N, Barbon C, Zaki A, et al. Intraductal papillary mucinous neoplasm (IPMN) with high-grade dysplasia is a risk factor for the subsequent development of pancreatic ductal adenocarcinoma. HPB (Oxford) 2016;18(3):236–46.

[45] Frankel TL, LaFemina J, Bamboat ZM, et al. Dysplasia at the surgical margin is associated with recurrence after resection of non-invasive intraductal papillary mucinous neoplasms. HPB (Oxford) 2013;15(10):814–21.

[46] Yogi T, Hijioka S, Imaoka H, et al. Risk factors for postoperative recurrence of intraductal papillary mucinous neoplasms of the pancreas based on a long-term follow-up study: proposals for follow-up strategies. J Hepatobiliary Pancreat Sci 2015;22(10):757–65.

[47] Marchegiani G, Mino-Kenudson M, Sahora K, et al. IPMN involving the main pancreatic duct: biology, epidemiology, and long-term outcomes following resection. Ann Surg 2015;261(5):976–83.

Advances in Surgery 52 (2018) 235–246

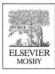

ADVANCES IN SURGERY

ELSEVIER
MOSBY

What Is the Best Pain Control After Major Hepatopancreatobiliary Surgery?

Bradford J. Kim, MD, MHS[a,b], Jose M. Soliz, MD[c],
Thomas A. Aloia, MD[a], Jean-Nicolas Vauthey, MD[a,*]

[a]Department of Surgical Oncology, The University of Texas MD Anderson Cancer Center, 1400 Herman Pressler Drive, Unit 1484, Houston, TX 77030, USA; [b]Department of Surgery, Indiana University School of Medicine, 545 Barnhill Drive, Indianapolis, IN 46202, USA; [c]Department of Anesthesiology and Perioperative Medicine, The University of Texas MD Anderson Cancer Center, 1400 Holcombe Boulevard, Unit 409, Houston, TX 77030, USA

Keywords

- Analgesia • Enhanced recovery • Epidural • ERAS • Hepatectomy
- Pancreatoduodenectomy • TAP

Key points

- The vast majority of hepatopancreatobiliary (HPB) surgery continues to be performed through an open approach, and the best modality to obtain adequate pain control continues to be a challenge.
- Currently, epidural analgesia is the most supported analgesic modality by high-level evidence (randomized clinical trials in liver surgery) for pain control, patient satisfaction, and minimization of total opiate use after HPB surgery.
- Historic concerns for analgesia-related events from epidural analgesia have not been observed in the most recent high-level studies.
- Randomized clinical trials comparing newer analgesic modalities (ie, transversus abdominis plane infiltration) versus epidural analgesia in the modern setting of enhanced recovery protocols after HPB surgery are currently on going.

Disclosure: B.J. Kim was supported by the National Institutes of Health grant T32CA009599; J.M. Soliz, T.A. Aloia, and J-.N. Vauthey have nothing to disclose.

*Corresponding author. Department of Surgical Oncology, University of Texas MD Anderson Cancer Center, 1400 Herman Pressler Drive, Unit 1484, Houston, TX 77030. E-mail address: jvauthey@mdanderson.org

https://doi.org/10.1016/j.yasu.2018.03.002

INTRODUCTION

In the modern era, hepatopancreatobiliary (HPB) surgery has become safe with significant reductions in morbidity and mortality at high-volume centers for both liver and pancreas surgery. Although laparoscopic surgery has provided a safe approach with superior pain control, laparotomy is still needed for most HPB operations. Inadequate pain control is not only associated with poor patient experience but also contributes to inferior outcomes. Specifically, inadequate pain control affects the neuroendocrine stress response, increases complication rates, and prolongs length of stay. Furthermore, there is an ongoing opioid epidemic, and all fields of medicine should strive to reduce narcotic use to limit transformation into chronic opiate dependence. As such, successful pain control after HPB surgery continues to be a challenge, and rigorous studies evaluating postoperative results are needed.

This article reviews the modalities debated to be the best strategies for pain control after major HPB surgery and discusses other important considerations when executing these plans.

Biologic effects of opiates

There are multiple reports in the literature on the negative effects opioids can have on patient function and on cancer biology [1,2]. Emerging data point to direct opioid-cellular interactions that explain these observations. Opiates have been reported to activate vascular endothelial growth factors, directly stimulating cancer growth and metastatic potential [1–3]. Moreover, worse survivals in patients with breast and lung cancer were reported when the tumors expressed certain polymorphism of the μ-opioid receptor (MOR) [4,5]. Additional studies focused on the effects of MOR on epithelial mesenchymal transition (EMT) [1], which is a necessary oncogenic process involving loss of cell-cell adhesion, subsequent loss of basoapical polarization, cytoskeletal remodeling, and increased cell motility and transcription factors for cancer cell growth and metastasis [6]. MOR regulates opioid and epidermal growth factor signaling, which is important for human cancer cell proliferation and migration. In addition, human cancer cells treated with opioids exhibited an increase (snail, slug, vimentin) and decrease in other (ZO-1 and claudin-1) protein levels consistent with an EMT phenotype [1]. Taken together, these results suggest that opioid-MOR interactions may have a direct effect on the proliferation, migration, and EMT transition for cancer progression. These findings have led to human clinical studies investigating the effects of analgesia agents on cancer outcomes, including recurrence and overall survival.

Opioid epidemic

Currently, the United States is suffering from a national crisis with opioid abuse with more than 600,000 deaths to date, and with a prediction of 180,000 additional mortalities by 2020 [7]. The opioid epidemic is accounting for an annual cost of more than $50 billion per year of treating prescription opioid use and abuse [8]. Moreover, opioid-naïve surgical patients are at high risk for becoming chronic opioid users [9], and minimizing the need for narcotics in the hospital and after discharge could aid in combating this major issue.

Intravenous patient-controlled analgesia

Intravenous patient-controlled analgesia (IV PCA) is one of the most common and "conventional" strategies for pain control postoperatively. Unfortunately, IV PCA alone can only provide short periods of pain relief; thus, it may not be the optimal method for extended pain control in the immediate postoperative recovery period. With this strategy alone, patients may consume larger amounts of opiates, increasing risk for nausea, vomiting, ileus, chronic opiate needs after discharge, delay in return of bowel function, and delay in postoperative mobilization. Now, many adjuncts (ie, continuous infiltrating wound catheters, nonsteroidal anti-inflammatory drugs [NSAIDs], transversus abdominis plane [TAP] infiltration) are used in conjunction with this modality or it is increasingly replaced by other strategies such as epidural analgesia (EA) to alleviate this concern.

Continuous infusion through a wound catheter

One retrospective study of 498 patients undergoing liver surgery comparing continuous infusion of bupivacaine through a wound catheter (CIWC) + IV PCA versus EA showed similar pain control, but lower amounts of opiate consumption in the CIWC + IV PCA group. However, this retrospective study was significantly weighted toward the CIWC + IV PCA group (n = 429) and was at high risk for selection bias [10]. Currently, a trial in the Netherlands is underway testing noninferiority of CIWC + IV PCA to EA after elective HPB surgery via laparotomy in an enhanced recovery (ER) setting [11]. The primary endpoint of this study is Overall Benefit of Analgesic Score, a composite endpoint of pain intensity, opioid-related adverse effects, and patient satisfaction during postoperative days 1 to 5. Secondary endpoints include length of stay, number of patients with severe pain, and the need for rescue medication.

Epidural analgesia

EA provides pain control through blockage of both visceral and somatic pain [12]. Historically, it was criticized by some because of the low-level evidence from retrospective studies reporting increased risk of epidural-related complications, including hypotension, intensive care unit readmissions, and a need for excessive fluid and blood product administration [13–15]. Sugimoto and colleagues [13] reported epidural dysfunction to be associated with an increase in overall complications ($P<.001$), pancreas-related complications ($P = .041$), and non-pancreas-related complications ($P = .001$). However, this study was retrospective, from a small cohort of patients (n = 72), and reported an abnormally high rate of epidural dysfunction (49%). In a larger retrospective study, 367 patients undergoing partial hepatectomy were examined and the study identified that the EA group (vs no EA) had a lower mean arterial pressure in recovery (86.6 mm Hg vs 94.5 mm Hg, $P<.001$), and higher percentage of patients receive packed red cells during the hospital course (44.5% vs 27.9%, $P<.001$), respectively. Subsequent multivariate analysis identified EA among many other variables (age >65 years, American Society of Anesthesiologists grade >2, starting hematocrit $<38\%$, operative time >300 minutes, blood loss >1 L) to be at increased odds for requiring blood transfusion. Of note, these data come outside of the modern era of striving for zero transfusions during hepatectomy [16] and reports an overall transfusion rate of 39%. Furthermore, the study's EA protocol used a high concentration of 0.1% bupivacaine, which is now typically started at significantly lower concentrations.

One large retrospective cohort study reviewed 8610 pancreatoduodenectomies (PD) in 2009 from a Nationwide Inpatient Sample from the Agency for Healthcare Research and Quality and identified that the use of EA was associated with a lower odds (odds ratio [OR] 0.61, confidence interval [CI] 0.37–0.99, $P = .044$) of complication including death [17]. This same analysis revealed that patients who received EA (vs no EA) also had a shorter length of stay (13.0 days vs 15.7 days, $P<.001$) and lower costs ($120,656 vs $152,905, $P<.001$), respectively. Subsequently, a more recent analysis from the same national database included all HPB operations performed in 53,712 patients between 2000 and 2012 [18]. Results showed that patients who received EA were less likely to have sepsis (OR 0.75, CI 0.61–0.94), postoperative hemorrhage (OR 0.79, CI 0.66–0.94), postoperative pneumonia (OR 0.73, CI 0.60–0.90), respiratory failure (OR 0.89, CI 0.79–0.99), and liver failure (OR 0.69, CI 0.49–0.98), all $P<.05$. No difference was observed with in-hospital mortality among patients who underwent hepatectomy, but a significant difference was observed in patients who received an EA versus no EA for pancreatic operations (2.1% vs 3.1%, $P<.001$, respectively). This study revealed a greater length of stay in patients who received an EA (8 days) versus those without EA (7 days) ($P<.001$).

More recent evidence has demonstrated EA to provide superior pain control based on 2 randomized controlled trials after HPB surgery [19,20]. The University of Edinburgh conducted a randomized clinical trial of CIWC + IV PCA versus EA following liver resection surgery that showed superior pain control in the epidural arm and lower overall use of narcotics, whereas overall complication rates were similar [20]. In contrast, in this small randomized study of 55 patients, the patients in the CIWC + IV PCA arm fulfilled discharge criteria faster than patients who received epidural (4.5 days vs 6.0 days, $P = .044$). Of note, this study did not include assessment of patient satisfaction and recovery through a validated patient-reported outcome tool.

At the University of Texas MD Anderson Cancer Center, a randomized clinical trial was conducted comparing EA versus IV PCA in a cohort of patients who underwent major HPB surgery (largely hepatic resection) [19]. Ultimately, this study of 140 patients reported EA (vs IV PCA) to be associated with superior area under the curve pain control scores (Fig. 1A: 78.6 pain-hours vs 105.2 pain-hours), less severe pain event rates, improved patient-reported outcomes (PRO), reduced total narcotic usage measured in oral morphine equivalents (Fig. 1B: 155.3 mg vs 429.8 mg), whereas having similar

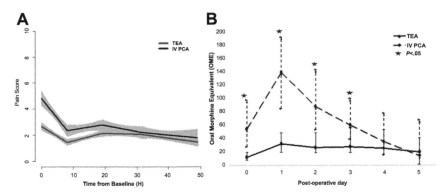

Fig. 1. (A) Pain scores over time in thoracic epidural analgesia (TEA) versus IV PCA. (B) Median oral morphine equivalent (with interquartile range) used on each postoperative day in TEA versus IV PCA. (*From* Aloia TA, Kim BJ, Segraves-Chun YS, et al. A randomized controlled trial of postoperative thoracic epidural analgesia versus intravenous patient-controlled analgesia after major hepatopancreatobiliary surgery. Ann Surg 2017;266(3):549; with permission.)

analgesia-related events, surgical complications, and length of stay. Of note, only one patient in the EA arm experienced transient renal insufficiency among the 13 patients who experienced analgesia-related events. Importantly, this trial used a lower concentration of bupivacaine (0.075%) to protect against clinically significant hypotension episodes while still maintaining adequate pain control, a balance that should be considered with all epidural protocols.

The use of EA has potential benefits beyond better pain control, patient-reported outcomes, and decreased narcotic use. In a study by Zimmitti and colleagues [21], the effect of EA on recurrence-free survival and overall survival was analyzed. In this study, 510 patients who had colorectal liver metastasis received either EA or IV PCA (Fig. 2). On multivariate analysis, the use of EA was an independent predictor of a longer recurrence-free survival (HR 0.76, CI 0.58–0.98; $P = .036$); however, the use of EA did not have a significant effect on overall survival (HR 0.72 CI 0.49–1.07; $P = .102$). In this study, length of hospital stay or postoperative complications were not affected by the use of EA.

Intrathecal analgesia

Intrathecal analgesia has long been a mainstay in providing analgesia for open abdominal surgery, although not extensively studied in HPB surgery. The risks involved with injection of intrathecal opioids or local anesthetics carry similar risks as that of epidural injection. One recent randomized controlled trial of 49 patients undergoing open HPB surgery compared intraoperative intrathecal morphine versus intravenous opioids during surgery (intravenous remifentanil infusion during surgery followed by intravenous bolus of morphine, 0.15 mg/kg before the end of surgery). The study showed pain scores to be significantly worse in patients who received intravenous opioids

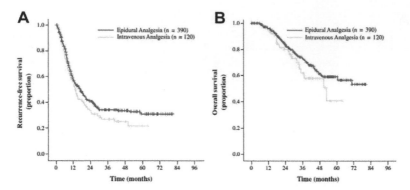

Fig. 2. Impact of analgesia type on recurrence-free survival (A) and overall survival (B). (*From* Zimmitti G, Soliz J, Aloia TA, et al. Positive impact of epidural analgesia on oncologic outcomes in patients undergoing resection of colorectal liver metastases. Ann Surg Oncol 2016;23(3):1008; with permission.)

at various time points until postoperative day 3 [22]. Although not examined in HPB surgery, one randomized study failed to demonstrate noninferiority of intrathecal morphine + IV PCA to EA with respect to pain control, ambulation, postoperative ileus, and pulmonary complications among patients undergoing gastrectomy [23].

Transversus abdominis plane infiltration

TAP infiltration is an emerging novel technique to provide analgesia to the anterior abdominal wall through coverage of somatic pain. The block is performed with the ultrasound-guided injection of local anesthetic into the fascial plane (TAP) separating the transverse abdominis and the internal oblique muscles (Fig. 3). Furthermore, the TAP block is associated with a lesser degree of perioperative hypotension when compared with EA and does not cause urinary retention. The procedure is easy to perform and safe and can be used in patients who are anticoagulated (unlike epidurals). Previously, a prolonged effect was impossible with this single-shot infiltration technique using conventional local anesthetic, but with the development of liposomal bupivacaine, an extended effect can now be provided [24].

Currently, there are few studies, all low-level evidence with limited power and retrospective in design, comparing TAP to EA [25–27]. Two of these studies showed comparable analgesia pain control between the 2 modalities, but all reported a larger use of total supplemental opioids in the TAP group [26,27]. Most recently, a study by Ayad and colleagues [25] conducted a noninferiority study comparing EA versus TAP versus IV PCA in patients undergoing major lower abdominal surgery. Among the 318 patients who were selected for analysis, TAP infiltration was noninferior to EA on both primary outcomes of pain scores and opioid consumption ($P<.001$). In addition, TAP

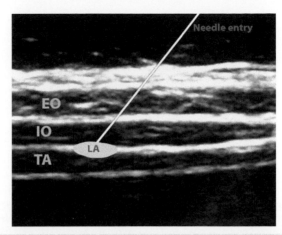

Fig. 3. Ultrasound image of transverse abdominis plane block. EO, external oblique muscle; IO, internal oblique muscle; LA, local anesthetic; TA, transverse abdominis muscle.

infiltration was noninferior to IV PCA on pain scores but was not superior on opioid consumption ($P = .37$). Last, the study did not find noninferiority of EA over IV PCA on pain scores ($P = .13$) nor was superiority observed on opioid consumption ($P = .98$). Furthermore, no studies to date have compared TAP to EA in the specific setting of HPB surgery.

Enhanced recovery

ER and fast-track protocols were initially implemented in the perioperative management of the surgical patient over 20 years ago. Although ER originated in colorectal surgery, it has been broadly adapted to most surgical specialties, including the field of HPB. Although there are many common ER end points that are routinely measured and improved with its utilization (shortened length of stay, improved functional outcomes, and decreased costs) [28], one of the most critical is effective pain control. Patient education and engagement are the foundation of all ER programs. Moreover, a multidisciplinary approach is necessary to support this foundation with 4 fundamental perioperative care principles that include early feeding, early ambulation, goal-directed fluid therapy, and opiate-sparing analgesia (Fig. 4) [29].

ER protocols commonly have an opiate-sparing analgesia principle that is achieved through a multimodal approach. One of these components includes the consideration of NSAIDs, which are commonly used in the authors' institution's ER liver surgery protocol. Use of NSAIDs has been shown to reduce overall narcotic use, reduce postoperative nausea/vomiting, and accelerate time to flatus/discharge [30]. A meta-analysis of 22 prospective, randomized, double-blind studies including 2307 patients showed NSAIDs to decrease postoperative nausea and vomiting by 30% and sedation by 29% [31]. Additional regression analysis demonstrated the incidence of nausea and vomiting was

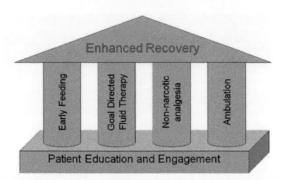

Fig. 4. ER sits on a foundation of patient education and engagement. Four perioperative fundamental strategies that support the program are early feeding, goal-directed fluid therapy, multimodal opiate limited analgesia, and ambulation. (*From* Kim BJ, Aloia TA. What is "enhanced recovery," and how can I do it? J Gastrointest Surg 2018;22(1):165; with permission.)

positively correlated with morphine consumption. However, one study observed that early administration of COX-2 inhibitors may be a risk factor for pancreatic fistula in patients who undergo PD [32]. In this study, use of nonselective inhibitors was not associated with an increase in pancreatic fistula, but COX-2 inhibitors were associated with increased pancreatic fistula (20.2% vs 10.5%, $P = .033$; OR 2.12, $P = .044$).

A meta-analysis of all randomized trials comparing EA to an alternative analgesic technique following open abdominal surgery within an ER setting recently identified 7 studies from 1966 to 2013 [33]. Overall, the analysis of 378 patients did not identify a difference in complication rate (OR 1.14, CI 0.49–2.64, $P = .76$), but a subanalysis between PCA versus EA showed a lower rate of complications (OR 1.97, CI 1.10–3.53, $P = .02$) in patients who received an IV PCA. Although EA was associated with a faster return of gut function and reduced pain scores, no difference in length of stay was observed. The vast majority of these randomized controlled trials were conducted in patients undergoing colorectal surgery, whereas only one trial was in patients who underwent open hepatic resection [20].

Additional high-level evidence regarding pain control is required in the context of ER for patients undergoing HPB surgery. Currently, the University of Texas MD Anderson Cancer Center is conducting a randomized clinical trial comparing TAP infiltration to EA in liver surgery patients in the setting of ER.

Patient-reported outcomes and return to intended oncologic therapy

Adequate pain control is the most common primary patient-centric outcome that is assessed in studies comparing analgesic modalities after surgery. However, other outcomes of patient satisfaction or functional recovery are rarely measured in the vast majority of high-level studies. Now, there are validated PRO tools to measure these important outcomes in surgical patients [34].

The MD Anderson Symptom Inventory-GI (MDASI-GI) is one example of a PRO tool that is composed of 24 questions broken into 3 sections (core, gastrointestinal, and symptom interference) used in patients with gastrointestinal cancer to assess functional recovery (Fig. 5) [35]. Using the MDASI-GI, Day and colleagues showed patients on an ER protocol after liver surgery was an independent predictor of return to baseline interference scores, a measure of functional recovery (OR 2.62, CI 1.15–5.94, $P = .021$). These important validated tools should be used in the assessment of patient recovery when determining the optimal analgesic modality in HPB surgery.

An additional outcome measure to consider in the domain of perioperative analgesia is the analgesic modality's impact on a patient's ability to return to intended oncologic therapy (RIOT). Divided into 2 components: first, a binary outcome (whether the patient did or did not initiate intended oncologic therapies after surgery), and second, the time between surgery and the initiation of these therapies [36]. Intended "adjuvant" therapies encompassing the current multimodality state of cancer care mandate beyond traditional adjuvant systemic therapy (ie, second-stage operations, interventional radiology, endoscopic cancer therapies, radiotherapy, biological and hormonal therapies). Implementation of the ER protocol at MD Anderson Cancer Center improved the rate of RIOT from 75% to 95% as well as a shorter time from 60.2 days to 44.7 days [35]. These data points suggest the clinical importance for establishing a paradigm for the association of perioperative medical care with long-term oncologic outcomes, and this measure of cancer care delivery should be included in the assessment of analgesic modalities in HPB surgery.

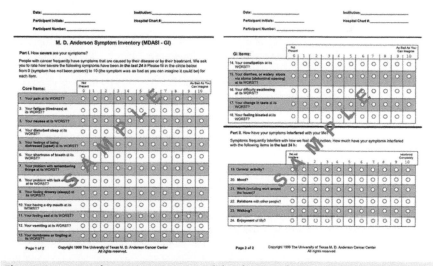

Fig. 5. University of Texas MDASI-GI. A validated PRO tool. (*From* Day RW, Cleeland CS, Wang XS, et al. Patient-reported outcomes accurately measure the value of an enhanced recovery program in liver surgery. J Am Coll Surg 2015;221(6):1030.e1–2; with permission.)

SUMMARY

Currently, EA is supported by high-level evidence, specifically in liver surgery, to be the most effective analgesic modality for pain control after HPB surgery. Additional high-level evidence for superior analgesic modalities after pancreatectomies is required. Subsequent randomized controlled trials are required to elucidate the effectiveness and safety of new strategies such as a TAP block compared with EA for both hepatectomies and pancreatectomies in the setting of ER. Beyond adequate pain control and total opiate consumption, PRO tools and the ability to RIOT in patients with cancer should be a secondary outcome measure in all future studies.

References

[1] Lennon FE, Mirzapoiazova T, Mambetsariev B, et al. The mu opioid receptor promotes opioid and growth factor-induced proliferation, migration and epithelial mesenchymal transition (EMT) in human lung cancer. PLoS One 2014;9(3):e91577.

[2] Lennon FE, Moss J, Singleton PA. The mu-opioid receptor in cancer progression: is there a direct effect? Anesthesiology 2012;116:940–5.

[3] Singleton PA, Lingen MW, Fekete MJ, et al. Methylnaltrexone inhibits opiate and VEGF-induced angiogenesis: role of receptor transactivation. Microvasc Res 2006;72(1–2):3–11.

[4] Bortsov AV, Millikan RC, Belfer I, et al. µ-Opioid receptor gene A118G polymorphism predicts survival in patients with breast cancer. Anesthesiology 2012;116(4):896–902.

[5] Wang S, Li Y, Liu XD, et al. Polymorphism of A118G in mu-opioid receptor gene is associated with risk of esophageal squamous cell carcinoma in a Chinese population. Int J Clin Oncol 2013;18(4):666–9.

[6] Iwatsuki M, Mimori K, Yokobori T, et al. Epithelial-mesenchymal transition in cancer development and its clinical significance. Cancer Sci 2010;101(2):293–9.

[7] Blau M. Opioids could kill nearly 500,000 Americans in the next decade. 2017. Available at: http://www.statnews.com/2017/06/27/opioid-deaths-forecast. Accessed October 1, 2017.

[8] Hansen RN, Oster G, Edelsberg J, et al. Economic costs of nonmedical use of prescription opioids. Clin J Pain 2011;27(3):194–202.

[9] Sun EC, Darnall BD, Baker LC, et al. Incidence of and risk factors for chronic opioid use among opioid-naive patients in the postoperative period. JAMA Intern Med 2016;176(9):1286–93.

[10] Wong-Lun-Hing EM, van Dam RM, Welsh FK, et al. Postoperative pain control using continuous i.m. bupivacaine infusion plus patient-controlled analgesia compared with epidural analgesia after major hepatectomy. HPB (Oxford) 2014;16(7):601–9.

[11] Mungroop TH, Veelo DP, Busch OR, et al. Continuous wound infiltration or epidural analgesia for pain prevention after hepato-pancreato-biliary surgery within an enhanced recovery program (POP-UP trial): study protocol for a randomized controlled trial. Trials 2015;16:562.

[12] Cederholm I, Anskar S, Bengtsson M. Sensory, motor, and sympathetic block during epidural analgesia with 0.5% and 0.75% ropivacaine with and without epinephrine. Reg Anesth 1994;19(1):18–33.

[13] Sugimoto M, Nesbit L, Barton JG, et al. Epidural anesthesia dysfunction is associated with postoperative complications after pancreatectomy. J Hepatobiliary Pancreat Sci 2016;23(2):102–9.

[14] Page A, Rostad B, Staley CA, et al. Epidural analgesia in hepatic resection. J Am Coll Surg 2008;206(6):1184–92.

[15] Choi DX, Schoeniger LO. For patients undergoing pancreatoduodenectomy, epidural anesthesia and analgesia improves pain but increases rates of intensive care unit admissions and alterations in analgesics. Pancreas 2010;39(4):492–7.

[16] Day RW, Brudvik KW, Vauthey JN, et al. Advances in hepatectomy technique: toward zero transfusions in the modern era of liver surgery. Surgery 2016;159(3):793–801.

[17] Amini A, Patanwala AE, Maegawa FB, et al. Effect of epidural analgesia on postoperative complications following pancreaticoduodenectomy. Am J Surg 2012;204(6):1000–4 [discussion: 1004–6].

[18] Amini N, Kim Y, Hyder O, et al. A nationwide analysis of the use and outcomes of perioperative epidural analgesia in patients undergoing hepatic and pancreatic surgery. Am J Surg 2015;210(3):483–91.

[19] Aloia TA, Kim BJ, Segraves-Chun YS, et al. A randomized controlled trial of postoperative thoracic epidural analgesia versus intravenous patient-controlled analgesia after major hepatopancreatobiliary surgery. Ann Surg 2017;266(3):545–54.

[20] Revie EJ, McKeown DW, Wilson JA, et al. Randomized clinical trial of local infiltration plus patient-controlled opiate analgesia vs. epidural analgesia following liver resection surgery. HPB (Oxford) 2012;14(9):611–8.

[21] Zimmitti G, Soliz J, Aloia TA, et al. Positive impact of epidural analgesia on oncologic outcomes in patients undergoing resection of colorectal liver metastases. Ann Surg Oncol 2016;23(3):1003–11.

[22] Dichtwald S, Ben-Haim M, Papismedov L, et al. Intrathecal morphine versus intravenous opioid administration to impact postoperative analgesia in hepato-pancreatic surgery: a randomized controlled trial. J Anesth 2017;31(2):237–45.

[23] Lee JH, Park JH, Kil HK, et al. Efficacy of intrathecal morphine combined with intravenous analgesia versus thoracic epidural analgesia after gastrectomy. Yonsei Med J 2014;55(4):1106–14.

[24] Chahar P, Cummings KC 3rd. Liposomal bupivacaine: a review of a new bupivacaine formulation. J Pain Res 2012;5:257–64.

[25] Ayad S, Babazade R, Elsharkawy H, et al. Comparison of transversus abdominis plane infiltration with liposomal bupivacaine versus continuous epidural analgesia versus intravenous opioid analgesia. PLoS One 2016;11(4):e0153675.

[26] Niraj G, Kelkar A, Hart E, et al. Comparison of analgesic efficacy of four-quadrant transversus abdominis plane (TAP) block and continuous posterior TAP analgesia with epidural analgesia in patients undergoing laparoscopic colorectal surgery: an open-label, randomised, non-inferiority trial. Anaesthesia 2014;69(4):348–55.

[27] Ganapathy S, Sondekoppam RV, Terlecki M, et al. Comparison of efficacy and safety of lateral-to-medial continuous transversus abdominis plane block with thoracic epidural analgesia in patients undergoing abdominal surgery: a randomised, open-label feasibility study. Eur J Anaesthesiol 2015;32(11):797–804.

[28] Stottmeier S, Harling H, Wille-Jorgensen P, et al. Pathogenesis of morbidity after fast-track laparoscopic colonic cancer surgery. Colorectal Dis 2011;13(5):500–5.

[29] Kim BJ, Aloia TA. What is "enhanced recovery," and how can I do it? J Gastrointest Surg 2018;22(1):164–71.

[30] Chen JY, Ko TL, Wen YR, et al. Opioid-sparing effects of ketorolac and its correlation with the recovery of postoperative bowel function in colorectal surgery patients: a prospective randomized double-blinded study. Clin J Pain 2009;25(6):485–9.

[31] Marret E, Kurdi O, Zufferey P, et al. Effects of nonsteroidal antiinflammatory drugs on patient-controlled analgesia morphine side effects: meta-analysis of randomized controlled trials. Anesthesiology 2005;102(6):1249–60.

[32] Behman R, Karanicolas PJ, Lemke M, et al. The effect of early postoperative non-steroidal anti-inflammatory drugs on pancreatic fistula following pancreaticoduodenectomy. J Gastrointest Surg 2015;19(9):1632–9.

[33] Hughes MJ, Ventham NT, McNally S, et al. Analgesia after open abdominal surgery in the setting of enhanced recovery surgery: a systematic review and meta-analysis. JAMA Surg 2014;149(12):1224–30.

[34] Wang XS, Williams LA, Eng C, et al. Validation and application of a module of the M. D. Anderson Symptom Inventory for measuring multiple symptoms in patients with gastrointestinal cancer (the MDASI-GI). Cancer 2010;116(8):2053–63.

[35] Day RW, Cleeland CS, Wang XS, et al. Patient-reported outcomes accurately measure the value of an enhanced recovery program in liver surgery. J Am Coll Surg 2015;221(6): 1023–30, e1–2.

[36] Aloia TA, Zimmitti G, Conrad C, et al. Return to intended oncologic treatment (RIOT): a novel metric for evaluating the quality of oncosurgical therapy for malignancy. J Surg Oncol 2014;110(2):107–14.

Advances in Surgery 52 (2018) 247–256

ADVANCES IN SURGERY

Are Opioids Overprescribed Following Elective Surgery?

Elizabeth B. Habermann, PhD, MPH

Departments of Surgery and Health Sciences Research, Mayo Clinic, 200 First Street Southwest, Rochester, MN 55905, USA

Keywords
• Opioid • Prescribing • Narcotic • Standardization • Surgery • Postoperative pain

Key points

- Recent legislation and proposed guidelines have suggested maximum amounts of opioid medications to prescribe for postoperative and/or acute pain.
- The evidence is clear: overprescribing of opioids following elective surgery exists. Unused opioids are not properly disposed and may be diverted to friends, family members, or the community.
- Despite evidence of overprescribing following elective surgery, recent initiatives to standardize and reduce opioid prescriptions are promising and may aid surgeons in reducing their role in the ongoing opioid epidemic in the United States.

INTRODUCTION

The opioid epidemic

A single-paragraph letter published in the *New England Journal of Medicine* in 1980 concluded that for hospitalized patients treated with narcotics, "the development of addiction is rare in medical patients with no history of addiction" [1]. Although this letter contained insufficient evidence to support its claim, hundreds of future research studies over the following decades cited it as evidence that addiction was rare in patients prescribed opioids [2], and opioid prescribing dramatically increased through 2012 [3]. These and other factors underlie the current opioid epidemic occurring in the United States.

Opioid misuse currently affects more than 2 million Americans [4] and is costly, with roughly one-quarter of the estimated $78.5 billion dollars spent annually on opioid overdose, abuse, or dependence attributed to increased

Disclosure: The author has nothing to disclose.

E-mail address: Habermann.elizabeth@mayo.edu

https://doi.org/10.1016/j.yasu.2018.03.003
0065-3411/18/© 2018 Elsevier Inc. All rights reserved.

health care or substance treatment costs [5]. In addition to its financial costs, opioid overuse and misuse lead to human costs: opioids were implicated in as many as 16,000 deaths in the United States in 2013 [5].

In response to the opioid epidemic, several individual states as well as the Centers for Disease Control and Prevention have passed legislation or drafted or established guidelines outlining suggested or mandated maximum limits for opioid prescriptions [6–10]. Most of these guidelines suggest a 7-day prescription as the maximum following acute pain or major surgery, whereas others use an amount defined using oral morphine equivalents (OME). The use of oral morphine equivalent units allows for a single number describing the amount of opioids prescribed regardless of the number or type of opioids prescribed. A description of common prescription drugs converted to OME using conversion factors published by the Centers for Medicare and Medicaid Services [11] is available in Table 1.

Given the growing number of initiatives aimed at limiting opioid prescribing, and in response to the opioid epidemic itself, it is essential to review the current and future state of opioid prescribing for surgical pain. More than one-third of all prescriptions written by surgeons are for opioids, and these surgeon-prescribed opioids comprise 10% of all opioids prescribed [12]. Therefore, opioid prescribing must be evaluated with the goals of addressing surgical pain while minimizing the risk of opioid dependence for surgical patients and the risk of diversion of opioids for use by others than to whom they were prescribed.

Risk of opioid dependence

One of the central risks of opioid prescribing for surgical patients is that of an opioid-naive patient becoming a longer-term user of opioids, or "opioid dependent." Studies have shown that although most patients present to surgery as opioid naive, estimates of opioid dependence following the perioperative period range widely, from less than 1% of opioid-naive spine surgery TRICARE beneficiaries [13] to 2% [14] of all surgical patients, 6% [15] of general surgical patients, 10% of cancer surgery patients [16], and 13% of hand surgery patients [17]. As noted above, opioid dependence results in significant medical and societal costs that underscore the need to reduce this risk for surgical patients.

Risk of opioid diversion

In addition to the risk of opioid dependence, which impacts the patients themselves, opioids prescribed for postsurgical pain may also result in potential

Table 1
Oral morphine mg equivalent conversion factors

Drug	Conversion factor	Prescriptions approximating 200 OME
Tramadol	0.1	40 tabs of 50 mg tramadol
Hydrocodone	1	40 tabs of 5 mg hydrocodone
Oxycodone	1.5	26.7 tabs of 5 mg oxycodone
Hydromorphone	4	25 tabs of 2 mg hydromorphone

harm to others through diversion of leftover opioids to friends, family, or other community members. In some cases, the surgical patient may be unaware of diversion (eg, a patient's leftover opioids are stolen), but evidence shows that most nonmedical users of opioids accessed them through prescriptions given to friends or family members [18]. Diversion can result in devastating consequences; up to 75% of heroin users report being first exposed to opioids through prescription opioids [19]. As opioids prescribed for surgery are rarely disposed of appropriately [20] and often remain in patients' homes [21], overprescribing opioids for surgical patients resulting in leftover opioids results in risks to our communities.

Opioid prescribing following surgery

Are patients overprescribed opioids following elective surgery? Whether overprescription is defined as exceeding guidelines or defined as patients being prescribed excess opioids they do not use, the evidence is astoundingly clear: Yes, opioids are overprescribed to surgical patients.

Although the literature on opioid prescribing for surgical patients was sparse during the initial years of the epidemic, recently several studies have been published evaluating the amounts and appropriateness of postsurgical opioid prescriptions, providing comparisons to recent prescribing guidelines.

In the author's study [8] conducted at Mayo Clinic, they found that across 25 common elective procedures in their 3 hospitals spread across 3 states, more than 80% of their opioid naive patients were prescribed in excess of the State of Minnesota's draft guideline maximum of 200 OME (Fig. 1).

Among the 25 procedures evaluated, the only 3 for which the median prescribing amount did not exceed guidelines were carotid endarterectomy, parathyroidectomy, and thyroid lobectomy. Overprescription was more common for the orthopedic procedures studied than for other specialties; the top 5 highest prescribing procedures included hip, knee, and shoulder arthroplasty, rotator cuff repair, and tonsillectomy. Maximum prescriptions in excess of 1000 OME, 5 times the suggested maximum, were observed for patients undergoing 13 of the 25 procedures. Not only were many patients prescribed above the suggested maximum amount but also large variation in amounts prescribed within each procedure type was observed and remained unexplained by patient and operative factors.

In another institutional study by Hill and colleagues [20] evaluating prescribing for 5 common outpatient general surgery procedures (partial mastectomy, partial mastectomy with sentinel node biopsy, laparoscopic cholecystectomy, and laparoscopic and open inguinal hernia repairs), overprescribing was also observed, with significant proportions of each procedure's patients receiving 26 or more 5-mg tabs of oxycodone (and therefore at or above a threshold of 200 OME).

These institutional studies are complemented by a recently published study that evaluated multi-institutional prescribing trends using OptumInsight claims data for patients [22]. The median OME prescribed exceeded 200 for each of the 5 major general surgical procedures studied (bariatric surgery, colectomy,

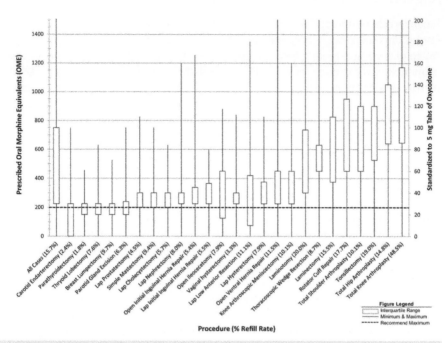

Fig. 1. Discharge opioid prescribing practices in opioid-naive patients across 25 common elective surgical procedures. Lap, laparoscopic. (*From* Thiels CA, Anderson SS, Ubl DS, et al. Wide variation and overprescription of opioids after elective surgery. Ann Surg 2017;266(4):567; with permission.)

incisional hernia repair, reflux surgery, and hysterectomy) and one of the minor procedures (hemorrhoidectomy). This study, as well as the 2 institutional studies described above [8,20], also noted wide ranges prescribed *within* each surgical procedure, with wide ranges across hundreds of OME observed.

Not only does evidence of widespread overprescribing exist when defined using guidelines, but the literature also shows overprescription is rampant when defined as patients having opioids remaining after their pain has been controlled [23]. For example, one study found that 45% of thoracic surgery patients took none or very few opioids prescribed [24]. Another study by Hill and colleagues [20] discovered that more than 70% of pills prescribed were not taken following the 5 common general surgery procedures studied. Other studies report similar proportions of opioids taken in upper extremity (34% utilization rate) [25,26], outpatient shoulder surgery (25%–67% utilization rate) [27], and urologic procedures (58% utilization rate) [21].

Refills

The above assessments of overprescribing have focused on initial prescriptions, but opioid refills must also be considered when evaluating opioid use following surgery. Indeed, surgeons contemplating reducing the amounts prescribed are concerned by whether patients will have difficulty accessing refill prescriptions when necessary [20]. Evidence shows refill rates range from 0% to 49% [8,20–22,28] (see Fig. 1 for procedure-specific refill rates available at Mayo Clinic). Interestingly, the amount of the index prescription has not been shown to correlate with the likelihood of a refill [8,22]. Although surgical prescribers may have concerns regarding patient satisfaction or administrative burden of providing refills, these are not sufficient reasons to overprescribe. Instead, institutions should support better systems for refilling prescriptions when needed. Unfortunately, even existing opportunities, such as electronic prescribing, although legal in most states, are currently underused [29], perhaps because of costs of implementation.

DISCUSSION

Given the opioid epidemic and the evidence demonstrating overprescription of opioids following surgery, it is clear that surgeons must take action. There are several specific strategies surgeons should take to optimize opioid prescribing for their patients.

First, surgeons should work with their surgical partners, their institutions, and their surgical societies to define best practices for opioid prescribing for their surgical practice. As noted above, although state and federal guidelines and legislation exist, to date these guidelines have generally recommended one maximum amount to prescribe regardless of specialty (eg, orthopedic, thoracic, gynecologic, or urologic surgery) or individual procedure's expected pain. It has been suggested that these guidelines should be more tailored to individual procedures [7,8], especially given the established wide variations of prescription amounts within individual surgical procedures.

In addition to better tailoring guidelines to specific surgical specialties or procedures, the needs or requirements for individual surgical patients must also be considered. Although the author's study of Mayo Clinic hospitals concluded that variations in prescribing were not explained by patient factors in available data [8], other patient characteristics have been found to be associated with increased needs or use of opioid medications. Within opioid-naive patients, those at higher risk of dependence, such as those with pain conditions, certain mental health issues, or substance abuse, should be recognized for their higher risk and counseled appropriately [15,30].

As surgeons define best practices for opioid prescribing for their surgical practices while considering the needs and requirements for individual surgical patients, they should continue to incorporate multimodal analgesia. Over the past few decades, the use of opioids has been the default choice for management of postsurgical pain, whether alone or as part of a multimodal regimen. Of note, the multimodal approach, combining opioids with nonsteroidal anti-inflammatory drugs and/or acetaminophen, is recommended [31] and has shown reduced opioid amounts used by surgical patients [32]. Other complementary or replacement approaches to postsurgical pain management, such as epidurals or Exparel, or even electrotherapy or acupuncture following total knee arthroplasty [33], may be considered. Furthermore, in some cases it is unclear whether opioids are necessary at all. Opioid-free surgery is increasingly discussed [34], although one study found it had no impact on opioid prescribing at discharge [35]. Finally, minor surgical procedures may not require any opioids for pain management.

In addition, surgeons may need to adapt their prescribing when operating on patients currently using opioids. Although studies have generally focused on opioid-naive patients [13–15,17,22,28], opioid users have been estimated to represent from 4% to 56% of various surgical populations [8,36–41]. These preoperative opioid users may have one of several previously noted underlying conditions [37], including psychological diagnoses, cancer, musculoskeletal pain, or other chronic pain. Because surgical outcomes vary for preoperative users, from less pain relief following surgery [42] to increased use of health care services [37,38,40] and higher expenditures [37,40], better understanding of how to prescribe opioids to these patients for surgical pain is needed.

Guidelines state either that guidelines do not apply to current users of opioids or those with chronic pain or palliative care or that similar amounts should be prescribed regardless of preoperative opioid use, but whether that is the best approach is yet to be determined. In the author's study of patients undergoing elective procedures at Mayo Clinic, patients taking opioids at the time of surgery were prescribed nearly double the amount of OME and received nearly double the amount of refills than those who were opioid naive, although procedure-specific data were not made available [8]. Another study found that of patients using chronic opioids before bariatric surgery, a higher number of morphine equivalents were consumed following surgery [41]. Whether and by how much standardized prescriptions for postsurgical opioids should be adjusted for opioid users is yet to be established.

Although the growing field of pharmacogenomics has been underrepresented in the surgical literature to date, it may offer a precision medicine–based approach to better match patient profiles to prescribing needs. One recent study demonstrated ease of pharmacogenetic testing in major abdominal surgery patients that resulted in improved analgesia and decreased opioid requirements [43]. As this testing becomes more widely available, its utility in informing opioid prescribing should continue to be assessed.

Once best practices are established, effectively communicating them to providers is necessary in light of busy surgical practices. An initiative focused on surgeon education at Dartmouth was deemed effective in reducing opioid prescription amounts and relative use of opioid alternatives [44] as was a study of education of hand surgeons [45]. Recognizing that the surgeon may or may not be the individual writing the discharge prescription for opioids, it is necessary for surgeons to coordinate care with their multidisciplinary teams during the perioperative period as well as patients' primary care and other medical providers to ensure appropriate pain management outside of the perioperative period. For surgeons who work with trainees, educating them is essential. Surgical residents reported lack of formal training in how to best prescribe opioids to patients, prescribing more opioids to patients than they believed necessary, and failing at instructing patients on proper opioid disposal [46]. Furthermore, it has been shown that involving pharmacists in reviews or consultations reduced the proportions and amounts of opioid prescribing following inpatient surgery [47].

Education of the patient

Although education of the surgeon and care team is necessary, it is also necessary that health care providers prompt discussions with patients regarding anticipated pain and approaches to pain management [29,31,48,49]. Given that surgery is a painful and traumatic experience by nature, patients expect pain, so reduction in opioid prescription should be done systematically and taking patient-reported data into consideration so the pendulum does not swing too far from the current direction. With this balance in mind, preoperative counseling may include discussions of pursuing optimal function rather than zero pain.

Even with development and application of appropriate postoperative opioid-prescribing guidelines, there will be leftover opioids for some patients. It is essential surgical providers focus not only on reducing the amount of leftover opioids but also on identifying safe storage and disposal practices that will be followed by surgical patients and on educating patients and their caregivers on these practices [46,49,50]. Although take-back programs, drug deactivation systems such as Deterra, and drop-off options should be encouraged, the US Food and Drug Administration (FDA) also endorses flushing pills down the toilet as a disposal option for many common opioid medications [51]. Unfortunately, fewer than 10% of patients follow FDA recommendations for opioid disposal [20,23], highlighting yet another opportunity for improved opioid stewardship and management.

Despite the evidence of the social and economic tolls of the opioid epidemic, the overprescription of opioids following surgery, and the need for further research in many patient and procedural populations and aspects of surgical care, there are some encouraging data and efforts signaling improvements in care. First, although opioid prescriptions increased over many years, they have plateaued and been decreasing since 2011 [52]. However, whether these decreases have been seen in surgical prescribing is unknown. Second, outside of state and federal guidelines, individual groups including researchers from Dartmouth [20] and the Michigan Opioid Prescribing Engagement Network [53] have published suggested maximums for prescribing following common general surgery procedures. Additional similar forms of guidance should be encouraged and disseminated to provide surgeons with easy-to-decipher instructions to guide their prescribing practices.

SUMMARY

The literature is clear: opioids have been overprescribed following surgery. Given the risks of overprescribing, including opioid dependence and potential diversion of opioids to persons other than the surgical patient, it is imperative that surgeons take action to address their practice patterns and contribution to the current epidemic in the United States. The increasing attention to this topic and growing body of literature on appropriate prescribing, accompanied by recent decreases in overall opioid prescribing [3], are encouraging, although trends specific to surgical prescribing are less clear. Further investigations and guidance are needed to minimize the role of surgeons and their prescribing to surgical patients in furthering the opioid epidemic.

References

[1] Porter J, Jick H. Addiction rare in patients treated with narcotics. N Engl J Med 1980;302(2):123.

[2] Leung PTM, Macdonald EM, Stanbrook MB, et al. A 1980 letter on the risk of opioid addiction. N Engl J Med 2017;376(22):2194–5.

[3] Center for Disease Control and Prevention. Annual surveillance report of drug-related risks and outcomes – United States, 2017. 2017. Available at: https://www.cdc.gov/drugoverdose/pdf/pubs/2017-cdc-drug-surveillance-report.pdf. Accessed November 10, 2017.

[4] Substance Abuse and Mental Health Services Administration. Reports and detailed tables from the 2016 National Survey on Drug Use and Health (NSDUH). 2017. Available at: https://www.samhsa.gov/samhsa-data-outcomes-quality/major-data-collections/reports-detailed-tables-2016-NSDUH. Accessed November 3, 2017.

[5] Florence CS, Zhou C, Luo F, et al. The economic burden of prescription opioid overdose, abuse, and dependence in the United States, 2013. Med Care 2016;54(10):901–6.

[6] Dowell D, Haegerich TM, Chou R. CDC guideline for prescribing opioids for chronic pain — United States, 2016. MMWR Recomm Rep 2016;65(1):1–49.

[7] Kaafarani HMA, Weil E, Wakeman S, et al. The opioid epidemic and new legislation in Massachusetts. Ann Surg 2017;265(4):731–3.

[8] Thiels CA, Anderson SS, Ubl DS, et al. Wide variation and overprescription of opioids after elective surgery. Ann Surg 2017;266(4):564–73.

[9] Liepert AE, Ackerman TL. 2016 state legislative year in review and a look ahead. Bull Am Coll Surg 2016;101(12):35–9.

[10] Fotsch R. States react to opioid crises with aggressive legislation aimed at saving lives. J Nurs Regul 2017;7(4):61–2.

[11] Centers for Medicare and Medicaid Services. Opioid oral morphine milligram equivalent (MME) conversion factors. 2016. Available at: https://www.cms.gov/Medicare/Prescription-Drug-Coverage/PrescriptionDrugCovContra/Downloads/Opioid-Morphine-EQ-Conversion-Factors-April-2017.pdf. Accessed November 3, 2017.

[12] Levy B, Paulozzi L, Mack KA, et al. Trends in opioid analgesic-prescribing rates by specialty, U.S., 2007-2012. Am J Prev Med 2015;49(3):409–13.

[13] Schoenfeld AJ, Nwosu K, Jiang W, et al. Risk factors for prolonged opioid use following spine surgery, and the association with surgical intensity, among opioid-naive patients. J Bone Joint Surg Am 2017;99(15):1247–52.

[14] Shah A, Hayes CJ, Martin BC. Factors influencing long-term opioid use among opioid naïve patients: an examination of initial prescription characteristics and pain etiologies. J Pain 2017;18(11):1374–83.

[15] Brummett CM, Waljee JF, Goesling J, et al. New persistent opioid use after minor and major surgical procedures in US adults. JAMA Surg 2017;152(6):e170504.

[16] Lee JS-J, Hu HM, Edelman AL, et al. New persistent opioid use among patients with cancer after curative-intent surgery. J Clin Oncol 2017;35(36):4042–9.

[17] Johnson SP, Chung KC, Zhong L, et al. Risk of prolonged opioid use among opioid-naïve patients following common hand surgery procedures. J Hand Surg Am 2016;41(10):947–57.e3.

[18] Jones C, Paulozzi L, Mack K. Sources of prescription opioid pain relievers by frequency of past-year nonmedical use: United States, 2008-2011. JAMA Intern Med 2014;174(5): 802–3, Author.

[19] Cicero TJ, Ellis MS, Surratt HL, et al. The changing face of heroin use in the United States. JAMA Psychiatry 2014;71(7):821.

[20] Hill MV, McMahon ML, Stucke RS, et al. Wide variation and excessive dosage of opioid prescriptions for common general surgical procedures. Ann Surg 2017;265(4): 709–14.

[21] Bates C, Laciak R, Southwick A, et al. Overprescription of postoperative narcotics: a look at postoperative pain medication delivery, consumption and disposal in urological practice. J Urol 2011;185(2):551–5.

[22] Sekhri S, Arora NS, Cottrell H, et al. Probability of opioid prescription refilling after surgery: does initial prescription dose matter? Ann Surg 2017; https://doi.org/10.1097/SLA. 0000000000002308.

[23] Bicket MC, Long JJ, Pronovost PJ, et al. Prescription opioid analgesics commonly unused after surgery. JAMA Surg 2017;1–6; https://doi.org/10.1001/jamasurg.2017.0831.

[24] Bartels K, Mayes LM, Dingmann C, et al. Opioid use and storage patterns by patients after hospital discharge following surgery. PLoS One 2016;11(1):1–10.

[25] Kim N, Matzon JL, Abboudi J, et al. A prospective evaluation of opioid utilization after upper extremity surgical procedures: identifying consumption patterns and determining prescribing guidelines. J Bone Joint Surg Am 2016;98 A(20):1–9.

[26] Rodgers J, Cunningham K, Fitzgerald K, et al. Opioid consumption following outpatient upper extremity surgery. J Hand Surg Am 2012;37(4):645–50.

[27] Kumar K, Gulotta LV, Dines JS, et al. Unused opioid pills after outpatient shoulder surgeries given current perioperative prescribing habits. Am J Sports Med 2017;45(3):636–41.

[28] Scully RE, Schoenfeld AJ, Jiang W, et al. Defining optimal length of opioid pain medication prescription after common surgical procedures. JAMA Surg 2018;153(1):37 43.

[29] Gawande AA. It's time to adopt electronic prescriptions for opioids. Ann Surg 2017;265(4):693–4.

[30] Hooten WM, St Sauver JL, McGree ME, et al. Incidence and risk factors for progression from short-term to episodic or long-term opioid prescribing: a population-based study. Mayo Clin Proc 2015;90(7):850–6.

[31] Chou R, Gordon DB, De Leon-Casasola OA, et al. Management of postoperative pain: a clinical practice guideline from the American Pain Society, the American Society of Regional Anesthesia and Pain Medicine, and the American Society of Anesthesiologists' Committee on Regional Anesthesia, executive committee, and administrative council. J Pain 2016;17(2):131–57.

[32] Wick EC, Grant MC, Wu CL. Postoperative multimodal analgesia pain management with nonopioid analgesics and techniques. JAMA Surg 2017;152(7):691.

[33] Tedesco D, Gori D, Desai KR, et al. Drug-free interventions to reduce pain or opioid consumption after total knee arthroplasty: a systematic review and meta-analysis. JAMA Surg 2017;94305(10):e172872.

[34] Kamdar NV, Hoftman N, Rahman S, et al. Opioid-free analgesia in the era of enhanced recovery after surgery and the surgical home. Anesth Analg 2017;125(4):1089–91.

[35] Brandal D, Keller MS, Lee C, et al. Impact of enhanced recovery after surgery and opioid-free anesthesia on opioid prescriptions at discharge from the hospital. Anesth Analg 2017;125(5):1784–92.

[36] Lee D, Armaghani S, Archer KR, et al. Preoperative opioid use as a predictor of adverse postoperative self-reported outcomes in patients undergoing spine surgery. J Bone Joint Surg Am 2014;96(11):e89, 1-8.

[37] Waljee JF, Cron DC, Steiger RM, et al. Effect of preoperative opioid exposure on healthcare utilization and expenditures following elective abdominal surgery. Ann Surg 2017;265(4): 715–21.

[38] Ben-Ari A, Chansky H, Rozet I. Preoperative opioid use is associated with early revision after total knee arthroplasty: a study of male patients treated in the veterans affairs system. J Bone Joint Surg Am 2017;99(1):1–9.

[39] Jiang X, Orton M, Feng R, et al. Chronic opioid usage in surgical patients in a large academic center. Ann Surg 2017;265(4):722–7.

[40] Cron DC, Englesbe MJ, Bolton CJ, et al. Preoperative opioid use is independently associated with increased costs and worse outcomes after major abdominal surgery. Ann Surg 2017;265(4):695–701.

[41] Raebel MA, Newcomer SR, Reifler LM, et al. Chronic use of opioid medications before and after bariatric surgery. JAMA 2013;310(13):1369.

[42] Smith SR, Bido J, Collins JE, et al. Impact of preoperative opioid use on total knee arthroplasty outcomes. J Bone Joint Surg Am 2017;99(10):803–8.

[43] Senagore AJ, Champagne BJ, Dosokey E, et al. Pharmacogenetics-guided analgesics in major abdominal surgery: further benefits within an enhanced recovery protocol. Am J Surg 2017;213(3):467–72.

[44] Hill MV, Stucke RS, McMahon ML, et al. An educational intervention decreases opioid prescribing after general surgical operations. Ann Surg 2018;267(3):468–72.

[45] Stanek JJ, Renslow MA, Kalliainen LK. The effect of an educational program on opioid prescription patterns in hand surgery: a quality improvement program. J Hand Surg Am 2015;40(2):341–6.

[46] Chiu AS, Healy JM, DeWane MP, et al. Trainees as agents of change in the opioid epidemic: optimizing the opioid prescription practices of surgical residents. J Surg Educ 2017;1–7; https://doi.org/10.1016/j.jsurg.2017.06.020.

[47] Tran T, Taylor SE, Hardidge A, et al. Impact of pharmacists assisting with prescribing and undertaking medication review on oxycodone prescribing and supply for patients discharged from surgical wards. J Clin Pharm Ther 2017;42(5):567–72.

[48] Peponis T, Kaafarani HMA. What is the proper use of opioids in the postoperative patient? Adv Surg 2017;51(1):77–87.

[49] Saluja S, Selzer D, Meara JG. The opioid epidemic: what can surgeons do about it? Individual strategies to combat the opioid epidemic. Bull Am Coll Surg 2017;102(7):13–8.

[50] Kennedy-Hendricks A, Gielen A, McDonald E, et al. Medication sharing, storage, and disposal practices for opioid medications among US adults. JAMA Intern Med 2016;176(7):1027.

[51] U.S. Food & Drug Administration. Flushing of certain medicines. 2017. Available at: https://www.fda.gov/Drugs/ResourcesForYou/Consumers/BuyingUsingMedicineSafely/EnsuringSafeUseofMedicine/SafeDisposalofMedicines/ucm576167.htm. Accessed November 1, 2018.

[52] Pezalla EJ, Rosen D, Erensen JG, et al. Secular trends in opioid prescribing in the USA. J Pain Res 2017;10:383–7.

[53] Michigan Opioid Prescribing Engagement Network. Opioid prescribing recommendations for opioid-naïve patients. Available at: https://opioidprescribing.info. November 10, 2017.

Advances in Surgery 52 (2018) 257–274

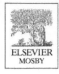

ADVANCES IN SURGERY

Contemporary Management of Critical Limb Ischemia

Jonathan R. Thompson, MD, Peter K. Henke, MD*

Section of Vascular Surgery, Department of Surgery, University of Michigan, Cardiovascular Center-5463, 1500 East Medical Center Drive, Ann Arbor, MI 48109-5867, USA

Keywords

- Critical limb ischemia • Rest pain • Peripheral arterial disease • Endovascular
- Angioplasty • Bypass graft

Key points

- Critical limb ischemia suggests extensive systemic atherosclerosis.
- Critical limb ischemia mandates aggressive medical management.
- Arterial revascularization may be indicated with endovascular or surgical techniques, depending on the specific arteries involved.
- Primary amputation is the best option for a select group of patients.

DEFINITION

Critical limb ischemia (CLI), sometimes referred to as severe limb ischemia or chronic CLI, is best defined by the Trans-Atlantic Inter-Society Consensus Document for the Management of Peripheral Arterial Disease [TASC II]. This definition states patients with CLI have (1) chronic ischemic rest pain (at night or at all times) or (2) tissue loss (ischemic skin lesions such as ulcers or gangrene) whose disease can be attributed to peripheral vascular disease [1]. There are 2 primary classification systems for identifying the severity of peripheral arterial disease (PAD): Fontaine classification stages and Rutherford classification categories (Table 1). A patient with CLI is classified into either stage III or IV for the Fontaine classification. Using the Rutherford system, a patient with CLI is in category 4, 5, or 6. It should be emphasized the TASC II definition includes chronic as a key element in the diagnosis. The

Disclosure Statement: The authors have nothing to disclose.

*Corresponding author. E-mail address: henke@umich.edu

https://doi.org/10.1016/j.yasu.2018.03.012

Table 1
Fontaine and Rutherford classifications for peripheral arterial disease, with critical limb
ischemia italicized

Fontaine		Rutherford		
Stage	Clinical Features	Grade	Category	Clinical
I	Asymptomatic	0	0	Asymptomatic
IIa	Mild claudication	I	1	Mild claudication
IIb	Moderate to severe claudication	I	2	Moderate claudication
		I	3	Severe claudication
III	Ischemic rest pain	II	4	Ischemic rest pain
IV	Ulceration or gangrene	III	5	Minor tissue loss
		III	6	Major tissue loss

Data from Fontaine R, Kim M, Kieny R. Surgical treatment of peripheral circulation disorders. Helv Chir Acta
1954;21:499–533. [in German]; and Rutherford RB, Baker JD, Ernst C, et al. Recommended standards for
reports dealing with lower extremity ischemia: revised version. J Vasc Surg 1997;26:517–38.

symptoms should be present for more than 2 weeks [1]. This helps distinguish
from acute limb ischemia, which is a surgical emergency. Acute limb ischemia
also has a Rutherford classification scheme and it should not be confused with
the classification for CLI.

DIAGNOSIS
At the center of a CLI diagnosis are history and physical examination. Patients
have a classic history of claudication that has progressed to pain at all times or
pain at night. Often, patients endorse getting up at night to either walk or
dangle their feet over the bed to relieve symptoms. Pain most often be
described in the distal aspect of the foot. The physical examination often reveals loss of hair over the distal extremity, ruborous and nonswollen extremities with delayed capillary refill, and, in severe cases, a wound. The ankle-
brachial index (ABI) and toe systolic pressure (to give a toe-brachial index)
are still the first recommended tests for patients with suspected ischemic
changes in their lower extremities. There is no consensus on absolute pressure
measurements for the diagnosis of CLI. TASC II does have general guidelines
to help. True ischemic rest pain is believed present when an absolute ankle
pressure drops below 50 mm Hg or a toe pressure is less than 30 mm Hg. If
these are not present, alternative diagnoses should be sought. With an ulcer
or wound is present, CLI is the diagnosis when the absolute ankle pressure
drops below 70 mm Hg or the toe pressure is less than 50 mm Hg [1].
Cross-sectional imaging with CT angiography or conventional angiography
provides specific information about areas of stenosis and occlusions. Duplex ultrasound and magnetic resonance angiography can also be used. Transcuta-
neous partial pressure of oxygen measurements can be helpful for predicting
wound healing (the critical level for healing is between 30 mm Hg and
40 mm Hg, depending on the vascular laboratory). Other studies (capillaro-
scopy and laser Doppler imaging) are used primarily in research settings [1].

WOUNDS

For patients with CLI and distal wounds, these wounds are classified either ulcers or gangrene. Gangrene affects the distal most aspect of the limb, the digits, first. For bedbound patients or those with prolonged periods of laying, the heel is affected [1]. Dry gangrene forms a dry eschar and occasional lead to autoamputation. Wet gangrene is often treated with urgent surgery in the form of débridement, guillotine amputation, or formal amputation, depending on the clinical scenario. Diabetics deserve special attention. They form wounds through the process of neuropathy and loss of sensation in conjunction with pressure points and activity [1]. Not all diabetic foot ulcers are ischemic in nature. Most are neuropathic in origin and form on the weight-bearing surfaces. Other diabetic wound origins are venous, mixed arterial and venous, skin infarction/embolization, and neuroischemic [1]. Ischemic ulcers are often painful with irregular margins in a cold, pale foot. Table 2 compares ischemic and neuropathic ulcers. Wound scoring systems, including the Society for Vascular Surgery Threatened Limb Classification System (wound, ischemia, and foot infection), have generated guidelines to help practitioners understand wound severity and help counsel patients on outcomes [2]. This has been validated in several studies to predict stenosis events, wound healing, and amputation [3–5].

EPIDEMIOLOGY

The yearly incidence of CLI is believed 50 to 100 cases per 100,000 [6,7]. For patients with PAD, the risk of progressing to CLI is believed only 1% to 3%. Diabetics are 4-fold and smokers are 3-fold more likely to progress to CLI. Age greater than 65 confers a 2-times increased risk for progression to CLI from PAD [1]. One-year mortality is 25% and amputation rate approaches 30% at 1 year in patients with CLI [1]. Five-year mortality in these patients

Table 2
Comparison between neuropathic and ischemic ulcers

Ischemic ulcer	Neuropathic ulcer
Painless	Painful
Normal pulses/ABIs	Absent pulses/abnormal ABIs
Regular margins with punched-out appearance	Irregular margins
Often on plantar aspect of foot	Often located on distal aspect of toes
Calluses present	Calluses infrequent
Loss of sensation, reflexes, and vibration	Variable sensory examination
Increased blood flow (arterio-venous shunting)	Decreased blood flow
Dilated veins	Collapsed veins
Dry, warm foot	Cold foot
Bony deformities	No bony deformities
Red appearance	Pale, cyanotic

From Norgren L, Hiatt WR, Dormandy JA, et al. Inter-society consensus for the management of peripheral arterial disease (TASC II). J Vasc Surg 2007;45(Suppl S):S5–67; with permission.

is greater than 50%, primarily related to other comorbidities, including cardiac, pulmonary, and cerebrovascular disease [1]. Overall, patients with CLI have much higher risk of limb loss, nonfatal vascular events, myocardial infarction, stroke, and death than those with claudication [1].

MEDICAL THERAPY

Patients with CLI are at particularly high risk for cardiovascular ischemic events. Excellent data exist on medical therapy for cardiovascular risk reduction in patients with PAD. There is level IA evidence to support single antiplatelet therapy (aspirin, 75–325 mg daily, or clopidogrel, 75 mg daily) in all symptomatic PAD patients to reduce rate of myocardial infarction, stroke, and vascular death [8]. The effectiveness of dual antiplatelet therapy in preventing cardiovascular ischemic events in symptomatic PAD is not well established [8]. Vorapaxar (Zontivity), a novel protease-activated receptor-1 antagonist, has unclear benefit in symptomatic PAD at reducing ischemic events but was associated with reduced need for revascularization [9]. All patients with PAD should be treated with statin medication (level IA evidence) [8]. One therapy often overlooked is strict hypertension management. Antihypertensive therapy is critical to reduce risk of myocardial infarction, stroke, heart failure, and cardiovascular death. Angiotensin-converting enzyme inhibitors or angiotensin-receptor blockers have level IIA evidence to support use for reducing cardiovascular ischemic events [8]. Smoking cessation is essential and should be discussed at every visit, with prescription of pharmacologic aids as indicated.

PAIN CONTROL

Providers who have taken care of patients with CLI may be frustrated by the lack of effective analgesic therapy. Treatment of the underlying ischemia with revascularization and reperfusion is best, but occasionally this is not immediately or ever possible. Scheduled acetaminophen and nonsteroidal anti-inflammatory medications are generally not effective. Narcotic medications are generally required [1]. Other adjuncts, such as magnesium oxide and γ-aminobutyric acid analogs, occasionally are effective [10]. Short-term pain control, on the order of minutes to hours, has been improved with both intravenous lidocaine and intravenous ketamine in 2 separate controlled trials [11,12]. For inpatient pain control, epidurals can be effective. The addition of transdermal buprenorphine improves the epidural's effect [13].

TREATMENT

All patients with CLI should receive some form of treatment of their symptoms. Treatment should focus on relieving ischemic pain, healing wounds, preventing amputation, improving quality of life, and prolonging survival [1].

REVASCULARIZATION

Revascularization is the objective for all patients amenable to intervention. The goal is to establish inline blood flow to the foot with either endovascular or open surgical means. The effectiveness, durability, and superiority of each procedure continues to be a hotly debated topic.

SURGICAL REVASCULARIZATION

Open surgical revascularization includes bypass and endarterectomy procedures. This approach is the gold standard with which endovascular procedures are compared. Aortoiliac disease, when present, is often addressed first or in conjunction with a femoropopliteal procedure, if this disease exists. The aortobifemoral bypass is a durable procedure for patients with aortoiliac occlusive disease. In a meta-analysis, 15-year limb-based patency rate for patients with ischemic lesions was 75.1% [14]. For open infrainguinal surgery, most of the clinical debate is in choosing the best conduit for bypass. Suitable autologous vein should be the primary conduit when bypass is planned to the popliteal or infrapopliteal arteries [8]. The first vein conduit option is ipsilateral great saphenous vein. Vein may be harvested through a single open continuous incision, skip incisions, or an endoscopic harvest technique. The latter has gained popularity among cardiac surgeons for coronary bypass conduits but remains less embraced by the vascular surgery community. Soft, compressible veins greater than 2.5 mm are considered a potential bypass conduit and should be explored. Poor-quality veins should not be used. The small saphenous vein in the posterior calf and arm vein (cephalic and basilic) can be alternative options but often require vein splicing. The techniques of reversed, in situ, and translocated nonreversed vein configurations are similar in terms of efficacy and are based on surgeon preference.

There are good data to suggest the superiority of vein graft over polytetrafluoroethylene (PTFE) for infrapopliteal bypasses [15]. Some investigators have argued efficacy between PTFE and autologous vein for above-the-knee popliteal bypasses. Lower long-term patency, infection risk, and an often limb-threatening presentation when the graft occludes, however, make this less appealing [16]. When prosthetic graft must be used, externally supported PTFE is generally favored. In CLI patients with open wounds, gangrene, or osteomyelitis, prosthetic graft should be avoided. Although Dacron has not been shown inferior to PTFE, most contemporary series evaluate PTFE compared with vein grafts. For tibial anastomoses, adjunct vein techniques at the distal anastomosis, such as a Miller cuff, Linton patch, Taylor patch, or St. Mary boot, have shown improved patency compared with PTFE alone in several trials [17,18].

A meta-analysis in CLI patients compared primary patency of femoral to above-the-knee popliteal bypass with vein, femoral to below-the-knee popliteal bypass with vein, and femoral to above-the-knee popliteal bypass with PTFE (Fig. 1) [19]. The pooled estimates of primary patency in this meta-analysis at 5 years were 69.4% and 68.9% for above-the-knee and below-the-knee bypasses with vein, respectively. The estimated 5-year patency rate for above-the-knee bypass with prosthetic graft in patients with CLI was 48.3%. Both above-the-knee and below-the-knee vein bypasses were superior to prosthetic conduit every year out to 5 years.

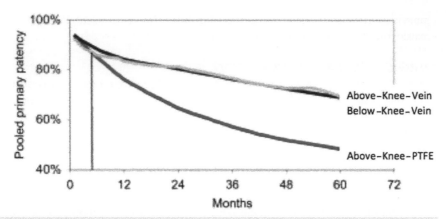

Fig. 1. Comparison of bypass patency in CLI patients with varied conduits. Used with permission. (*From* Pereira CE, Albers M, Romiti M, et al. Meta-analysis of femoropopliteal bypass grafts for lower extremity arterial insufficiency. J Vasc Surg 2006;44:510–7; with permission.)

All patients who have undergone a bypass procedure should be on antiplatelet therapy in the form of aspirin, 81 mg or 325 mg daily. There are data to support the use of Plavix therapy solely for improved lower extremity bypass patency. The use of systemic anticoagulation for the indication of bypass graft patency seems generally provider specific based on graft characteristics. The Dutch Bypass Oral Anticoagulants or Aspirin trial randomized patients to an anticoagulation arm and an aspirin alone arm. This trial, with 2690 lower extremity bypass patients, did not show a significant difference. Subgroup analysis favored oral anticoagulation to improve vein graft patency and antiplatelet therapy (aspirin) to improve prosthetic graft patency [20–22]. A Veterans Affairs study reached a different conclusion [23], because vein bypass graft patency was not improved with anticoagulation. Prosthetic bypass graft patency was improved with anticoagulation but had twice the risk of bleeding complications. Another small study evaluated anticoagulation in high-risk grafts, defined as poor arterial runoff, marginal vein conduit, and redo bypasses [24]. At 3 years, patency was higher in the anticoagulation plus aspirin compared with the aspirin alone group but at the expense of bleeding complications. Most vascular surgeons support anticoagulation for high-risks grafts, even though high-quality data are lacking.

ENDOVASCULAR REVASCULARIZATION
Endovascular techniques have revolutionized the care of patients with CLI. The 2016 American Heart Association lower extremity peripheral artery disease consensus document recommends endovascular revascularization in patients with wounds to establish inline blood flow to the foot (grade IA evidence) [8]. If a patient only has ischemic rest pain, a staged approach is appropriate (grade IIA evidence) [8]. This involves addressing inflow disease first, followed by an outflow procedure if pain persists. The TASC II document

provides excellent recommendations for the use of endovascular therapy based on lesion type for both aortoiliac lesions and femoral-popliteal lesions [1]. Table 3 summarizes this classification scheme. For aortoiliac lesions, endovascular therapy is recommended first for TASC A lesions, and open surgery is recommended first for TASC D lesions. For TASC B lesions, endovascular therapy is preferred and open surgery is preferred for TASC C lesions. For TASC B and C lesions, however, patient comorbidities and patient preference should be used when deciding on therapy. Similarly, for femoral popliteal lesions, TASC A lesions should be treated by endovascular techniques and D lesions should be treated with open surgical intervention. TASC B and TASC C lesions should be treated with endovascular and open techniques, respectively. As with aortoiliac disease, patient comorbidities, operator experience, and patient preference should be considered when determining the best treatment plan for a patient.

STANDARD ANGIOPLASTY

Standard percutaneous transluminal [balloon] angioplasty (PTA) has been around for many years and has been used with success for treating a range of vascular lesions throughout the body. PTA can be used prior to adjunct therapy (such as stenting) or as primary therapy. For isolated aortoiliac disease at 1 year, patency rates were between 47% and 63% [25]. Five-year patency rate was between 26% and 45%. Three-year patency rate for primary PTA of femoropopliteal lesions in patients with CLI was 43% for stenoses and only 30% if completely occluded [26].

DRUG-COATED BALLOON ANGIOPLASTY

The advent and subsequent approval of drug-coated balloons (DCBs) has increased the use of balloon angioplasty as primary therapy. All DCBs have 3 features: a balloon, an antiproliferative drug, and an excipient, or carrier, which transfers the drug to the arterial wall. As can be imagined, the specific differences in these 3 components are the features companies use to promote their specific balloon. Three DCBs are currently approved for femoropopliteal disease: the Lutonix 035 D B (Bard), the IN.PACT Admiral DCB (Medtronic, Minneapolis, MN), and the Stellarex DCB (Spectranetics). All 3 of these balloons have paclitaxel for the antiproliferative drug.

The Lutonix Paclitaxel-Coated Balloon for the Prevention of Femoropopliteal Restenosis (LEVANT I) trial compared the Lutonix DCB to standard PTA on new or restenotic femoropopliteal lesions. This study was performed in Germany and enrolled 101 patients. The primary endpoint was angiographic late lumen loss out to 24 months. Primary patency rate at 24 months was 57% in the DCB group and 40% in the uncoated balloon group, although these were not compared with statistical analysis [27]. The similar LEVANT 2 study, also investigating the Lutonix DCB, enrolled 316 patients into the DCB arm and 160 patients in the standard PTA arm. Most patients had severe claudication. Only 8% in each arm would be categorized as CLI. No patients had wounds. Primary endpoints were patency at

Table 3
TASC classification for aortoiliac and femoral popliteal lesions

TASC classification	Aortoiliac lesions	Femoral popliteal lesions
Type A lesions	Unilateral or bilateral stenoses of CIA Unilateral or bilateral single short (≤3 cm) stenosis of EIA	Single stenosis ≤10 cm in length Single occlusion ≤5 cm in length
Type B lesions	Short (≤3 cm) stenosis of infrarenal aorta) Unilateral CIA occlusion Single or multiple stenosis totaling 3–10 cm involving the origins of internal iliac or CFA Unilateral EIA occlusion not involving the origins of internal iliac or CFA	Multiple lesions (stenoses or occlusions), each ≤5 cm Single stenosis or occlusion ≤15 cm not involving the infrageniculate popliteal artery Single or multiple lesions in the absence of continuous tibial vessels to improve inflow for a distal bypass Heavily calcified occlusion ≤5 cm in length Single popliteal stenosis
Type C lesions	Bilateral CIA occlusions Bilateral EIA stenoses 3–10 cm long not extending into the CFA Unilateral EIA stenosis extending into the CFA Unilateral EIA occlusion that involves the origins of internal iliac and/or CFA Heavily calcified unilateral EIA occlusion with or without involvement of origins of internal iliac and/or CFA	Multiple stenoses or occlusions totaling >15 cm with or without heavy calcification Recurrent stenoses or occlusions that need treatment after 2 endovascular interventions
Type D lesions	Infrarenal aortoiliac occlusion Diffuse disease involving the aorta and both iliac arteries requiring treatment Diffuse multiple stenoses involving the unilateral CIA, EIA, and CFA Unilateral occlusions of both CIA and EIA Bilateral occlusions of both CIA and EIA Iliac stenoses in patients with AAA requiring treatment and not amenable to endograft placement or other lesions requiring open aortic or iliac surgery	Chronic total occlusions of CFA or SFA (>20 cm, involving the popliteal artery) Chronic total occlusion of popliteal artery and proximal trifurcation vessels

Abbreviations: AAA, abdominal aortic aneurysm; CFA, common femoral artery; CIA, common iliac artery; EIA, external iliac artery.

From Norgren L, Hiatt WR, Dormandy JA, et al. Inter-society consensus for the management of peripheral arterial disease (TASC II). J Vasc Surg 2007;45(Suppl S):S5–67; with permission.

12 months assessed via ultrasound evaluation and freedom from target-lesion revascularization (another angiographic intervention treating the same lesion). Primary patency rate at 12 months was 65.2% in the DCB group and 52.6% (*P* = .02) in the standard angioplasty group (Fig. 2) [28].

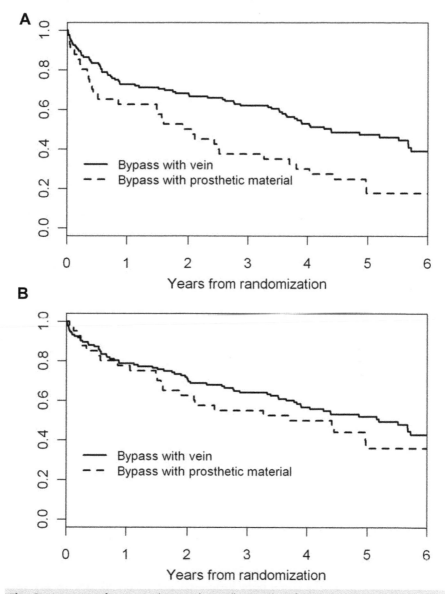

Fig. 2. Amputation-free survival (*A*) and overall survival (*B*) for patients undergoing bypass with vein versus prosthetic in the BASIL trial. (*From* Bradbury AW, Adam DJ, Bell J, et al. Bypass versus angioplasty in severe ischaemia of the leg (BASIL) trial: analysis of amputation free and overall survival by treatment received. J Vasc Surg 2010;51:18S–31S; with permission.)

The Medtronic IN.PACT Admiral DCB was evaluated in the IN.PACT SFA trial. The design is similar to the LEVANT 2 trial, with most patients having severe claudication and only 5% having ischemic rest pain; 331 patients were randomized 2:1 (DCB to standard PTA). The primary endpoint was patency at 24 months. Patency was defined as freedom from clinically driven target vessel revascularization (CD-TLR) (reintervention at the lesion due to symptoms or decrease in ABI >20% or >0.15) or freedom from restenosis via duplex ultrasound. Primary patency rate of the group treated with the IN.-PACT Admiral DCB was 78.9% at 24 months compared with 50.1% in the PTA-alone group. This difference was seen at 12 months and continued through the endpoint of 24 months [29]. The ILLUMENATE Pivotal trial, evaluating the Stellarex DCB, primarily enrolled patients at facilities in the United States. Similar to the IN.PACT SFA trial, 300 patients were randomized 2:1 DCB:PTA. The primary endpoint was patency at 12 months with similar requirements as the IN.PACT SFA trial (duplex criteria and CD-TLR). At 12 months, patency was 82.3% in the DCB group and 70.9% in the PTA group [30].

Criticisms of these trials relate to the comparison groups. All patients treated with DCBs were compared with patients treated with standard balloon angioplasty alone. Other adjuncts, such as stenting and atherectomy, may improve patency when used in combination with PTA. This was not accounted for in these trials. It seems, however, as though there is a real clinical benefit. From a financial perspective, DCBs cost approximately $1500. A recent cost-effectiveness analysis in the IN.PACT SFA II trial suggests the cost at 2 years for patients treated with a DCB is $1200 less than the cost of those patients treated with standard PTA, essentially offsetting the cost of the balloon. The authors suggest this benefit will persist at longer follow-up points, making the IN.PACT Admiral DCB a cost-effective option [31].

STENTING

There are 2 basic types of stents, balloon-expandable (cobalt chromium or stainless steel) and self-expanding (nickel-titanium, known as nitinol). Each of these can be either bare metal or covered. Balloon-expandable stents are often used for accurate deployment, particularly in the common iliac artery. Self-expanding stents are generally placed in the external iliac and superficial femoral arteries.

Although some practitioners are still placing flexible stents in the popliteal artery, the risk of stent fracture and occlusion makes this a poor treatment strategy. Stents placed in this area may compromise bypass options for the patient when it is needed in the future. Furthermore, endovascular therapy for the common femoral artery has been promoted [32]. This technique is fraught with danger and generally not recommended. Stenting in this vessel places a foreign device in a highly mobile artery, placing the stent at risk for fracture and occlusion. Angioplasty has a risk of dissection, which could occlude the profunda femoris artery. This may occlude an important source of collaterals and hamper wound healing. Any intervention also increases the inflammation and scar tissue in this region. Subsequent open surgical intervention is appreciably more difficult. Endarterectomy and patch angioplasty remain the gold standard for common femoral artery disease in any patient with PAD, specifically the patient with CLI.

There have been no data to support improved patency of stenting over PTA for short (<4.5 cm) femoropopliteal lesions [32]. For longer lesions, stenting does have benefit. Schillinger and colleagues [33] evaluated PTA alone versus placement of self-expanding bare metal stents. For long lesions, greater than 9 cm, stenting was better than angioplasty alone at 12 months. Restenosis on duplex was 37% compared with 63% for the stent and PTA groups, respectively. In the RESILIENT trial, less than 15 cm superficial femoral artery (SFA) and proximal popliteal lesions treated with a LifeStent self-expanding nitinol stent (Bard, Tempe, AZ) had superior outcomes at 12 months compared with PTA alone [34]. Approximately 12.5% of patients in the DURABILITY I trial had CLI. Long SFA lesions, mean length 96.4 mm, were treated with the ev3 EverFLex self-expanding stent. At 12 months, 72.2% of patients had less than 50% stenosis. At 1 year, 91% of patients improved at least 1 Rutherford category and 82.5% had improved ABIs [35].

New drug-eluting stents (DESs), similar to DCBs, are coated with an antiproliferative drug to reduce neointimal hyperplasia. The SIROCCO II trial, conducted with primarily claudicants, failed to demonstrate any statistical benefit with the sirolimus-eluting S.M.A.R.T. nitinol self-expanding stent (Cordis, Milpitas, CA) compared with a bare metal stent in patients with greater than 4-cm SFA occlusions [36]. The Zilver PTX DES (Cook, Bloomington, IN) is a paclitaxel-coated DES Food and Drug Administration (FDA) approved for SFA lesions. In the subgroup analysis for patients in Rutherford categories 4 to 6, the restenosis hazard ratio for SFA lesions treated with DES compared with PTA and provisional bare metal stent at 5 years was 0.32 (CI, 0.13–0.82) [37]. This seems to favor the Zilver PTX DES for SFA lesions in CLI patients.

INFRAPOPLITEAL INTERVENTIONS

As endovascular technology is improving and the technical skill base is growing, so is the willingness to aggressively treat tibial vessels. There is a paucity of level I data for endovascular treatment in this region for both claudication and CLI. Most of these interventions are performed on Rutherford category 4 to 6 patients. Schmidt and colleagues [38] performed a retrospective study of 58 consecutive patients with at least 1 infrapopliteal vessel successfully treated with PTA. Patients were either Rutherford category 4 or 5. At 3 months, 31.2% lesions had a greater than 50% occlusion and 37.6% of lesions were reoccluded. Despite this, at 15 months, minor amputation rate was 8.1% and limb salvage rate was 100%. A large retrospective review from the Czech Republic analyzed 1445 limbs with infrapopliteal angioplasty as a primary procedure. Impressively, more than 50% of these interventions were for lower extremity gangrene, Rutherford category 6. Overall primary limb salvage rate at 1 year was 76.1% whereas secondary limb salvage was 84.4% [39].

Donas and colleagues [40] reported their series of patients treated with stent placement for below-the-knee lesions after suboptimal angioplasty. At 24 months, primary and secondary patency was 75.5% and 88.7%, respectively. Although not a primary therapeutic modality, this study demonstrated safety of stenting as a bailout procedure if needed. DESs have also been evaluated in infrapopliteal lesions. A German study by Rastan and colleagues [41] randomized 161 patients with below-the-knee popliteal lesions to receive a sirolimus-coated stent or bare metal stent. CLI was present in 46.6% of patients. At 1 year, primary patency was 80.6% for the sirolimus stent group and 55.6% for the bare metal stent group. Rates of death, minor amputation, and major amputation, however, were not different between the groups. Although primary stenting for infrapopliteal lesions is not recommended, this study suggests that if it is required it may be beneficial to use a DES. Unfortunately, these smaller stents are not available in the United States.

ATHERECTOMY

Atherectomy devices are designed to debulk plaque and allow for full expansion of endovascular interventions, such as PTA and stenting. There are several mechanisms of action for atherectomy devices, including orbital, photoablative (laser), rotational/aspirational, and excisional/directional [32]. The LACI trial evaluated laser-assisted angioplasty in CLI patients not amenable to open surgical intervention. At 6 months, limb salvage rate was approximately 92% [42]. In the CONFIRM trials, orbital atherectomy systems were investigated. The mean Rutherford category was 3.68 in 3785 patients. Unfortunately no long-term data are presented in this trial, but the systems were successful at decreasing lesion percent stenosis immediately after the procedure. Dissection rate was as high as 14% and frequency of embolism was up to 3.2% [43]. The TRUE study evaluated the Jetstream G2 rotational atherectomy device (Pathways Technology, Kirkland, WA) in 18 patients with severe claudication or CLI. At 1 year, only 2 patients (11%) required reintervention on the lesion of interest (freedom from target lesion revascularization) [44]. The SilverHawk device (Medtronic, Minneapolis, MN) was studied in the DEFINITIVE LE trial on patients with claudication and CLI. There was no control group. Primary patency at 12 month for CLI patients was 71%. Secondary patency was 88% in this same cohort. Limb salvage was an impressive 95% at 12 months for patients with CLI [45]. Atherectomy seems a good option for patients with CLI who are not candidates for open surgical intervention.

OPEN VERSUS ENDOVASCULAR REVASCULARIZATION

The UK Bypass versus Angioplasty in Severe Ischemia of the Leg (BASIL) trial is the largest prospective randomized trial to compare patients with CLI who were assigned an endovascular-first strategy compared with a surgery-first strategy. In the initial analysis, there was no difference between the endovascular-first group and surgery-first group for amputation-free survival and overall survival at 1 year and 3 years. However, 6 months after intervention there seemed to be a trend toward improved survival (amputation-free survival and overall survival) with surgical revascularization [6]. In a more in-depth analysis of the BASIL trial data, investigators concluded an angioplasty-first strategy is best in patients expected to live less than 2 years whereas a surgery-first strategy should be used in those expected to live longer than 2 years [46]. An ongoing study being performed in the United States, the Best Surgical Therapy in patients with CLI (BEST-CLI) trial hopes to expand on the BASIL results. One main criticism of the BASIL trial was the endovascular cohort was treated with angioplasty alone. Tools outside of standard balloon angioplasty are available to optimize endovascular therapy [47].

Special mention should be made to the observation in several trials where bypass after peripheral endovascular interventions have worse outcomes. The Vascular Study Group of New England performed a retrospective cohort analysis of all CLI patients undergoing infrainguinal bypass procedures (n = 1880). Prior peripheral endovascular interventions were performed in 134 patients. One-year mortality was not different between those with prior endovascular intervention compared with those without any prior intervention (open or endovascular), but 1-year amputation was higher in patients with prior endovascular procedures compared with those without any prior intervention (34% vs 20%, respectively). Graft occlusion at 1 year was also higher: 28% versus 18% for prior endovascular procedure compared with no prior interventions [48]. Similarly in the BASIL trial, amputation-free survival and overall survival were better at 6 years in patients treated with initial bypass compared with those treated with bypass after failed angioplasty (see Fig. 2) [49].

AMPUTATION

Amputation can be an effective primary treatment strategy for certain patients. The BASIL trial investigators acknowledge many of the study participants may have benefited from an amputation-first strategy followed by aggressive rehabilitation [46]. There is agreement for primary amputation in patients with extensive, unsalvageable foot wounds, nonreconstructable arterial disease, life-threatening sepsis from a foot wound, and a diagnosis of a terminal illness. Furthermore, most nonambulatory patients should not be considered for revascularization but instead amputation as a destination therapy [50]. For patients with severe comorbidities and CLI, surgeons should not shy away from offering amputation as a palliative surgery. When done under controlled conditions, any toe, foot, or leg amputation can be safely performed on most patients under spinal or regional anesthesia with minimal blood loss, particularly if a tourniquet is used.

SPECIAL POPULATIONS—END-STAGE RENAL DISEASE

PAD is present in up to 40% of patients on hemodialysis [51]. In a subgroup analysis of the German CRITISCH trial, treatment strategies for CLI patients with end-stage renal disease (ESRD) were compared with non-ESRD patients. Patients with ESRD had higher rate of in-hospital amputation or death compared with those without ESRD [51]. A meta-analysis of lower extremity bypass for CLI in patients with ESRD demonstrated a 50.4% graft patency at 5 years and 66.6% limb salvage at 5 years but only 27.5% patient survival at 5 years [52]. A Japanese study demonstrated for those treated with bypass, limb salvage rate for ESRD patients was lower compared with non-ESRD patients treated with bypass [53].

Patients with ESRD and CLI consistently perform worse with all treatment modalities. This does not mean these patients should not be offered

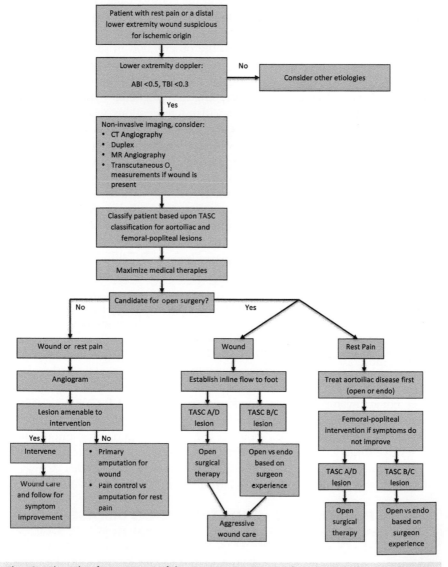

Fig. 3. Algorithm for treatment of the patient presenting with suspected CLI. MR, magnetic resonance; TBI, toe brachial index.

interventions; they should be informed about the increased risk of complications, progression to amputation, and death. Studies have supported both endovascular-first and bypass-first treatment modalities [51,53]. Twelve-month amputation-free survival is improved when revascularization is offered compared to best medical therapy in ESRD patients with CLI [54].

ALTERNATIVE THERAPIES

Hyperbaric oxygen therapy has been used for chronic wounds, including ischemic wounds of the lower extremities. There are good data to support its use in adequately perfused diabetic wounds. Regardless, it is a reasonable therapy to attempt when all other modalities have been exhausted [55]. Angiogenesis as a treatment of CLI initially showed promise, but recent results have been disappointing. Fibroblast growth factor, vascular endothelial growth factor, and hepatocyte growth factor have been delivered by a variety of means directly to patients not eligible for open or endovascular intervention. These growth factors failed to show consistent benefit [56,57]. Stem cell therapy from peripherally derived stem cells or bone marrow have shown decreased amputation rates in small trials, but larger trials are needed [50,58]. It is likely these therapies will be important adjuncts in the next decade but no treatments have been FDA approved outside a trial setting.

SUMMARY

CLI is a significant health burden to our society with an estimated cost burden approaching $4 billion dollars annually. The aggressiveness of treatment is dependent on the patient. In healthy patients with minimal health history, aggressive therapy is warranted. With multiple comorbidities, CLI is often treated through a palliative approach. Most patients, however, fall into a middle group where risks and benefits are weighed next to their overall fitness and ability to tolerate a specific intervention. If a patient will tolerate an open intervention, the authors believe this is still the most durable solution. As technology advances, the options for patients with CLI will likely become better and less invasive. Fig. 3 offers a proposed treatment algorithm for patients with suspected CLI.

References

[1] Norgren L, Hiatt WR, Dormandy JA, et al, TASC II Working Group. Inter-society consensus for the management of peripheral arterial disease (TASC II). J Vasc Surg 2007;45(Suppl S): S5–67.
[2] Mills JL Sr, Conte MS, Armstrong DG, et al, Society for Vascular Surgery Lower Extremity Guidelines Committee. The Society for Vascular Surgery lower extremity threatened limb classification system: risk stratification based on wound, ischemia, and foot infection (WIfI). J Vasc Surg 2014;59:220–34.e1-2.
[3] Darling JD, McCallum JC, Soden PA, et al. Predictive ability of the Society for Vascular Surgery Wound, Ischemia, and foot Infection (WIfI) classification system following infrapopliteal endovascular interventions for critical limb ischemia. J Vasc Surg 2016;64:616–22.
[4] Causey MW, Ahmed A, Wu B, et al. Society for Vascular Surgery limb stage and patient risk correlate with outcomes in an amputation prevention program. J Vasc Surg 2016;63: 1563–73.e2.

[5] Beropoulis E, Stavroulakis K, Schwindt A, et al. Validation of the wound, ischemia, foot Infection (WIfI) classification system in nondiabetic patients treated by endovascular means for critical limb ischemia. J Vasc Surg 2016;64:95–103.

[6] Adam DJ, Beard JD, Cleveland T, et al, BASIL trial participants. Bypass versus angioplasty in severe ischaemia of the leg (BASIL): multicentre, randomised controlled trial. Lancet 2005;366:1925–34.

[7] European Stroke Organisation, Tendera M, Aboyans V, et al, ESC Committee for Practice Guidelines. ESC Guidelines on the diagnosis and treatment of peripheral artery diseases: document covering atherosclerotic disease of extracranial carotid and vertebral, mesenteric, renal, upper and lower extremity arteries: the task force on the diagnosis and treatment of peripheral artery diseases of the European Society of Cardiology (ESC). Eur Heart J 2011;32:2851–906.

[8] Gerhard-Herman MD, Gornik HL, Barrett C, et al. 2016 AHA/ACC guideline on the management of patients with lower extremity peripheral artery disease: a report of the American College of Cardiology/American Heart Association task force on clinical practice guidelines. Circulation 2017;135:e726–79.

[9] Bonaca MP, Scirica BM, Creager MA, et al. Vorapaxar in patients with peripheral artery disease: results from TRA2{degrees}P-TIMI 50. Circulation 2013;127:1522–9, 1529.e1–6.

[10] Morris-Stiff G, Lewis MH. Gabapentin (Neurontin) improves pain scores of patients with critical limb ischaemia: an observational study. Int J Surg 2010;8:212–5.

[11] Vahidi E, Shakoor D, Aghaie Meybodi M, et al. Comparison of intravenous lidocaine versus morphine in alleviating pain in patients with critical limb ischaemia. Emerg Med J 2015;32:516–9.

[12] Mitchell AC, Fallon MT. A single infusion of intravenous ketamine improves pain relief in patients with critical limb ischaemia: results of a double blind randomised controlled trial. Pain 2002;97:275–81.

[13] Laoire AN, Murtagh FEM. Systematic review of pharmacological therapies for the management of ischaemic pain in patients with non-reconstructable critical limb ischaemia. BMJ Support Palliat Care 2017;1–11.

[14] de Vries SO, Hunink MG. Results of aortic bifurcation grafts for aortoiliac occlusive disease: a meta-analysis. J Vasc Surg 1997;26:558–69.

[15] Veith FJ, Gupta SK, Ascer E, et al. Six-year prospective multicenter randomized comparison of autologous saphenous vein and expanded polytetrafluoroethylene grafts in infrainguinal arterial reconstructions. J Vasc Surg 1986;3:104–14.

[16] Jackson MR, Belott TP, Dickason T, et al. The consequences of a failed femoropopliteal bypass grafting: comparison of saphenous vein and PTFE grafts. J Vasc Surg 2000;32:498–504, 504–5.

[17] Stonebridge PA, Prescott RJ, Ruckley CV. Randomized trial comparing infrainguinal polytetrafluoroethylene bypass grafting with and without vein interposition cuff at the distal anastomosis. The Joint Vascular Research Group. J Vasc Surg 1997;26:543–50.

[18] Yeung KK, Mills JL Sr, Hughes JD, et al. Improved patency of infrainguinal polytetrafluoroethylene bypass grafts using a distal Taylor vein patch. Am J Surg 2001;182:578–83.

[19] Pereira CE, Albers M, Romiti M, et al. Meta-analysis of femoropopliteal bypass grafts for lower extremity arterial insufficiency. J Vasc Surg 2006;44:510–7.

[20] Tangelder MJ, McDonnel J, Van Busschbach JJ, et al. Quality of life after infrainguinal bypass grafting surgery. Dutch Bypass Oral Anticoagulants or Aspirin (BOA) Study Group. J Vasc Surg 1999;29:913–9.

[21] Tangelder MJ, Algra A, Lawson JA, et al. Optimal oral anticoagulant intensity to prevent secondary ischemic and hemorrhagic events in patients after infrainguinal bypass graft surgery. Dutch BOA Study Group. J Vasc Surg 2001;33:522–7.

[22] Oostenbrink JB, Tangelder MJ, Busschbach JJ, et al, Dutch Bypass Oral anticoagulants or Aspirin Study Group. Cost-effectiveness of oral anticoagulants versus aspirin in patients after infrainguinal bypass grafting surgery. J Vasc Surg 2001;34:254–62.

[23] Johnson WC, Williford WO. Benefits, morbidity, and mortality associated with long-term administration of oral anticoagulant therapy to patients with peripheral arterial bypass procedures: a prospective randomized study. J Vasc Surg 2002;35:413–21.

[24] Sarac TP, Huber TS, Back MR, et al. Warfarin improves the outcome of infrainguinal vein bypass grafting at high risk for failure. J Vasc Surg 1998;28:446–57.

[25] Johnston KW. Factors that influence the outcome of aortoiliac and femoropopliteal percutaneous transluminal angioplasty. Surg Clin North Am 1992;72:843–50.

[26] Muradin GS, Bosch JL, Stijnen T, et al. Balloon dilation and stent implantation for treatment of femoropopliteal arterial disease: meta-analysis. Radiology 2001;221:137–45.

[27] Scheinert D, Duda S, Zeller T, et al. The LEVANT I (Lutonix paclitaxel-coated balloon for the prevention of femoropopliteal restenosis) trial for femoropopliteal revascularization: first-in-human randomized trial of low-dose drug-coated balloon versus uncoated balloon angioplasty. JACC Cardiovasc Interv 2014;7:10–9.

[28] Rosenfield K, Jaff MR, White CJ, et al. Trial of a paclitaxel-coated balloon for femoropopliteal artery disease. N Engl J Med 2015;373:145–53.

[29] Laird JR, Schneider PA, Tepe G, et al, IN.PACT SFA Trial Investigators. Durability of treatment effect using a drug-coated balloon for femoropopliteal lesions: 24-month results of IN.PACT SFA. J Am Coll Cardiol 2015;66:2329–38.

[30] Krishnan P, Faries P, Niazi K, et al. Stellarex drug-coated balloon for treatment of femoropopliteal disease: twelve-month outcomes from the randomized ILLUMENATE pivotal and pharmacokinetic studies. Circulation 2017;136:1102–13.

[31] Salisbury AC, Li H, Vilain KR, et al. Cost-effectiveness of endovascular femoropopliteal intervention using drug-coated balloons versus standard percutaneous transluminal angioplasty: results from the IN.PACT SFA II trial. JACC Cardiovasc Interv 2016;9:2343–52.

[32] Shishehbor MH, Jaff MR. Percutaneous therapies for peripheral artery disease. Circulation 2016;134:2008–27.

[33] Schillinger M, Sabeti S, Loewe C, et al. Balloon angioplasty versus implantation of nitinol stents in the superficial femoral artery. N Engl J Med 2006;354:1879–88.

[34] Laird JR, Katzen BT, Scheinert D, et al. Nitinol stent implantation versus balloon angioplasty for lesions in the superficial femoral artery and proximal popliteal artery: twelve-month results from the RESILIENT randomized trial. Circ Cardiovasc Interv 2010;3:267–76.

[35] Bosiers M, Torsello G, Gissler HM, et al. Nitinol stent implantation in long superficial femoral artery lesions: 12-month results of the DURABILITY I study. J Endovasc Ther 2009;16:261–9.

[36] Duda SH, Bosiers M, Lammer J, et al. Sirolimus-eluting versus bare nitinol stent for obstructive superficial femoral artery disease: the SIROCCO II trial. J Vasc Interv Radiol 2005;16:331–8.

[37] Dake MD, Ansel GM, Jaff MR, et al. Durable clinical effectiveness with paclitaxel-eluting stents in the femoropopliteal artery: 5 year results of the zilver PTX randomized trial. Circulation 2016;133:1472–83 [discussion: 1483].

[38] Schmidt A, Ulrich M, Winkler B, et al. Angiographic patency and clinical outcome after balloon-angioplasty for extensive infrapopliteal arterial disease. Catheter Cardiovasc Interv 2010;76:1047–54.

[39] Peregrin JH, Koznar B, Kovac J, et al. PTA of infrapopliteal arteries: long-term clinical follow-up and analysis of factors influencing clinical outcome. Cardiovasc Intervent Radiol 2010;33:720–5.

[40] Donas KP, Torsello G, Schwindt A, et al. Below knee bare nitinol stent placement in high-risk patients with critical limb ischemia is still durable after 24 months of follow-up. J Vasc Surg 2010;52:356–61.

[41] Rastan A, Tepe G, Krankenberg H, et al. Sirolimus-eluting stents vs. bare-metal stents for treatment of focal lesions in infrapopliteal arteries: a double-blind, multi-centre, randomized clinical trial. Eur Heart J 2011;32:2274–81.

[42] Laird JR, Zeller T, Gray BH, et al. Limb salvage following laser-assisted angioplasty for critical limb ischemia: results of the LACI multicenter trial. J Endovasc Ther 2006;13:1–11.

[43] Das T, Mustapha J, Indes J, et al. Technique optimization of orbital atherectomy in calcified peripheral lesions of the lower extremities: the CONFIRM series, a prospective multicenter registry. Catheter Cardiovasc Interv 2014;83:115–22.

[44] Singh T, Koul D, Szpunar S, et al. Tissue removal by ultrasound evaluation (the TRUE study): the Jetstream G2 system post-market peripheral vascular IVUS study. J Invasive Cardiol 2011;23:269–73.

[45] McKinsey JF, Zeller T, Rocha-Singh KJ, et al, DEFINITIVE LE Investigators. Lower extremity revascularization using directional atherectomy: 12-month prospective results of the DEFINITIVE LE study. JACC Cardiovasc Interv 2014;7:923–33.

[46] Bradbury AW, BASIL trial Investigators and Participants. Bypass versus angioplasty in severe ischaemia of the leg (BASIL) trial in perspective. J Vasc Surg 2010;51:1S–4S.

[47] Farber A, Rosenfield K, Menard M. The BEST-CLI trial: a multidisciplinary effort to assess which therapy is best for patients with critical limb ischemia. Tech Vasc Interv Radiol 2014;17:221–4.

[48] Nolan BW, De Martino RR, Stone DH, et al, Vascular Study Group of New England. Prior failed ipsilateral percutaneous endovascular intervention in patients with critical limb ischemia predicts poor outcome after lower extremity bypass. J Vasc Surg 2011;54: 730–5 [discussion: 735–6].

[49] Bradbury AW, Adam DJ, Bell J, et al. Bypass versus angioplasty in severe ischaemia of the leg (BASIL) trial: analysis of amputation free and overall survival by treatment received. J Vasc Surg 2010;51:18S–31S.

[50] Farber A, Eberhardt RT. The current state of critical limb ischemia: a systematic review. JAMA Surg 2016;151:1070–7.

[51] Meyer A, Lang W, Borowski M, et al, CRITISCH collaborators. In-hospital outcomes in patients with critical limb ischemia and end-stage renal disease after revascularization. J Vasc Surg 2016;63:966–73.

[52] Albers M, Romiti M, De Luccia N, et al. An updated meta-analysis of infrainguinal arterial reconstruction in patients with end-stage renal disease. J Vasc Surg 2007;45:536–42.

[53] Yamamoto S, Hosaka A, Okamoto H, et al. Efficacy of revascularization for critical limb ischemia in patients with end-stage renal disease. Eur J Vasc Endovasc Surg 2014;48: 316–24.

[54] Ortmann J, Gahl B, Diehm N, et al. Survival benefits of revascularization in patients with critical limb ischemia and renal insufficiency. J Vasc Surg 2012;56:737–45.e1.

[55] Kranke P, Bennett MH, Martyn-St James M, et al. Hyperbaric oxygen therapy for chronic wounds. Cochrane Database Syst Rev 2015;(6):CD004123.

[56] Belch J, Hiatt WR, Baumgartner I, et al, TAMARIS Committees and Investigators. Effect of fibroblast growth factor NV1FGF on amputation and death: a randomised placebo-controlled trial of gene therapy in critical limb ischaemia. Lancet 2011;377:1929–37.

[57] Morishita R, Makino H, Aoki M, et al. Phase I/IIa clinical trial of therapeutic angiogenesis using hepatocyte growth factor gene transfer to treat critical limb ischemia. Arterioscler Thromb Vasc Biol 2011;31:713–20.

[58] Moazzami K, Moazzami B, Roohi A, et al. Local intramuscular transplantation of autologous mononuclear cells for critical lower limb ischaemia. Cochrane Database Syst Rev 2014;(12):CD008347.

Advances in Surgery 52 (2018) 275–286

ADVANCES IN SURGERY

The Use of Lavage for the Management of Diverticulitis

Cyrus Jahansouz, MD[a], Mary R. Kwaan, MD, MPH[b],*

[a]Department of Surgery, University of Minnesota, 420 Delaware Street. SE, MMC 195, Minneapolis, MN 55455, USA; [b]Department of Surgery, Division of General Surgery, UCLA, 10833 Le Conte Avenue, CHS 72-253, Los Angeles, CA 90095, USA

Keywords

- Diverticulitis • Laparoscopic peritoneal lavage • Purulent peritonitis
- Sigmoid resection

Key points

- Complicated diverticulitis is a disease with potential for significant morbidity and mortality.
- The gold standard for the treatment of diverticulitis Hinchey stage III, characterized as perforated purulent peritonitis, has been immediate operative intervention with colonic resection and proximal diversion to avoid primary anastomosis in a contaminated field. More than 30% of patients, however, never have their colostomy reversed, which leads to reduced quality of life.
- Over the past 20 years, laparoscopic peritoneal lavage emerged as an alternative with reduced morbidity without the need for diversion. Initial studies were promising, but results have been mixed.
- Although laparoscopic peritoneal lavage offers a less invasive means of damage control surgery, this treatment modality must be considered on an individualized basis as criteria for patient selection continue to be delineated.

INTRODUCTION

Diverticular disease is increasing in incidence in North America and Europe [1]. It is characterized by outpouchings of the colon at sites of vascular penetration. The most common site of involvement is the sigmoid colon, involved in 70% to 90% of cases, followed by the descending colon [2,3]. Although the incidence of

Disclosure Statement: The authors have nothing to disclose.

*Corresponding author. Department of Surgery, Division of General Surgery, UCLA, 10833 Le Conte Avenue, CHS 72-253, Los Angeles, CA 90095. E-mail address: MKwaan@mednet.ucla.edu

https://doi.org/10.1016/j.yasu.2018.03.004

diverticular disease increases with age (present in approximately 50% of the population aged 60 years or older), other contributory factors include genetics, smoking, and nonsteroidal anti-inflammatory drug use and those factors associated with developed countries, in particular obesity and the sedentary lifestyle [4].

Diverticular disease only becomes problematic for 10% to 25% of people who harbor diverticula, with the most common manifestation characterized by an acute episode of inflammation, or diverticulitis [3]. Traditional symptoms of uncomplicated diverticulitis are that of left lower quadrant pain and changes in bowel habits (constipation or diarrhea). Urinary symptoms may also be present depending on the proximity of diseased colon to the bladder. Physical examination usually yields variable left lower quadrant tenderness to palpation. Laboratory tests often reveal leukocytosis [5]. Evaluation by CT scanning, the most valuable imaging modality, usually shows diverticula with colonic wall thickening and pericolic fat stranding at least. Complicated diverticulitis manifests with greater acuity and is accompanied by the presence of abscess, fistula, obstruction, or perforation into the abdomen as identified by CT scan. The Hinchey classification, first described in 1978, is commonly used to describe the severity of complicated diverticulitis, as determined during intraoperative evaluation, in 4 stages: stage I describes colonic inflammation with localized microperforation and abscess; stage II as colonic inflammation with an associated pelvic abscess; stage III as perforation with intraperitoneal dissemination of abscess (purulent peritonitis); and stage IV as perforation with intraperitoneal dissemination of feculence (feculent peritonitis) [6]. Treatment of complicated diverticulitis is dependent on Hinchey stage, taking into account patient comorbidities, and has consisted of either resection with immediate anastomosis or resection with diversion (Hartmann procedure). Over the past decade, there has been some controversy regarding the optimal surgical management of Hinchey stage III. Although Hartmann procedure has been the gold standard of care for its avoidance of a primary anastomosis in a contaminated field, more than 30% of patients never have their colostomy reversed and subsequently experience reduced quality of life [7,8]. Thus, other less drastic options for surgical management have emerged for consideration. These include resection with primary anastomosis or laparoscopic peritoneal lavage and drainage. These strategies have emerged as safe alternatives that result in reduced stoma rate after initial hospitalization [9]. This review focuses on laparoscopic lavage with drainage for the treatment of Hinchey stage III.

EARLY STUDIES

Laparoscopic peritoneal lavage with drainage as a treatment alternative for perforated purulent peritonitis was initially described by O'Sullivan and colleagues [10] in Ireland in 1996. This small series (n = 8) described the initial management of patients presenting with generalized peritonitis secondary to perforated diverticular disease of the left colon diagnosed at the time of laparoscopic evaluation (Hinchey III). All patients were managed by lavage, intravenous fluids, and antibiotics, and average length of stay was 10 days. No patient required further surgical intervention beyond lavage. These encouraging results prompted more widespread evaluation of this approach, and 3 subsequent case series affirmed the promising observations from Ireland [11–13]. Franklin and colleagues [11] (n = 18, Hinchey II and III) reported excellent outcomes with average length of stay of 7.5 days and resolution of leukocytosis and fevers by postoperative day 4. Among these 18 patients, no one required further surgical intervention during initial hospitalization beyond initial lavage. Faranda and colleagues [12] (n = 18, Hinchey stages III and IV) reported successful treatment in all patients as well. All patients presented with generalized peritonitis and leukocytosis and received intravenous fluids, broad-spectrum antibiotics, and laparoscopic lavage with 15 L of saline. Biologic fibrin glue was spread on pathologic areas of colon and 2 drains were left in place. Average length of stay was 8 days. Taylor and colleagues [13] (n = 14, Hinchey stage II, III, or IV) reported a successful treatment rate of 79%. All patients were managed with broad-spectrum antibiotics, at least 3 L of lavage, and 1 or 2 peritoneal drains. The 2 patients in the study presenting with Hinchey stage IV and 1 of the 10 patients with Hinchey stage III did not improve and required subsequent colon resection during the initial hospitalization. Median length of stay was 6.5 days but considerably longer for the 3 patients requiring resection, as expected. A majority of patients in these initial studies underwent interval elective resections completed laparoscopically without the use of a stoma.

In these early studies, preoperative imaging modality was not uniformly implemented, which limits generalizability to modern United States. In the study by O'Sullivan and colleagues [10], no imaging was performed as per hospital practice at the time; patients presenting with generalized peritonitis were taken to the operating room (OR) for diagnostic laparoscopy. In the 18 patients who underwent lavage, Franklin and colleagues [11] reported diagnostic laparoscopy performed as initial assessment without imaging in 14 patients, whereas a combination of CT, ultrasonography, and water-soluble contrast study per rectum was diagnostic in the remaining 4 patients. Faranda and colleagues [12] assessed patients by radiography and/or ultrasonography (not CT) and Taylor and colleagues [13] evaluated patients by radiography and/or CT. The lack of standard CT imaging in these series raises the question of whether these patients are equivalent to those seen in the acute setting in modern United States practice, the vast majority of whom have been assessed with CT.

FOLLOW-UP STUDIES

Building on this experience, larger studies were subsequently performed. In a prospective multi-institutional study of 100 patients in Ireland, Myers and colleagues [14] once again assessed the feasibility of laparoscopic lavage alone for patients presenting with generalized peritonitis secondary to perforated diverticulitis. All patients had evidence of perforation on preoperative imaging on either upright plain chest radiography (n = 43) or CT scan (n = 57). Importantly, patients diagnosed with feculent peritonitis (n = 8) underwent a Hartmann procedure. Otherwise, all patients underwent peritoneal lavage with

4 L of saline and placement of 2 Penrose drains (n = 92). All patients received at least 72 hours of intravenous antibiotics and then converted to oral antibiotics for 1 week. Among the 92 patients, 67 were Hinchey stage III and 25 were Hinchey stage II. Morbidity was 4% with 2 patients requiring pelvic drain placement for recurrent abscesses and 1 of these patients requiring a Hartmann procedure. Mortality was 3% (n = 3); 2 patients were immunosuppressed secondary to renal transplantation and 1 patient died of pulmonary embolism. Median times to discharge among patients with Hinchey stage II and stage III were 8 days and 10 days, respectively. Thus, this larger prospective study supported the earlier smaller studies, giving further credence to the use of lavage, particularly for Hinchey stage III diverticulitis. It is remarkable, however, that the interval between publication of the small and the larger series was 13 years. To accrue 100 patients over such a long time period suggests that the appropriate diverticulitis case for this operative approach may have been uncommon.

Bretagnol and colleagues [15] reported their experience in 24 patients (Hinchey grade II: n = 5; Hinchey grade III, n = 18; and Hinchey grade IV, n = 1) with an initial laparoscopic approach to acute sigmoid diverticulitis. Their approach consisted of full lavage of the abdomen with at least 10 L of irrigation, drainage of pus without lysis of any adhesions surrounding the sigmoid colon, placement of a pelvic drain, and medical treatment with antibiotics and bowel rest for at least 21 days. Operation was indicated for clinical diffuse peritonitis, septic shock, or no clinical improvement after 48 hours of medical treatment. Notably, 5 patients had radiologic evidence of pneumoperitoneum and 10 patients had diffuse intraperitoneal fluid. No conversions to laparotomy were required, morbidity was 8% with 2 patients requiring postoperative radiology guided drains for abscesses, and median hospital stay was 12 days. Elective sigmoid resection was performed in all patients with an open conversion rate of 16%.

Karoui and colleagues [16] prospectively collected data on 35 patients who underwent lavage and a comparison group of 24 patients who underwent open resection with defunctioning stoma. All patients were Hinchey stage III, and both groups were similar in age, American Society of Anesthesiologists score, body mass index, history of open abdominal surgery, and number of prior attacks of diverticulitis. Similar to Bretagnol and colleagues, adhesions to the colon were left untouched. Obvious perforations discovered at time of laparoscopy in 6 patients were closed by suture and fibrin glue. On average, 15 L of fluid was used for irrigation. There were no conversions to laparotomy or mortalities. However, 30-day morbidity was 26%; 1 patient required laparotomy on postoperative day 7 for colonic fistula, 1 patient underwent postoperative drain placement for pelvic abscess, and 6 patients had extra-abdominal complications. Average median hospital length of stay was 8 days; 25 of the 34 patients managed successfully by lavage underwent elective sigmoid resection at a median of 4 months after lavage. All but 1 underwent successful laparoscopic resection, and morbidity was 12% with no leaks and no mortalities. Among the comparison group of patients who underwent open surgery, 42% (n = 10) experienced complications, including abscesses, fluid collections, and obstructions, without leaks or mortalities. Median length of hospital stay in the comparison cohort was 17 days. Stoma closures occurred in all at a median time of 3 months after surgery; complication rate was 8%. Overall, a comparison of the 2 cohorts indicated a significantly shorter cumulative length of stay and reduced morbidity in the lavage group (inclusive of elective sigmoidectomy) relative to the 2 open procedures in the control group, all the while avoiding the need for a stoma.

White and colleagues [13,17] performed an audit of 35 cases of perforated diverticulitis treated by lavage as a follow-up to their initial published observations. Patients presented with 4-quadrant peritonitis and free air on imaging or 2-quadrant peritonitis with collections greater than 3 cm on CT. All patients had failed initial conservative medical management. Their surgical approach was mobilization of all attachments to the sigmoid colon, followed by débridement and suction aspiration of abscess contents. For Hinchey III cases, saline lavage of usually no more than 1 L was used. Drains were placed in all cases adjacent to the colon. The air leak test, in which the sigmoid colon is submerged in irrigation fluid and then insufflated per rectum with a rigid sigmoidoscope, was implemented toward the end of the study. A second-look laparoscopy was performed in patients who were septic; 8 (20%) of the 35 lavage patients required surgical resection during index hospitalization (n = 6 Hartmann procedure; n = 2 resection with primary anastomosis) due to fistula formation (n = 2), obstructing malignancy (n = 1), ongoing phlegmon (n = 3), and missed collections (n = 2). Importantly, 8 of the initially 27 successfully managed patients developed recurrent symptoms within a mean of 6 months due to either persistent phlegmons, colovesical fistula formation, or reperforation. The lone reperforation was again successfully managed by washout. Early in the series, 8 elective resections were performed at 3 months after successful washout before symptom recurrences. Later in the series, patients were observed until symptoms recurred.

RANDOMIZED CONTROLLED TRIALS

The emergence of lavage as an alternative to sigmoid resection for the treatment of Hinchey stage III in these early and follow-up studies necessitated more rigorous evaluation in larger, randomized controlled trials (RCTs).

The Ladies trial, a multicenter, parallel-group, randomized open-label trial conducted in Belgium, Italy, and the Netherlands, included the LOLA (LaparOscopic LAvage and drainage) group, which compared laparoscopic lavage versus sigmoidectomy for purulent peritonitis, whereas the DIVA (perforated DIVerticulitis: sigmoid resection with or without Anastomosis) group compared Hartmann procedure versus primary anastomosis in sigmoidectomy patients [18]. Inclusion criteria for the trial were patients with signs of generalized peritonitis due to suspected perforated diverticulitis, and radiologic examination by radiography or CT scan (n = 84; 95%) indicating diffuse free intraperitoneal air or fluid. Of note, 21% of the patients had 1 previous episode of diverticulitis. Patients were excluded if they had a history of dementia, previous sigmoidectomy, pelvic irradiation, steroids (>20 mg/d), age less than 18 or greater than

85 years, and preoperative shock requiring pressor support. Hinchey stage I or II were excluded, and Hinchey stage IV patients were included in the DIVA study. Patients with purulent peritonitis without overt perforation (on intraoperative evaluation) were included within the LOLA group and randomized to receive either laparoscopic lavage, sigmoidectomy without primary anastomosis, or sigmoidectomy with primary anastomosis (with or without defunctioning ileostomy) in a ratio of 2:1:1, respectively. For lavage, adherent tissue was dissected unless they were firmly adherent to the sigmoid colon. Irrigation was performed with up to 6 L of saline, and a drain was left in place. Elective sigmoidectomy was not recommended for patients after lavage, and stoma reversal was offered in the sigmoidectomy group if patients were fit and willing to undergo surgery. Primary endpoint was a composite of major morbidity, including surgical reintervention, and mortality within 12 months; 46 patients were included in laparoscopic lavage and 42 patients in sigmoidectomy for final analysis. Surprisingly, the trial was ended at 33% of its recruitment due to a high rate of morbidity in the lavage group; 37 major morbidity events were recorded in the lavage group versus 10 in the sigmoidectomy group ($P = .0005$); 28 surgical reinterventions were required in the lavage group (overall 20% of patients had a surgical reintervention) versus 11 in the sigmoidectomy group ($P = .02$). Morbidity after lavage occurred in 18 patients (39%) compared with 8 (19%) after sigmoidectomy ($P = .04$). This difference was primarily driven due to persistent sepsis in the lavage group because 9 patients required surgical reintervention. During the 12-month follow-up period, no differences was reported in primary composite endpoint. Lavage showed long-term success in 24 patients (52%), defined as survival with no acute or elective reoperation, and 35 patients (76%) never required a stoma. No statistically significant differences were apparent in quality-of-life assessments (SF-36 [Short-Form 36-item questionnaire], GIQLI [Gastrointestinal Quality of Life Index], and EuroQol EQ-5D) between both cohorts. The apparently high failure rate of lavage to control sepsis, relative to previous studies, may have been attributable to the misdiagnosis of feculent peritonitis as well as presence of underlying cancer. One important observation of the LOLA trial was that despite the high reintervention rate after lavage, mortality remained low (2 of 46 patients), suggesting that failure is salvageable.

The Scandinavian Diverticulitis (SCANDIV) trial, the second RCT, was an open-labeled multicenter study conducted in Sweden and Norway [19]. The clinical indication for operative intervention was the presence of clinical peritonitis. Inclusion criteria were CT scan indicating free air and findings compatible with perforated diverticulitis. Hinchey stage was confirmed after entry into the abdomen, with grade III defined as pneumoperitoneum on preoperative CT scan and intraoperative findings of localized or generalized pus in the abdominal cavity. Exclusion criteria were bowel obstruction and pregnancy. A Hartmann procedure was performed on patients with feculent peritonitis or a visible defect in the colon wall; 199 patients were randomized to either lavage (n = 101) or primary colon resection (n = 98). In lavage, all quadrants were rinsed before placing drains on each side of the pelvis. Colon resection included the choices of laparoscopic versus open resection and Hartmann versus primary resection and anastomosis and were determined by surgeon preference. The abdomen was rinsed with greater than or equal to 4 L of saline or until drainage was clear. Adhesions to the sigmoid were not dissected, which was different from the LOLA trial, where adherent tissue to the sigmoid colon was dissected unless firmly adherent. The primary outcome was having any complication which was Clavien-Dindo classification grade IIIa or greater (interventions requiring general anesthesia, a life-threatening organ dysfunction, or death) at 90 days. This did not differ between patients randomized to lavage (31/101) or resection (25/96; $P = .53$). Death rate was a surprising 13.9% in lavage and 11.5% after resection ($P = .67$). Secondary surgical procedures were required more frequently after lavage (20%) than in resection (6%; $P = .01$) due to a higher rate of secondary peritonitis and intra-abdominal infections in the lavage group. Lavage was associated, however, with shorter OR times and less blood loss. Resection did result in a much higher stoma rate after resection (69%) than lavage (16%; $P<.001$) as well. Neither hospital stay nor quality of life was different between the 2 cohorts. Several limitations were noted in the study. Despite the inclusion criteria, the spectrum of abdominal contamination varied greatly, and determination of Hinchey stage was not straightforward. Leaving adhesions in place may have served to either seal small perforations but also could have hidden larger defects unlikely to seal. Thus, although impact of adhesiolysis remains unclear, it may be hypothesized that even dissecting loosely adherent tissue may result in a worse outcome, as observed in the LOLA study [18].

The third RCT was DIverticulitis-LAparoscopic LAvage versus resection (DILALA) which randomized patients with acute diverticulitis with peritonitis to either laparoscopic lavage (n = 39) or open resection (n = 36) [20,21]. Inclusion criteria consisted of intraabdominal fluid or gas on imaging and a decision to proceed with operative intervention. Immunosuppressed patients were not specifically excluded. Patients were randomized intraoperatively after diagnostic laparoscopy confirmed Hinchey III disease. This is contrast to the SCANDIV and LOLA trials, which randomized patients prior to laparoscopy. Patients with Hinchey grades I, II, or IV were excluded from the study. Lavage was performed with at least 3 L of saline until clear fluid was returned. A drain was placed in the pelvis of all patients and left for at least 24 hours. Primary outcome was reoperation within 12 months postoperatively. Reoperations in this study included stoma reversal and did not consider percutaneous drain placement as a surgical intervention. This was an important difference in comparison to the other 2 trials. In contrast to the other randomized trials, at 12 months, fewer patients in the lavage group (27.9%) underwent reoperations than in the Hartmann group (62.5%; $P = .004$). The majority (75%) of reoperations in the lavage group were for colon resection or abscess and for patients in the Hartmann group, 21 of 25 (84%) of surgical interventions were stoma takedowns. In the lavage group, 26% of patients had postoperative abscess compared with 15% in the Hartmann group. Patients undergoing lavage had significantly shorter OR times and shorter hospital length of stay (6 days vs 9 days). No differences were observed in overall morbidity within 30 days or mortality within 90 days. Morbidity and mortality did not differ at this time point, whereas patients in the lavage cohort had an overall reduced number of hospital days at 12 months (14 days vs 18 days; $P = .047$) than the Hartmann cohort. No differences in quality of life (EQ-5D and SF-36) were observed at 6 months and 12 months.

ADDITIONAL CONSIDERATIONS

The future of lavage as a treatment of perforated diverticulitis remains unclear. The Clinical Practice Guidelines Task Force of the American Society of Colon and Rectal Surgeons set forth practice parameters in 2014 prior to the completion of the RCTs, and, at that time, the safety of lavage for purulent or feculent peritonitis was unclear and it was not recommended as an appropriate alternative to colectomy [22]. Three RCTs performed thus far have directly compared lavage against Hartmann procedure for Hinchey III diverticulitis overall with mixed results [18–21].

Patient selection remains of paramount importance. When early case series of laparoscopic lavage were published, many investigators wondered whether many of these patients, who were not evaluated with a CT scan on presentation, could have been successfully managed either nonoperatively or with percutaneous drains. White and colleagues [17] from Australia acknowledged that "improvements in the availability and reliability of percutaneous drainage have also been welcomed in our institution and cases of simple abscess without peritonitis that were successfully managed by laparoscopic lavage before 2005 would now be referred for attempted percutaneous drainage." As research progressed to randomized trials, mitigating the effect of selection bias that is often seen in case series, most of these patients were evaluated with a CT scan, enriching cohorts in patients with Hinchey III disease. For the most part, it seems that a 20% reoperation rate can be expected after lavage, with most of these interventions needed to control intraabdominal infection. In contrast, United States data from the National Surgical Quality Improvement Program shows a reoperation rate of 9% to 11% after sigmoid resection for contaminated or dirty (Hinchey III or IV) sigmoid resections. Given the current data, surgeons who perform lavage should counsel patients about the high reintervention rate and should monitor them closely to detect and address persistent sepsis promptly.

If lavage is to be a successful treatment of patients, further work on selecting ideal patients for this technique is essential. Currently, there are no studies that incorporate CT scan features predictive of successful lavage. Perforations that cause pneumoperitoneum without significant contamination, although uncommon, may be subject to a decision for nonoperative management versus lavage, as discussed later in more detail.

Pneumoperitoneum without peritonitis

In a retrospective review of 136 patients, Dharmarajan and colleagues [23] evaluated the efficacy of nonoperative management of patients presenting with complicated diverticulitis defined as having an associated abscess or free air on CT scan at the time of admission. The primary endpoint of the retrospective study was the success of nonoperative management and the need for surgery in the acute setting. Failure of nonoperative management was defined as failure of patient improvement or the development of hemodynamic instability. CT scans were stratified according to the following grading system:

- Grade 1: localized free air (pericolonic) without abscess (n = 19)
- Grade 2: small (<2 cm) collections of distant free air or small (<4 cm) abscess (n = 45)
- Grade 3: large (>2 cm) collections of distant free air or large (>4 cm) abscess (n = 66)
- Grade 4: free air with nonloculated free fluid in the peritoneal cavity (feculent peritonitis; n = 6)

All patients deemed appropriate for nonoperative management were resuscitated with IV fluids and started on broad-spectrum IV antibiotics. Patients with abscesses greater than 4 cm were treated with percutaneous drain placement. In total, 124 of 131 patients were successfully treated with nonoperative management in the acute setting. Notably, 25 of 27 patients with pneumoperitoneum were successfully managed nonoperatively; 10 of these patients had concomitant abscesses treated with percutaneous drainage. Of the 98 patients with abscesses, 38 were treated with percutaneous drain placement; 5 of 6 patients presenting with grade 4 required emergent surgery for presenting with generalized peritonitis.

The success of aggressive nonoperative management of perforated diverticulitis without generalized peritonitis evident in this study complicates, and may even mitigate, the role lavage may potentially have in this population. Even patients with pneumoperitoneum may be successfully managed without surgery or drain placement.

It is likely that certain intraoperative findings (other than Hinchey IV) could be described to prompt immediate conversion to colonic resection. Use of intraoperative flexible sigmoidoscopy, for example, could identify patients with large perforations that may not be appropriate for lavage. In the DILALA study, 50% of patients randomized to the Hartmann procedure were found to have an obvious visible perforation in the colon intraoperatively. Other factors that may have an impact on outcome after lavage have not been explored, such as the degree of adhesions and angulation of the bowel, as assessed on endoscopic evaluation, or the degree of fecal loading proximal to diseased colon, either seen on preoperative CT scan or in the OR.

Once in the OR, the proper manner of addressing loculated abscesses is not clear, with some investigators breaking apart [17,18] pericolic adhesions to achieve source control and others leaving adhesions intact to facilitate occlusion of small microperforations [15,16,19]. Perforations that are discovered to be lentiform, perhaps loosely contained in the leaves of the mesentery, may be safest to dissect, whereas dense adhesions without obvious pus might be best left untouched.

Beyond intraoperative considerations, patient comorbidities may play an important role in lavage versus resection as well. As expected, operative time is shorter in lavage given the more extensive nature of open resection. Additionally, in a meta-analysis performed by Penna and colleagues [24], cardiac complications are lower in patients undergoing lavage. Thus, lavage may be more suitable in complex patients with medical comorbidities to reduce operative risk.

Immunosuppression

Data to support lavage in patients on immunosuppression remains sparse. A recent series from France reported 71 patients managed with laparoscopic lavage. Hemodynamically stable patients were candidates for this procedure if Hinchey III disease was considered likely on CT scan and confirmed on laparoscopy. Perforations were identified and sutured in 13% of patients. A 20% lavage failure was noted, and immunosuppression was the only significant risk factor on multivariable analysis (odds ratio: 17) [25]. Although the 3 RCTs did not specifically exclude immunosuppressed patients, the LOLA trial did exclude patients on greater than 20 mg of steroids [18–20]. Outcomes of immunosuppressed patients from these trials are unclear. From the follow-up study of 100 patients performed by Myers and colleagues [14], 2 of the 3 patients who died were on immunosuppression as required for a prior history of renal transplantation. Of the 2 patients on immunosuppression in the study by Dharmarajan and colleagues [23], both received ostomies due to concerns for healing. Given concerns for sealing potential in the setting of immunosuppression, patients on immunosuppression are not candidates for lavage.

Interval surveillance

An important consideration for the use of lavage remains missed diagnoses of cancer. Thus, interval colonoscopy should be performed in all patients. A majority of studies reported some degree of missed malignancy in patients treated by lavage. In their study of 100 patients, Myers and colleagues [14] reported missed cancer in 1 of 88 patients undergoing interval colonoscopy at 6 weeks. White and colleagues reported 1 missed cancer among 35 patients, the LADIES trial reported 11% (5/46) cancers in lavage patients, the SCANDIV trial reported 5% (4/74) patients with cancer, and the DILALA trial also reported a 5% (4/83) rate of cancer. [17–20]. It is possible that leaving cancer in these patients until elective colonoscopy and resection may result in adverse oncologic outcomes in the future.

Interval resection

Resection after complicated diverticulitis is strongly recommended, and primary resection in the setting of peritonitis has been shown to result in fewer reoperations and shorter hospital stay [26]. Thus, patients who have been successfully managed by lavage are best served by interval resection of the diseased colon. Mortality in patients undergoing lavage and patients undergoing resection seems similar at 30 days and 90 days, suggesting that delayed resection after a failure of lavage does not necessarily increase the risk of mortality [24,27]. Among the advantages of lavage is the possibility of approaching resection laparoscopically as opposed to laparotomy potentially offering lower morbidity [28]. Several studies highlighted a high rate of success of delayed laparoscopic resection without conversion to open in patients treated by lavage [11–13,16]. The risk remains that during delay; however, persistent or recurrent sepsis may necessitate urgent surgery.

Given these considerations, it is important to longitudinally compare outcomes of patients treated by lavage and interval resection with those having undergone Hartmann procedure with interval takedown of their ostomy. A trend toward reduced stoma has been reported after lavage [24,27]. Hartmann reversal is associated with up to 50% morbidity and approximately 30% of patients are never reversed, which diminishes quality of life [7,8].

SUMMARY

As with most pathologies, patients must be considered on an individualized basis. Lavage offers a less invasive means of damage control surgery and allows for interval laparoscopic resection of diseased colon without a stoma, whereas standard of care remains sigmoid resection, either with primary anastomosis and diversion or Hartmann procedure. RCT data have put a considerable damper on enthusiasm for this procedure by highlighting the high surgical reintervention rate in lavage patients. Criteria that continue to require further delineation include patient selection and surgical approach to lavage, including amount of irrigation, approach to adhesions, and performance of flexible sigmoidoscopy at time of surgery.

References

[1] Hall J, Roberts P, Ricciardi R, et al. Long-term follow-up after an initial episode of diverticulitis: what are the predictors of recurrence? Dis Colon Rectum 2011;54(3):283–8.

[2] Rezapour M, Ali S, Stollman N. Diverticular disease: an update on pathogenesis and management. Gut Liver 2017; https://doi.org/10.5009/gnl16552.

[3] Stollman NH, Raskin JB. Diagnosis and management of diverticular disease of the colon in adults. Ad Hoc Practice Parameters Committee of the American College of Gastroenterology. Am J Gastroenterol 1999;94(11):3110–21.

[4] Weizman AV, Nguyen GC. Diverticular disease: epidemiology and management. Can J Gastroenterol 2011;25(7):385–9.

[5] Sirany AE, Gaertner WB, Kwaan MR, et al. Diverticulitis diagnosed in the emergency room: is it safe to discharge home? J Am Coll Surg 2017;225(1):21–5.

[6] Hinchey EJ, Schaal PG, Richards GK. Treatment of perforated diverticular disease of the colon. Adv Surg 1978;12:85–109.

[7] Van De Wall BJ, Draaisma WA, Schouten ES, et al. Conventional and laparoscopic reversal of the Hartmann procedure: a review of literature. J Gastrointest Surg 2010;14(4):743–52.

[8] Banerjee S, Leather AJM, Rennie JA, et al. Feasibility and morbidity of reversal of Hartmann's. Colorectal Dis 2005;7(5):454–9.

[9] Agha MSA, Gundling WHF, Iesalnieks PSI. Damage control strategy for the treatment of perforated diverticulitis with generalized peritonitis. Tech Coloproctol 2016;20(8): 577–83.

[10] O'Sullivan GCO, Murphy D, Brien MGO, et al. Laparoscopic management of generalized peritonitis due to perforated colonic diverticula. Am J Surg 1995;171:432–4.

[11] Franklin M Jr, Dorman JP, Jacobs M, et al. Is laparoscopic surgery applicable to complicated colonic diverticular disease? Surg Endosc 1997;11:1021–5.

[12] Faranda C, Barrat C, Catheline J. Two-stage laparoscopic management of generalized peritonitis due to perforated sigmoid diverticula: eighteen cases. Surg Laparosc Endosc Percutan Tech 2000;10(3):135–8.

[13] Taylor CJ, Layani L, Ghusn M, et al. The perforated diverticulitis managed by laparoscopic lavage. ANZ J Surg 2006;76:962–5.

[14] Myers E, Hurley M, Sullivan GCO, et al. Laparoscopic peritoneal lavage for generalized peritonitis due to perforated diverticulitis. Br J Surg 2008;95(1):97–101.

[15] Bretagnol F, Pautrat K, Mor C, et al. Emergency laparoscopic management of perforated sigmoid diverticulitis: a promising alternative to more radical procedures. J Am Coll Surg 2008;206(4):654–7.

[16] Karoui M, Ph D, Champault A, et al. Laparoscopic peritoneal lavage or primary anastomosis with defunctioning stoma for Hinchey 3 complicated diverticulitis: results of a comparative study. Dis Colon Rectum 2009;4:609–15.

[17] White SI, Frenkiel B, Martin PJ. A ten-year audit of perforated sigmoid diverticulitis: highlighting the outcomes of laparoscopic lavage. Dis Colon Rectum 2010;11:1537–41.

[18] Vennix S, Musters GD, Mulder IM, et al. Laparoscopic peritoneal lavage or sigmoidectomy for perforated diverticulitis with purulent peritonitis: a multicentre, parallel-group, randomised, open-label trial. Lancet 2015;386:1269–77.

[19] Shultz J, Yaqub S, Wallon C, et al. Laparoscopic lavage vs primary resection for acute perforated diverticulitis: the SCANDIV randomized clinical trial. JAMA 2016;314(13):1364–75.

[20] Angenete E, Thornell A, Burcharth J, et al. Laparoscopic lavage is feasible and safe for the treatment of perforated diverticulitis with purulent peritonitis: the first results from the randomized controlled trial DILALA. Ann Surg 2016;263(1):117–22.

[21] Thornell A, Angenete E, Bisgaard T, et al. Laparoscopic lavage for perforated diverticulitis with purulent peritonitis. Ann Intern Med 2017;164(15):137–46.

[22] Feingold D, Steele SR, Lee S, et al. Practice parameters for the treatment of sigmoid diverticulitis. Dis Colon Rectum 2014;57:284–94.

[23] Dharmarajan S, Hunt SR, Birnbaum EH, et al. The efficacy of nonoperative management of acute complicated diverticulitis. Dis Colon Rectum 2011;54(6):663–71.

[24] Penna M, Markar SR, Mackenzie H, et al. Laparoscopic lavage versus primary resection for acute perforated diverticulitis: review and meta-analysis. Ann Surg 2017; https://doi.org/10.1097/SLA.0000000000002236.

[25] Greilsammer T, Abet E, Meurette G, et al. Is the failure of laparoscopic peritoneal lavage predictable in Hinchey III diverticulitis management? Dis Colon Rectum 2017;60(9):965–70.

[26] Zeitoun G, Laurent A, Rouffet F, et al. Multicentre, randomized clinical trial of primary versus secondary sigmoid resection in generalized peritonitis complicating sigmoid diverticulitis. Br J Surg 2000;87(10):1366–74.

[27] Marshall JR, Buchwald PL, Gandhi J, et al. Laparoscopic lavage in the management of Hinchey Grade III diverticulitis: a systematic review. Ann Surg 2017;265(4):670–6.

[28] Cirocchi R, Farinella E, Trastulli S, et al. Elective sigmoid colectomy for diverticular disease. laparoscopic vs open surgery: a systematic review. Colorectal Dis 2011;14:671–83.

Moving?

Make sure your subscription moves with you!

To notify us of your new address, find your **Clinics Account Number** (located on your mailing label above your name), and contact customer service at:

Email: journalscustomerservice-usa@elsevier.com

800-654-2452 (subscribers in the U.S. & Canada)
314-447-8871 (subscribers outside of the U.S. & Canada)

Fax number: 314-447-8029

Elsevier Health Sciences Division
Subscription Customer Service
3251 Riverport Lane
Maryland Heights, MO 63043

*To ensure uninterrupted delivery of your subscription, please notify us at least 4 weeks in advance of move.

CPI Antony Rowe
Chippenham, UK
2018-09-27 14:18